# HEALTH PSYCHOLOGY

## Biological, Psychological, and Sociocultural Perspectives

**Margaret Konz Snooks, PhD**
School of Human Sciences and Humanities
University of Houston–Clear Lake

JONES AND BARTLETT PUBLISHERS
*Sudbury, Massachusetts*
BOSTON    TORONTO    LONDON    SINGAPORE

*World Headquarters*

Jones and Bartlett Publishers
40 Tall Pine Drive
Sudbury, MA 01776
978-443-5000
info@jbpub.com
www.jbpub.com

Jones and Bartlett Publishers
Canada
6339 Ormindale Way
Mississauga, Ontario L5V 1J2
Canada

Jones and Bartlett Publishers
International
Barb House, Barb Mews
London W6 7PA
United Kingdom

Jones and Bartlett's books and products are available through most bookstores and online booksellers. To contact Jones and Bartlett Publishers directly, call 800-832-0034, fax 978-443-8000, or visit our website www.jbpub.com.

Substantial discounts on bulk quantities of Jones and Bartlett's publications are available to corporations, professional associations, and other qualified organizations. For details and specific discount information, contact the special sales department at Jones and Bartlett via the above contact information or send an email to specialsales@jbpub.com.

**Production Credits**
Acquisitions Editor: Shoshanna Goldberg
Associate Editor: Amy L. Flagg
Editorial Assistant: Kyle Hoover
Production Manager: Julie Champagne Bolduc
Production Assistant: Jessica Steele Newfell
Marketing Manager: Jessica Faucher
V.P., Manufacturing and Inventory Control: Therese Connell
Composition: Publishers' Design and Production Services, Inc.
Cover Design: Kristin E. Ohlin
Assistant Photo Researcher: Meghan Hayes
Cover Images: (*clockwise from top left*) © 2734725246/ShutterStock, Inc.; © Andresr/ShutterStock, Inc.; © Liv friis-tarsen/ShutterStock, Inc.; © Tan Wei Ming/ShutterStock, Inc.; © digitalskillet/ShutterStock, Inc.
Printing and Binding: Malloy, Inc.
Cover Printing: Malloy, Inc.

**Library of Congress Cataloging-in-Publication Data**
Snooks, Margaret K.
    Health psychology / by Margaret Konz Snooks.
        p. ; cm.
    Includes bibliographical references and index.
    ISBN-13: 978-0-7637-4382-6
    ISBN-10: 0-7637-4382-8
    1. Clinical health psychology.    I. Title.
    [DNLM: 1. Behavioral Medicine.    2. Attitude to Health.    3. Disease—psychology.    4. Health Behavior.
WB 103 S673h 2010]
    R726.7.S66 2010
    616.001'9—dc22
                                                                                              2008043348
6048

Printed in the United States of America
12  11  10  09  08    10  9  8  7  6  5  4  3  2  1

*This book is dedicated to my husband and*
*our three wonderful daughters.*

# CONTENTS

## Chapter 8   The Reciprocal Effects of Stress on Illness and Injury    189

## Chapter 9   Coping and Stress Management    209

**Chapter 13** **Applications of Health Psychology to Chronic Illness**     **321**

**Chapter 14** **Applications of Health Psychology to Diversity Issues**     **347**

# PREFACE

The purpose of this text is to show students how biological, psychological, and sociocultural perspectives influence an individual's overall health. It is meant to guide students through common health psychology topics and motivate them to make positive changes that are based on current health research.

A major frustration for faculty members is that their students do not bother to read assigned textbooks. This is unfortunate because the experience of reading a textbook reinforces what a student hears in lecture and provides valuable content for a student's research and studies.

This book was written specifically to encourage students to read it. Words used, order of chapters, examples, and emphases are geared toward traditional, nontraditional, and diverse college students' interests and experiences. For example, there is not a separate chapter on biology; instead, biology is included where appropriate within a chapter topic so that students can relate biology to specific health issues and be able to better understand it if they don't have a science background. The same approach was used for careers in health psychology. Throughout the book references are made to the work of health psychologists within chapter topics so that students can relate to the theories and be better able to apply them. Exercise and nutrition are discussed near the beginning of the text to provide an early opportunity for students to think about applications of health psychology theories and models within familiar topic areas.

## Special Features

- **Learning Objectives** at the beginning of each chapter give students an idea of what they will learn as they read the chapter.

- **Bolded Key Terms** with definitions give students a quick reference for easier understanding of important terms.

- **Think About It** boxes encourage students to think more about specific topics related to health psychology.

- **Summaries** at the end of each chapter provide a brief recap of the chapter's most important topics.

- **Review Questions** correspond with the chapter's learning objectives and encourage critical thinking and review of important chapter topics.

- **Student Activities** at the end of each chapter encourage students to use material presented in the chapter for more active learning.

## Interactive Web Site: http://health.jbpub.com/psychology

The web site that accompanies this text includes resources for both students and instructors. Students can access animated flashcards, crossword puzzles, an interactive glossary, practice quizzes, and web links, all of which help to reinforce important topics covered in the text. Instructors will find helpful teaching tools including an instructor's manual, PowerPoint presentations, and a TestBank.

## Acknowledgments

The author gratefully acknowledges the foresight, patience, and support of the editorial, production, and marketing staff at Jones and Bartlett Publishers. Boundless thanks are given with enormous respect to Sherran Saladino, our wonderful and intelligent suite secretary, and to the many library staff members at the University of Houston–Clear Lake who gave me valuable and gracious assistance over the past several years.

The author would also like to thank the many reviewers who provided valuable feedback throughout the manuscript process:

Justin P. Bailey, PhD, Framingham State College

Thomas L. Flagg, PhD, Adrian College

John P. Garofalo, PhD, Washington State University Vancouver

Nancy A. Hamilton, University of Kansas

Elissa Koplik, PhD, Bloomfield College

Beth Krone, MS, Rutgers University at Newark

Catherine Salmon, PhD, University of Redlands

Judith Skala, RN, PhD, Washington University

Holly E. Tatum, PhD, Randolph College

Zaje A. T. Harrell, PhD, Michigan State University

# Chapter 1

# Introduction to Health Psychology

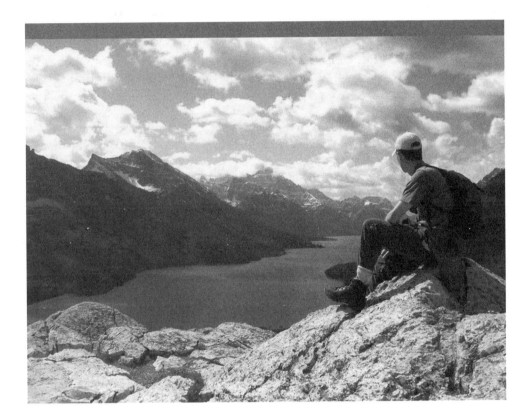

## Learning Objectives

After studying this chapter students will have the knowledge and skills to be able to:

1. Define health psychology as a field of scientific investigation within psychology and discuss its applications.

2. Contrast the biomedical and biopsychosocial models of health and explain varying outcomes from each perspective.

3. Explain systems theory and its relationship to the biopsychosocial approach to health.

4. Compare perspectives on health in ancient times to the biomedical approach and to the biopsychosocial approach to health.

5. Define health and give examples of the physical, emotional, social, and cultural dimensions of health.

6. Explain three major factors affecting health characteristics of everyone.

1

## Introduction

As a college student, you will have little difficulty relating to the field of **health psychology**, because you already know about the importance of **health** and ways to preserve and improve your own health. In addition, you have experienced both illness and injury, so you will appreciate and recognize many of the concepts and examples used in this textbook. You are also aware that biology is not always responsible for your physical ailments. For example, most college students experience headaches and stomachaches. These rarely indicate cancer or other serious biological problems. Most of the time they are consequences of emotional reactions or stress, which is psychological, or problems with relationships, which are social and cultural.

Health psychology, a division within the American Psychological Association (APA), is a specialty applying psychological principles to the scientific study of health, illness, and health-related behaviors. It is empirically based, which means its vast and growing research literature is the outcome of scientific methods. It is specifically aimed toward a broader understanding of health, illness, injury, recovery, and the impact of each on human lives. Knowledge developed in this field includes psychological, social, and cultural influences on diagnosis, treatment, and rehabilitation of ill and injured people. Health psychologists are also interested in the prevention of illness and injury and in health policy formation (American Psychological Assocation, 2008).

Health psychology formally began in the 1970s when the behavioral sciences began to contribute more to the understanding of health problems (Schwartz & Weiss, 1977). Medicine had long included psychiatry, and clinical psychology was a specialty within general psychology. **Clinical psychologists** are mental health professionals with backgrounds in counseling and health psychology. Health psychology grew in relation to behavioral med-

---

**health psychology** A specialty applying psychological principles to the scientific study of health, illness, and health-related behaviors. It is specifically aimed toward a broader understanding of health, illness, injury, recovery, and the impact of each on human life. Knowledge developed in this field includes psychological, social, and cultural influences on the development, diagnosis, treatment, and rehabilitation of ill and injured people. Health psychologists are also interested in the prevention of illness and injury and in health policy formation. It is a field of study within the general discipline of psychology.

**health** Soundness of body and mind: a state of physical, emotional, and social well-being.

**clinical psychologist** A mental health professional with a background in counseling and health psychology.

icine as physicians began to include patient education in their medical practices. **Behavioral health** is a subfield within the field of behavioral medicine; it emphasizes the maintenance of health, including prevention of both physical and emotional illness (Matarazzo, 1980).

The origins of health psychology rest in a combination of biology, medicine, physiology, philosophy, and social science. Health psychology interfaces with the fields of epidemiology and public health and contributes to improvements in health by increasing knowledge about how health can best be achieved. The work of clinical health psychologists sometimes intersects with the fields of nursing, social work, exercise science, and other disciplines aimed toward understanding and changing health-related behavior. The fields of medical sociology and anthropology add to the subject by exploring the impact of social and cultural factors on health and illness. Health psychology is a science as well as a profession. It is rooted in clinical psychology, social psychology, and psychophysiology. Clinical health psychology has specific educational, training, and credentialing requirements (Papas, Belar, & Rozensky, 2004).

Those working in the field of health psychology recognize that each individual bears some responsibility for his or her health; the government and communities also have social responsibilities. As a science, the field includes health behavior research that focuses on physical, social, and emotional issues. For example, many psychologists focus on understanding how behavior modification can be helpful in changing problem behaviors such as alcohol abuse, drug addictions, and overeating. They recognize that emotions are linked closely to health and in turn, that physical health affects emotional states. One simple example is the way strong emotions, such as anger or fear, cause increases in heart rates and blood pressure. **Cognition**, or what people believe, and **emotion**, or how they feel about events and ideas, also influence health (Baum, Perry, & Tarbell, 2004).

Health and healing are also affected by social factors, including ethnicity and socioeconomic conditions such as poverty. Other influences on health are cultural beliefs, including religious and spiritual convictions. Human behavior has a tremendous impact on the development and progression of diseases, particularly those linked to lifestyle choices such as

**behavioral health** A subfield of behavioral medicine emphasizing the maintenance of health including prevention of both physical and emotional illnesses. Behavioral medicine combines work in the biomedical and behavioral sciences.

**cognition** The act or process of knowing, and products of the process such as problem solving. In health psychology, cognitions affect perception of stressors. Cognitive restructuring refers to methods of changing ones thinking about a stressor.

**emotion** Affective consciousness including feelngs such as joy, sadness, fear, and hate. In health psychology, emotional support from others is helpful in recovery from illness and injury, and emotion-focused coping is a way to manage stress.

smoking, overeating, alcohol abuse, and failing to exercise. Health psychologists research hundreds of topics and clinicians work with patients in hospital and clinical settings to change lifestyles. Other examples of clinical work are helping patients manage the distress of illness and teaching them techniques to alter their physiological responses to stressors. Some psychologists specialize in pain management, including the idea that taking a pre-emptive approach or preventing pain is more effective than dealing with it after the fact (Turk, 2002). Patients, family members, and even friends are included in efforts to manage the stress of medical treatments. Through scientific research, health psychologists even de-vised ways to prevent the conditioned vomiting associated with chemotherapy treatments for cancer (Redd, DuHamel, Vickberg, et al., 2001). Health psychologists also work in pub-lic health, patient education, nursing, and diet therapy.

The APA established the division of health psychology "to advance contributions of psy-chology to the understanding of health and illness through basic and clinical research, edu-cation, and service activities, and encourage the integration of biomedical information about health and illness with current psychological knowledge" (American Psychological Associa-tion, 2008). The division publishes a bimonthly scholarly journal, *Health Psychology*, and a newsletter, *The Health Psychologist*. In addition to college courses in the United States, health psychology is taught at colleges and universities in Canada, Europe, Australia, New Zealand, and Asia (Jansen & Weinman, 1991; Morrow, Hankivsky, & Varcoe, 2007). An International Society of Health Psychology was formed in 1996. A major thrust of work in health psychol-ogy throughout the world is interdisciplinary collaboration (Belar & McIntyre, 2004).

There are more than 20 journals focusing on health psychology and behavioral medicine, including the *British Journal of Health Psychology*, and the journals *Behavioral Medicine* and *Psy-chosomatic Medicine*. Health psychology is a broad field, and psychologists may specialize in a variety of areas including pediatrics, pain management, cardiovascular diseases, cancer, diabetes patient care, addictions, and disease prevention.

Appropriate education and training programs are paramount to becoming a health psy-chologist (McDaniel, Belar, Schroeder, Hargrove, & Freeman, 2002). Among suggested areas of competence are knowledge of the biological, cognitive-affective, social, and developmen-tal bases of health and specific diseases; the necessary knowledge and skills to assess and in-tervene in illness and injury; and an understanding of ethical, legal, policy, professional, and multicultural issues associated with practice specific to patients' problems (Belar, Brown, Hersch, et al., 2001).

## The Study of Human Health

### Two Scientific Viewpoints

You may wonder how using a science-based perspective affects the study of a topic. Perspec-tives are important because they influence explanations that guide thinking, research, and problem solving in specific fields. There are at least two contrasting viewpoints about health. One approach, with which you are more familiar, is called the **biomedical model of health**. This perspective includes the idea that illness and injury are biological problems with biomedical solutions. People who hold this view assume that when someone is ill or injured only the physical self is affected and must be treated.

A second viewpoint, and the model used in this course, is known as the **biopsychosocial model of health**. This model assumes that illness and injury have biological, psychological, and sociocultural components. From this perspective, diagnosis and treatment decisions should take into account all three aspects.

The biomedical model is most characteristic of medicine as it is practiced in the United States. Great advances are made using this model. It is most successful against infectious agents, but less successful against lifestyle-related diseases such as heart disease and some cancers. The biomedical view is more mechanistic or mechanical than the biopsychosocial model and is based in molecular biology. One limitation is that it ignores psychological and sociocultural factors that are important in diagnosis, treatment, and recovery. Clearly, health is related to attitudes, emotions, and personality characteristics, as well as to exposure to viruses or bacteria.

The biopsychosocial model of health represents the guiding perspective used in health psychology courses and professions. This broader view allows analyses, diagnoses, and treatments of illnesses and injuries to incorporate multiple factors that might influence patients and their recovery. Using this wider viewpoint about patients' health problems generally improves healing. For example, the health psychology approach includes patients' families and friends as sources of social support important to patient progress. The cultures in which people grew up and in which they now live also affect actions about health and patients' emotional states and motivations to heal.

One major advantage of the biopsychosocial approach used in health psychology is that it searches for multiple causes and multiple solutions to health problems and appreciates the complexity of health, disease, injury, and healing. This approach encourages students to expand their thinking away from the more limited biological and physiological perspectives. The biopsychosocial approach means that we will consider more than one explanation

**biomedical model of health** A narrow perspective that includes the idea that illness and injury are biological problems with biomedical solutions. People who hold this view assume that when someone is ill or injured only the physical self is affected and must be treated.

**biopsychosocial model of health** The perspective that illness and injury have biological, psychological, and sociocultural components. From this perspective diagnosis and treatment decisions should take into account all three aspects.

when discussing causes of health problems in this textbook. We will look for multiple contributing factors to explain injury and illness. In a similar manner, we will investigate multiple solutions to illness and injury. Causes of health problems, as well as their resolution, are located in biological, psychological, and sociocultural contexts.

## The Relationship of Emotional and Physical Health

Emotions, which are basically psychological, can cause changes in the body's biological system. This is most easily seen in the study of the effects of stress on health. For example, people die of cardiac arrest when facing fearful situations. Severe jealousy and anger can contribute to strokes. Asthma and colitis attacks are more likely when people are under stress. Other examples of mind–body connections are fainting or psychogenic shock, developing fever or high body temperatures in response to social situations, and hyperventilating when stressed. When someone smokes a cigarette near you, you are also smoking. Your biological, emotional, and social states are all affected. This also happens when someone talks on a cell phone near you at a concert or cuts in front of you on the freeway. Stress causes physical changes in your body.

Thoughts, emotions, and bodily functions affect the brain, nervous system, and endocrine and immune systems (Baum, Perry, & Tarbell, 2004). The reverse is also true. Physical changes are accompanied by emotional reactions. Growth is one example. Due to beliefs based in the culture, most young males are pleased when their feet grow bigger, but most young females are not. Many adults are frustrated when they weigh themselves because they usually do not want to gain weight. On the other hand, football-playing high school students are delighted to step on a scale and discover a weight gain, but wrestlers would not be happy. Reactions to physical changes vary from person to person and reflect individual and social factors.

## Origins of the Biopsychosocial Approach to Health

For this course and textbook, the concept of health is defined in the broadest possible terms. Health includes biological, psychological, and sociocultural components. This inclusive theoretical approach is basic to health psychology. The fundamental principle is that health both reflects and generates psychological and sociocultural issues along with the biological. By examining the history of any illness or injury, we can usually discover the presence of all three factors. All three also affect recovery of those who are ill or injured. The biopsychosocial approach used in health psychology can be applied before an illness or injury occurs for preventive purposes, during recovery efforts, and to any after-effects in the lives of patients and their loved ones.

## Systems Theory

The biopsychosocial approach is based in what is known as a **systems theory** approach (Engel, 1977; Schwartz, 1982). Human events, such as injury and illness, exist within several interconnected systems. Each system influences the others. For example, most humans are brought up in a network of relationships with parents, caregivers, teachers, babysitters, neighborhood and school friends, and even strangers. The larger social and cultural system is layered on top of what we learn through individual and group social relationships. The media, including books, television programs, DVDs, movies, music, newspapers, magazines, and blogs, are other social and cultural influences on human health and development. Systems range from the general global culture to more narrow national, state, and community cultures in which families and individuals reside. There is constant interchange or feedback among system components. This interchange means that an entire system is more than just a collection or a sum of each part. A change in one part of the system changes other parts of the system. Systems theory includes the idea that medical providers, patients, family members, and friends need to consider the total situation and think about many different factors when dealing with illness or injury. Engel (1977) emphasized this when he wrote that patients should be viewed in their social contexts and physicians should use patients' social support systems to aid in treatment.

## One Example of Biopsychosocial Analysis

Here is one example of the interplay of biopsychosocial factors and the use of the systems approach. Imagine your 70-year-old grandmother falls and breaks her hip. The origin of the break lies in biological, psychological, and sociocultural causes, and healing and preventing a repetition of the injury improve when using a systems perspective. Your grandmother's bones are weak due to osteoporosis, reflecting the lack of calcium in her diet over many years. She probably stopped drinking milk because she thought it would make her gain weight. Most women in this culture want to avoid obesity at all costs. Aging also reflects biological changes due to social and cultural effects. Her lack of doing weight-bearing or bone-strengthening exercises throughout her life reflects the outdated sociocultural idea that women should not sweat because it is unladylike. Further, part of aging is often being socially isolated and lonely. Perhaps your grandmother fell while eagerly rushing to the phone

**systems theory** An approach to human events, such as injury and illness, including the idea that events occur and exist within several interconnected systems. Each system influences the others. Systems theory in health psychology includes the idea that medical providers, patients, family members, and friends need to consider the total situation and think about many different factors when dealing with an illness or injury.

thinking you were calling. The causes of her fall and injury are biological, psychological, and sociocultural in origin.

Her recovery also depends on biological, psychological, and sociocultural elements. She broke the femur. This may appear to be only a biological problem that can be solved with medical care, including setting and splinting the break. A second biological issue is pain control. The femur is a big bone with many nerve endings. She will be in great pain until sedated for surgery and splinting. Later the bone will ache. After the bone knits, your grandmother will need rehabilitation to ensure that she will walk again and avoid being limited to a wheelchair for the rest of her life. Physical therapists will supervise her rehabilitation and encourage her to make every effort to recoup her previous level of fitness. She will also need care and encouragement from family and friends. Following treatment, your grandmother may be discouraged about her future life, possible disability, and she probably fears falling again and breaking another bone. She may even become depressed and feel helpless and hopeless. These feelings or emotions are psychological, but they influence her struggle to walk again and her ability to maintain her health. Her recovery depends also on her social relationships. Recovery is more likely when friends and family members help by bringing meals, doing household chores, and transporting her to the doctor and rehabilitation facility. Research indicates that social support from family members and friends encourages healing (Baron, Cutrona, Hicklin, Russel, & Lubaroff, 1990).

## Historical Perspectives on Health and Healing

### Perceptions of Health and Healing

Human beliefs about the causes of illness and injury vary from age to age. In Neolithic times (ca. 8000–9000 BC), illness and injury were probably common and attributed to natural events or to some higher powers that also controlled climate changes and other events in nature. Evil forces, including curses, were often blamed for sickness and accidents. Incantations, songs, sacred objects, and healing ceremonies were developed to soothe evil spirits and cure patients. A Greek healer, Hippocrates (ca. 460–360 BC), is called the father of medicine, because he wrote recommendations for health and healing based on his own experiences and work with other people (Hippocrates, trans. 1952). Galen (ca. 200–130 BC), a Greek physician, referred to disease-causing organisms (Galen, trans. 1952). Today, ideas about causes of illnesses are somewhat similar. We use the term **pathogens** to refer to bacteria, viruses, and other infectious agents. In later times, illness and injury were also viewed as consequences of evil acts for which people must atone. Max Weber (1864–1920) suggested that part of the Protestant ethic in the United States was the idea that being wealthy and healthy meant you had earned God's good graces (Weber, trans. 1930). Even today there is a strong

---

**pathogen** Microorganism capable of producing illness or disease.

relationship between wealth and health, because education and wealth provide resources for medical treatment.

Other cultures viewed health and healing differently. Some early Christians prayed for illness and suffering in order to be closer to God. In early Christian times, many people also believed that prayer and good acts would result in healing. This may sound very much like "the power of positive thinking" that we hear about today. This view is partially reflected when sick or injured people are told they must rest and relax in order to get well. Durkheim (1858–1917) studied suicide rates and demonstrated how the presence or absence of close relationships to other people and ties to one's culture affected the probability of suicide (1897/1997). Sigmund Freud (1856–1939) contributed the idea that physical symptoms such as blindness could result from emotional problems and harmful social relationships (Freud, trans. 1952). Many physicians now acknowledge that emotional stress affects one's physical health and that recovery depends in part on the social support given to patients by family and friends. An area of special interest to some researchers and physicians is how the quality of the interaction between doctors and patients can promote healing (Delbanco, 1993).

## The Biomedical Approach to Health

For much of the past hundred years in the United States, health and healing were narrowly attributed to medical care and biological solutions. This perspective relies upon the basic sciences of biochemistry and anatomy to diagnose and treat health problems. Physiology is viewed as the most important cause for illness and injury. A biomedical viewpoint tends to ignore the influence of patients' minds or mental states, their social relationships, and their cultural backgrounds.

**René Descartes** (1596–1650), a French philosopher and mathematician, is generally considered one of the first to write in terms of the body being apart from or separated from the influence of the mind (Descartes, trans. 1952). He believed physicians should concentrate on physical aspects of illness and injury. Some physicians and medical schools continue to emphasize the biomedical approach to healing rather than taking a more holistic approach such as the biopsychosocial model. The biomedical approach is a powerful influence on new physicians, and many doctors still accept this narrow view of health and healing.

One limitation of using the biomedical model exclusively is the assumption that there is only one cause or contributing factor for any health problem. In most cases it is assumed that a correct diagnosis as to cause will lead directly to a specific biological solution, such as prescribing an antibiotic, surgically removing a growth, or putting a splint or cast on an injured arm. Relying on one cause and one cure often means other aspects of problems are

**René Descartes** A French philosopher and mathematician generally considered one of the first to write in terms of the body being apart from or separated from the influence of the mind (1596–1650).

## Think About It!

**Explain This!**

1. College graduates are three times more likely to describe their health as excellent than those who had not graduated from high school.

2. People with family incomes above $75,000 are twice as likely to describe their health as excellent than those with incomes of less than $20,000.

3. Of the people whose ages fall between 18 and 44, 10 out of every 1,000 describe themselves as limited by mental illness.

4. Of the people whose ages fall between 18 and 44, 15 out of every 1,000 describe themselves as limited by arthritis or other musculoskeletal problems.

*Source:* Centers for Disease Control and Prevention, National Center for Health Statistics, National Health Interview Survey.

ignored, such as in cases of child abuse or syndromes with multiple symptoms. Patients' problems often reappear, indicating there was neither a single medical cause nor just one cure.

Medical treatments also can damage patients' health. **Iatrogenic illnesses** are illnesses caused by diagnostic procedures or treatments. For example, Cushing's syndrome is the result of medical treatments using excessive amounts of corticosteroids. Patients being treated in rehabilitation centers sometimes experience burns due to excessive heat applied to the skin. Limbs or joints may be reinjured because of overly vigorous exercise (overuse injuries). **Nosocomial infections** are those specifically acquired during hospital stays.

After practicing medicine for a few years, many physicians begin to appreciate the fact that healing and good health are not just the result of medical treatments such as surgery or antibiotics. It becomes increasingly clear that patients' psychological states, and the attention and care provided by family and friends, also influence outcomes. Many medical care providers eventually recognize the connections among patients' bodies, their minds, and their social relationships. Psychological factors and social relationships play an important role in health and healing. This is what is meant by the connection of the body, the mind, and the sociocultural. Each is a system connected to other systems. Health, illness, injury, and death are linked to emotional and sociocultural aspects of patients' lives, not just to biological aspects.

**iatrogenic illness** A condition occurring as a result of medical diagnostic procedures, medical treatments, or exposure while in a medical facility.

**nosocomial infection** Infection acquired during a hospital stay.

## Benefits of Using the Biopsychosocial Model of Health

In addition to hours of credit towards a degree, students taking this course will gain knowledge and insight into their own health and the health of others. At least two factors make taking a course in health psychology more worthwhile than ever before. One factor is that the most common causes of illness, injury, and deaths have changed. Earlier in history the major causes of death were infectious diseases that were difficult to control. Two examples are plagues and influenza epidemics. Today, the major causes of illness and premature death in industrialized countries are chronic diseases related to lifestyle choices or human behavior. A second major change is the cost of health care. At this time the costs of medical care are rising rapidly and increasing much faster than the rate of inflation. Millions of adults and children have no medical insurance in the United States. To add to these issues, life expectancy is greater than ever before. This is due to the control of infections, fewer infant deaths, and advances in medical treatment.

Health psychology emphasizes the beneficial role played by healthy lifestyles and positive mental attitudes in the prevention and treatment of illness and injury. Students will learn how to choose better options for exercise, eating patterns, and managing stress. Students will also learn theories of behavior change and how to help themselves and others develop healthy lifestyles and discontinue unhealthy behaviors. Three chapters are about the effects of psychological stress on illness and injury. Students will come to understand that recovery from illness and injury is more likely when psychological and sociocultural factors are taken into account along with the biological. Our health depends on biological, psychological, and sociocultural factors (see **Figure 1.1**).

**Figure 1.1**
Our health depends on
biological, psychological,
and sociocultural factors.

*Source:* Edlin, G., & Golanty, E.
(2007). *Health and wellness* (9th
ed.) (p. 7). Sudbury, MA: Jones
and Bartlett Publishers.

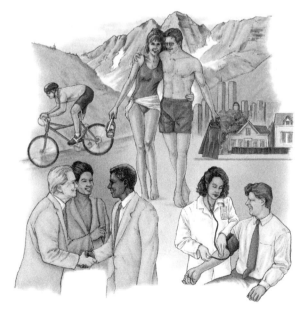

This course also will improve students' communication skills about health issues. People who are knowledgeable about health care issues are more effective in discussions with medical providers, family members, friends, and coworkers. For example, students will understand how to ask more precise questions and give more accurate and useful answers to medical care providers. Adherence to health care recommendations may also increase, because students will participate more actively in their own medical care and the medical care of those important to them. By taking a broader view of health, students will be more effective in helping significant others recover from injury or illness. The knowledge and skills covered in this course will empower students and help them develop greater self-confidence about their ability to affect their own health and the health of others. Students also will learn to think critically about health and health-related recommendations.

## Important Concepts in Health Psychology

When taking a college course, it is important to understand the precise meaning of key words and concepts. Agreement on meanings of commonly used terms ensures students will understand the textbook, the professor, and each other when talking or writing about topics in this course.

### Health

In this class, health is defined broadly and refers to physical, psychological, and sociocultural well-being. Health psychology takes its perspective from the World Health Organization (WHO). In 1948, WHO stated, "Health is a state of complete physical, mental, and social well-being and not merely the absence of disease or infirmity. The enjoyment of the highest attainable standard of health is one of the fundamental rights of every human being without distinction of race, religion, political beliefs, economic or social condition" (p. 1).

You may be in good health physically, but in poor health psychologically or socially. The reverse is also possible. For example, if you are an international student who has just arrived in the United States, you are probably physically healthy, but psychologically and socially lonely. You miss friends and family members you left to come to this campus. Socially you are feeling isolated. You may not know anyone on campus and are reluctant or shy about introducing yourself to others because you are not sure about customs or the right way to do things. At the same time, you are experiencing what is called **culture shock**. Familiar sights, smells, and sounds are missing. Perhaps you came from a rural area and now you are

**culture shock** Emotional upheaval and even illness due to significant changes in living conditions. It particularly occurs when people experience a drastic change in their surroundings due to immigration or forced migration to new geographical areas. Another example is moving from a rural area to an urban area.

living in a city. The area seems very noisy, and the food tastes strange. Many of the foods you really like are not offered in the campus cafeteria. You must communicate with and learn from teachers speaking a language different from the one you first learned as a child. You studied English in school and practiced speaking it, but everyone here talks very fast and many accents are difficult to understand.

Culture shock occurs when New Yorkers immigrate to Botswana and when Botswanians immigrate to New York. Culture shock happens to students from the United States attending colleges in Asia, Africa, South America, Australia, or Europe. Some international students return to their homes because culture shock is too hurtful and distressing. Some become physically ill due to their efforts to work and study in a different culture.

## Evaluating Your Physical Health

One way to evaluate your own health at any given time is to locate yourself on a **continuum**. Think of a continuum as a line with extremes of some concept at either end. There can be many variations between the extremes or ends of a continuum. We use continuums to assess muscle strength (strong to weak) or elasticity (flexible to stiff). Some health books also include intellectual health and spiritual health. Find yourself on each continuum after reading the discussion below.

How do you feel right now? Are you healthy or sick? Do you have lots of energy or are you tired most of the time? Are you in pain or are you free of pain? Would you describe yourself as ill or well? Maybe you have the flu or your back is hurting and you can hardly walk. Some people can be sick and not know it, because there are no outward signs of physical problems. For example, high blood pressure is a risk factor for stroke. Unfortunately, many people with high blood pressure do not know they have it, because there are no outward signs. The way people find out about hypertension is by having someone measure their blood pressure. Find your current location on the continuum for **physical health** in **Figure 1.2**.

## Evaluating Your Psychological Health

Do you like the way your life is going? Are you happy and content, or sad and dissatisfied with your life? Are you worried about something? Are you afraid or anxious? Do you think that someone is out to get you? Are you so sad you often lie down and stare at the ceiling of your bedroom? Do you cry a lot? How healthy are you from a psychological perspective? Look at **Figure 1.3** and decide the current state of your **psychological health**.

**continuum** Illustrative figure such as a line with two extreme conditions of some phenomenon located at either end of the line.

**physical health** Positive physical functioning.

**psychological health** Positive emotional functioning.

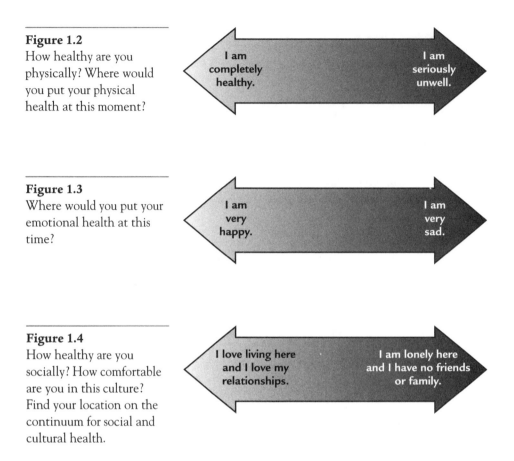

**Figure 1.2**
How healthy are you physically? Where would you put your physical health at this moment?

**Figure 1.3**
Where would you put your emotional health at this time?

**Figure 1.4**
How healthy are you socially? How comfortable are you in this culture? Find your location on the continuum for social and cultural health.

## Evaluating Your Social and Cultural Health

Do you have many satisfactory relationships? Are there people you can count on when you want to talk about something important to you? Do you have positive relationships with family members? Are there good friends you can call upon when you need help? Do you feel relaxed most of the time, or tense? Do you like where you live, your workplace, your school campus, and community or do you feel alienated from those around you? Look at **Figure 1.4** and locate yourself on the continuum of **social and cultural health**.

> **social and cultural health** Normal functioning within a culture including having friends and family members for interaction and social support.

## Outcomes of Your Beliefs About Health

Health psychology is a behavioral science. Today most of the leading causes of premature death are due to behaviors such as smoking, overeating, lack of exercise, abusing alcohol or other substances, and participating in unsafe or reckless behaviors. These behaviors reflect your beliefs about health. By using a continuum, you clarified the state of your physical, emotional, and sociocultural health. Now ask yourself about the behavioral factors affecting your health.

First, think about behaviors directly connected to health and safety. Do you exercise, eat healthily, get adequate sleep, use sunscreen , and wear a seat belt? When you play sports, do you wear protective gear? Do you smoke tobacco or abuse alcohol or other substances? Do you take other risks with your physical health? What about your emotional health? Do you feel depressed, angry, frustrated, or guilty or are you generally happy, calm, friendly, and satisfied with your life? Do you have good relationships with family and friends, or are you isolated from others? Do you argue with everyone you meet? Do you think people are out to take advantage of you? Do you feel alienated from most of the people around you? Actions, feelings, and attitudes are behavioral and are measures of physical, mental, and social health. You might think of the three kinds of health as conditions or as processes, because health is both a condition (like a snapshot) and an ongoing process (like a video). Health is a process requiring neverending effort. We work all our lives to stay healthy and to avoid physical, emotional, and relational problems.

## Illness

Arriving at a suitable definition of illness is difficult. There are scientific descriptions and medical diagnoses for specific diseases. Being ill means you are not in good health. Most of us tolerate some unwellness, such as spring allergies, but do not say we are ill enough to seek medical care. Other people go to school or work when they are very ill. They feel terrible and suffer from severe colds or the flu. These acute illnesses are usually short term and treatable. Chronic illnesses such as heart disease and cancer may go on silently for long periods of time and endure until we die.

Whether or not we are ill is in part subject to our personal perceptions about illness and may reflect how we are feeling at the time. Sometimes illness cannot be measured objectively. For example, have you ever felt terrible, but you did not have an elevated body temperature or any other symptoms? Other people cough, sneeze, and experience watering of their eyes, but they insist they feel fine. Sometimes people ignore symptoms or signs of illness when there is something they really want to do, such as participate in athletic competitions, school plays, band performances, or go on important dates such as proms. Emotional states and social relationships play an important role in how illnesses are perceived as well as how difficult or easy recovery is for us.

The words *illness* and *sickness* are often used in a variety of ways in our culture. Have you ever said to someone, "You make me sick"? Did you mean the person made you physically ill, or were you talking about emotional or relational illness? When watching a news report on television, have you ever said, "That makes me sick"? Sometimes we talk about being sick at heart, meaning our emotional health is disturbed by something we saw or heard. We might also say we are heartsick when a romance ends.

Health psychology sometimes makes a distinction between **illness behaviors** and actual illness. Recent research indicates that fear, anxiety, and depression may be connected to rising blood pressure levels, with stroke and death as a result, while in other cases neuroticism and negative affect predict heart attacks (Smith & Ruiz, 2004, pp. 168–169). The Sickness Impact Profile (SIP) measures ambulation, mobility, social interaction, alertness, emotional behaviors, communication, sleeping and rest, eating, work, home management, recreation, and pastimes (Bergner, Bobbit, Carter, & Gibson, 1981). Other checklists assess psychosocial adjustment to illness.

## Pregnancy

Many people still treat pregnant women as if expecting a baby is an illness. Being pregnant is not the same thing as being ill, although some pregnant women experience nausea and vomiting in the early months. In the later stages of pregnancy, doctors advise women to avoid activities that might result in falls or cause body heat to rise to very high levels. Either situation could endanger the pregnancy. It is true that pregnant women should be aware of what they eat or drink, because everything affects the fetus.

## People with Disabilities

Having a disability is not the same thing as having an illness. (Later chapters discuss chronic illness and disabilities.) How would you assess the health of a person you think has different abilities than you do? Some people experience limitations due to the effects of chronic illnesses such as cardiovascular, pulmonary, or metabolic diseases. People with immune system limitations due to lupus, AIDS/HIV, or cancer treatments may be socially restricted to avoid being infected by others. Many people live with anemia, clotting disorders, organ transplants, and fibromyalgia. **Orthopedic disabilities** include arthritis, lower back pain, osteoporosis, and amputations, especially of the lower limbs. **Neuromuscular disorders** include strokes and other types of brain injuries, spinal cord injuries, epilepsy, muscular dystro-

---

**illness behavior** Actions taken by people who believe they are ill to discover causes and solutions to their situation.

**orthopedic disabilities** Physical limitations due to damage to the bones, joints, muscles, ligaments, and tendons.

**neuromuscular disorder** Illness or injury relating to nerves and muscles.

phy, multiple sclerosis, polio, cerebral palsy, and Parkinson's disease. There are also persons with cognitive, psychological, and sensory disabilities. These include mental illness, limited hearing, visual impairment, Alzheimer's disease, and mental retardation. Most persons with physical or mental disabilities are physically healthy, but face some limitations. For example, people who experience heart attacks may be troubled with chest pain or angina when they exercise in very hot or cold weather. Have you ever met persons who appear to be limited socially? There are persons who are unable to tolerate or relate to other people, perhaps as a result of childhood experiences, traumatic experiences, or an autism-spectrum disorder, or perhaps with no obvious cause.

### Injuries

Being injured is different from being ill. **Injury** is usually viewed as a temporary condition. Injuries include damage to bones, muscles, or other soft tissues, such as tendons and ligaments; our skin can be injured by bruising, cuts, and burns. Insect and animal bites may result in serious illnesses, such as anaphylactic shock or infections such as rabies or Lyme disease. Injuries occur during car wrecks, sports events, and fights. People who recover from injuries often report they are "as good as new," although they frequently experience lingering side effects.

## Responsibility for Health

Another important question in health psychology is how much responsibility individuals bear for their health. Some people assume that their health is out of their control and decide to let nature take its course. At the other end of the spectrum are those who work constantly to improve their physical, emotional, and social-relational well-being. They eat healthily and exercise regularly. If they are depressed, they seek therapeutic care. If they are having trouble with relationships, they get counseling. These are people who believe their behavior has a major effect on their health and that they can offset genetic limitations by following healthy lifestyles. Look at the continuum in **Figure 1.5** and decide how accountable you believe you are for your health.

Very few people would put themselves at either extreme on this continuum, because most people think they are born with some limitations. Nevertheless, most people take some responsibility for their health. They wash their hands, brush their teeth, and try to get adequate rest to avoid illness. They drive carefully and warm up before exercise to prevent injuries. Others believe they have little effect on their health and are careless in much of what they do. Some people believe that national, state, and local governments will protect their health and safety. They expect the Food and Drug Administration (FDA) to protect them from

**injury** Damage to some component of the body.

**Figure 1.5**
How responsible do you
think you are for your
health?

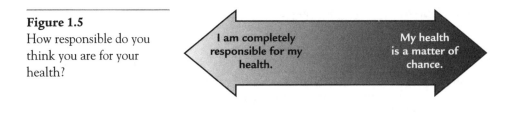

I am completely
responsible for my
health.

My health
is a matter of
chance.

harmful food and medications. They believe the Environmental Protection Agency (EPA) will keep the air clean and stop global warming. They may also believe the Occupational Safety and Health Administration (OSHA) will protect them at work. It is true these agencies exist for our protection, but they are often underfunded and cannot do everything or be everywhere. A great deal about our health and safety is up to us.

## Outcomes of Beliefs About Responsibility for Health

Your beliefs about your responsibility for your health are the most important of all. If your behavior matches your beliefs, then you are consistent. For example, Careless Caroline does not believe she has any control over illness or injury so she does whatever she feels like doing. She eats what she wants to eat, does not brush her teeth, avoids making friends, has temper tantrums when she does not get what she wants, drives recklessly, avoids exercise, and never gets medical checkups. She smokes, abuses alcohol, and uses a variety of illegal drugs. When she has sexual relationships with men she does not insist that her partner wear a condom. There is consistency between her behavior and her attitudes. Statistically she will die prematurely, probably in a car accident or as a result of a crime.

On the other end of the continuum is Healthy Hannah, who exercises aerobically 30 minutes a day. She does strength training and flexibility exercises. Hannah eats a balanced diet and maintains a normal weight. She attends college and studies often, but takes time to relax with friends. She gets adequate sleep, drives carefully, wears a seatbelt, does not smoke, and seldom drinks alcoholic beverages. Hannah sees her physician for checkups and her dentist every 6 months. She also values her family and spends time with them.

Most of us are somewhere in between Healthy Hannah and Careless Caroline. Find yourself on the continuum in Figure 1.5, and think about how much responsibility you take for your health. Inventory your current lifestyle including sleep, eating, exercise, management of stress, and use of substances. Wearing a seat belt, using sunblock, and taking other kinds of precautions are important behaviors. Maintaining good social relationships is part of good health practices too. All behaviors, both healthy and unhealthy, become even more important if we are injured or become ill. The healthier we are physically, emotionally, and socially, the more likely we are to recover from illness and injury, regardless of the cause.

# Factors Affecting Health

Several factors affect health. Think about which you believe to be the most important factors in your case. Do you believe that your genetic background is the most important factor affecting you health?

## Genetic Background

Genes are basic units of biological or family inheritance. In biology, you probably learned that some of your characteristics such as eye and skin color reflect genetic heritage. Scientists do not completely understand all the factors affected by genetics, but people at risk of some genetic disorders can be counseled about risks. Scientists are trying to discover how genes affect health. For example, two genes are believed to be related to breast cancer, but not everyone who develops breast cancer carries those genes, and many people with those genes never develop breast cancer. Some health-related factors are genetic, but other factors are probably more important. Genes can also be altered by exposure to radiation, drugs, viruses, and other factors. Eventually, nanotechnology, biotechnology, and information technology may result in very personalized medicine, but at this time it is most helpful to think about our behavior as the major cause of illness and injury.

## Environmental Factors During Childhood

Environments, both physical and social, affect health. This includes everything from the air we breathe to the thousands of social encounters and relationships we experience during our lives. Our health is also influenced by government policies affecting education, occupation, insurance, and access to health care. Our own health is affected by the health of our biological parents at the time of our conception. After being conceived, fetuses live about 9 months in their mother's uterus or womb. Their blood is interchanged with their mother's, so infants take in the same substances ingested by the mother. We know that smoking, alcohol, other substances, and radiation exposure prior to birth can affect fetal and infant health.

During childhood and adolescence, the behavior of caregivers as well as the behavior of young people themselves influences biological, emotional, and social health. Important factors include living in a loving home and safe shelter, eating nutritious meals, getting adequate sleep, receiving good medical care, and developing educationally, intellectually, emotionally, and spiritually. Values, attitudes, and beliefs of caregivers play an important part in children's health. What early childhood experiences had the greatest effect on your health?

## Behavior During Adulthood

Infectious diseases are still the major cause of death in most of the world (WHO, 2006). This was once true in the United States and other industrialized nations, but now the most influential factor for health is human behavior. In the 1970s researchers began to show

how specific lifestyle choices such as patterns of sleeping, eating, exercising, smoking, and alcohol use affected the likelihood of death (Belloc & Breslow, 1972). The greater the number of positive health behaviors a person practiced, the longer they were likely to live. People make many choices affecting their health throughout their lives. In fact, the majority of deaths in the United States are a result of behavioral risk factors (United States Department of Health and Human Services [USDHHS], 2004). The leading cause of death is cardiovascular disease, which is exacerbated or even caused by smoking, high-fat and high-caloric eating patterns, and little exercise. Cancer is the second leading cause of death, and it is often related to all of the factors mentioned above, plus alcohol and other substances, following unsafe sexual practices, contact with carcinogenic substances, and excessive exposure to sunlight and tanning beds. People younger than 24 years are more likely to die in motor vehicle collisions, which are labeled "unintentional" causes of death to distinguish them from suicides and homicides. Many of these collisions are due to alcohol abuse and reckless driving. Maintaining a stressful lifestyle is probably related to all of the above, but "stress" does not appear on death certificates.

## Summary

This chapter introduces students to the field of health psychology located within the scientific discipline of general psychology. Health psychology applies psychological principles toward a broader understanding of health, illness, and injury. It uses a systems approach to health rather than a more limited biomedical approach. The biopsychosocial model of health psychology includes biological, psychological, and sociocultural components of health in any analysis. Beliefs about influence on health vary from age to age. Health psychologists use information from a variety of fields, including behavioral medicine, epidemiology, medical sociology, and cultural anthropology. Completing a course in health psychology will result in students developing a better understanding of the multiple factors affecting their health and healing following an illness or injury. Students are asked to assess their attitudes about the state of their own physical, emotional, and sociocultural health as well as their level of responsibility for maintaining their health. Genetic background, environmental factors, and behaviors also affect health. For most of us, the most important health-related factor is our own behavior. The major causes of death in the United States in the 21st century are the result of human behaviors such as smoking, substance abuse, overeating, neglect of exercise, and risky behaviors.

## Review Questions

1. Write a brief description of the main goals of the field of health psychology.

2. What is different about health and life expectancy today than was true in the past?

3. List and briefly explain five benefits of completing a course in health psychology in addition to college credit.

4. Describe the biomedical approach to health and its limitations.

5. Explain advantages and disadvantages of taking a biopsychosocial approach to health.

6. What is systems theory? How does it help in the analysis of health issues?

7. Describe and give examples of the physical, emotional, and sociocultural dimensions of health.

8. If an individual is pregnant or has a disability, do you think of them as ill? Explain your answer.

9. Discuss three important factors affecting your health.

10. Write a brief summary of how your behavior affects your health.

## Student Activity

1. Write a sentence explaining your personal view of health. Clarify whether your view is closer to the biomedical or the biopsychosocial approach.

2. Write an evaluation of your location on the three continuums of health. Are you physically well and emotionally happy at this time? Are your relationships satisfactory? Very few people are completely healthy in all three areas studied by health psychology.

3. Now describe what actions you could take to move yourself toward complete health on each of the three health continuums.

4. Analyze your most recent illness or injury using the biopsychosocial approach. Write about biological, psychological, and sociocultural factors that contributed to the illness or injury.

5. Explain what biopsychosocial factors contributed to your recovery.

## References

American Psychological Association, Division 38-Health Psychology, Division Description. Retrieved January 24, 2008 from http://www.apa.org/about/division/div38.html

Baron, R., Cutrona, C., Hicklin, D., Russel, D., & Lubaroff, D. (1990). Social support and immune function among spouses of cancer patients. *Journal of personality and social psychology, 59,* 344–352.

Baum, A., Perry, N. W., & Tarbell, S. (2004). The development of psychology as a health science. In R. G. Frank, A. Baum, & J. L. Wallender (Eds.), *Handbook of clinical health psychology: Vol. 3, Models and perspectives in health psychology* (pp. 9–28). Washington, DC: American Psychological Association.

Belar, C. D., & McInyre, T. (2004). Professional issues in health psychology. In S. Sutton, A. Baum, & M. Johnston (Eds.), *The Sage hand-book of health psychology* (pp. 402–419). London: Sage.

Belar, C. D., Brown, R. A., Hersch, L. E., Hornyak, L. M, Rozensky, R. H., Sheridan, E. P., Brown R. T., & Reed, G. W. (2001). Self-assessment in clinical health psychology: A model for ethical expansion of practice. *Professional Psychology: Research and Practice, 32,* 135–141.

Belloc, N. B., & Breslow, L. (1972). Relationship of physical health status and health practices. *Preventive Medicine, 1,* 409–421.

Bergner, M., Bobbit, R. A., Carter, W. B., & Gibson, B. S. (1981). The Sickness Impact Profile: Development and final revision of a health status measure. *Medical Care, 19,* 787–805.

Delbanco, T. (1993). The healing roles of doctor and patient. In B. Moyers, *Healing and the mind* (pp. 7–23). New York: Doubleday.

Descartes, R. (1952). Meditations on the first philosophy in which the existence of God and the distinction between mind and body are demonstrated by Rene Descartes. (E. S. Haldane & G. R. T. Ross, Trans.). In *Great books of the western world* (Vol. 31, pp. 75–103). Chicago: Encyclopedia Britannica.

Durkheim, E. (1997). *Suicide.* New York: The Free Press.

Engel, G. L. (1977). The need for a new medical model: A challenge for biomedicine. *Science, 196,* 129–136.

Freud, S. (1952). Selected papers on hysteria. The major works of Sigmund Freud (A. A. Brill Trans.). In *Great books of the western world* (Vol. 54, pp. 25–118). Chicago: Encyclopedia Britannica.

Galen (1952). On the natural faculties by Galen (A. J. Brock, Trans.). In *Great books of the western world* (Vol. 10, pp. 166–215). Chicago: Encyclopedia Britannica.

Hippocrates (1952). Hippocratic writings (F. Adams, Trans.). In *Great books of the western world* (Vol. 10, pp. 1–166). Chicago: Encyclopedia Britannica.

Jansen, M. S., & Weinman, J. (Eds.) (1991). *The international development of health psychology.* New York: Harwood Academic.

Matarazzo, J. D. (1980). Behavioral health and behavioral medicine: Frontiers for a new health psychology. *The American Psychologist, 35* (9) 807–817.

McDaniel, S. H., Belar, C. D., Schroeder, C., Hargrove, D. S., & Freeman, E. L. (2002). A training curriculum for professional psychologists in primary care. *Professional Psychology: Research and Practice, 33,* 65–72.

Morrow, M., Harnkivsky, O. & Varcoe, C. (Eds.), (2007). *Women's health in Canada.* Toronto: University of Toronto Press.

Papas, R. K., Belar, C. D., & Rozensky, R. H., (2004). The practice of clinical health psychology: Professional issue. In R.G. Frank, A. Baum, & J. L. Wallander (Eds.), *Handbook of clinical health psychology, Volume 3* (pp. 293–319).

Washington, DC: American Psychological Association.

Redd, W. H., DuHamel, K. N., Vickberg, S. M. J., Ostroff, J. L., Smith, M. Y., Jacobson, P. B., et al. (2001). Long-term adjustment in cancer survivors: Integration of classical conditioning and cognitive processing models. In A. Baum & B. Anderson (Eds.), *Psychosocial interventions for cancer* (pp. 77-97). Washington, DC: American Psychological Association.

Schwartz, G. E., & Weiss, S. M. (1977). *Proceedings of the Yale conference on behavioral medicine.* New Haven, CT: U. S. Department of Health, Education, and Welfare, Public Health Service, National Institutes of Health.

Schwartz, G. E. (1982). Testing the biopsychosocial model: The ultimate challenge facing behavioral medicine? *Journal of Consulting and Clinical Psychology, 50,* 1040–1053.

Smith, T. W., & Ruiz, J. M. (2004). Personality theory and research in the study of health and behavior. In R. G. Frank, A. Baum, & J. L. Wallander (Eds.), *Handbook of Clinical Health Psychology, Volume 3* (pp. 143–199). Washington, DC: American Psychological Association.

United States Department of Health and Human Services (USDHHS), National Center for Health Statistics, National Vital Statistics reports, 56, (5). Deaths: Leading Causes for 2004. Retrieved January 24, 2008 from http://www.cdc.gov

Turk, D. C. (2002). Clinical effectiveness and cost effectiveness of treatments for chronic pain. *Clinical Journal of Pain, 18,* 355–365.

Weber, M. (1930). *The Protestant ethic and the spirit of capitalism* (T. Parsons Trans.) New York: Scribner's Sons.

World Health Organization (1948). *Constitution of the World Health Organization.* Geneva: Author; also *Basic Documents,* 45th ed, October 2006 (Supplement).

World Health Organization (2006). Mortality Data, November 17, 2006 Update. Retrieved October 9, 2007 from http:www.who.org

# Chapter 2

# Conducting and Evaluating Research in Health Psychology

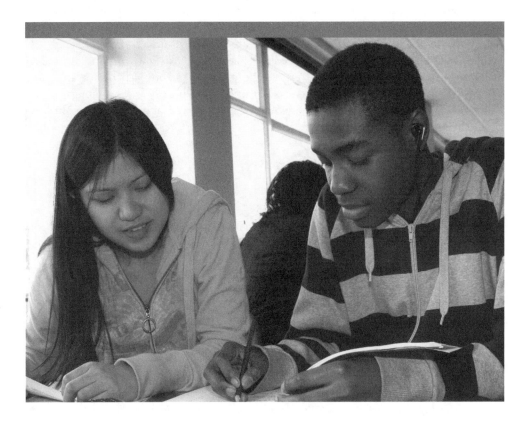

## Learning Objectives

After studying this chapter students will have the knowledge and skills to be able to:

1. Explain advantages of using scientific methods to gain knowledge.
2. Clarify differences between qualitative and quantitative research methods in health psychology.
3. Describe and explain the reasons for important aspects of scientific methods.
4. Define and give examples of experimental research methods.

5. Define and give examples of research methods that use correlations.
6. Evaluate reports of research studies in health psychology.
7. Design a health psychology research study on a topic of interest.

## Introduction

A great deal of what we learn when we are young is a result of **experiential learning**. In infancy we discover, explore, and learn through observation and experimentation. For example, we learned to avoid scalding water because of the pain we experienced the first time we touched it. The people taking care of us socialized us so we learned which behaviors were expected of us, including many of the health-related behaviors discussed in this textbook. Perhaps we tried experimenting with different behaviors, such as smoking, and noticed reactions from caregivers and peers. We learned about the world from every person and thing we saw, heard, and did. We spent many years learning and eventually learned enough to gain admission to college. Congratulations! Now we learn a great deal by reading and hearing about the world around us.

## Scientific Research: Another Way to Learn About the World

Scientific news is reported on television, the Internet, and in newspapers and magazines. It is important to understand scientific methods in order to evaluate those reports. When studies are well designed, well implemented, and accurately interpreted, they are probably worth applying in our lives. Scientific findings can help us make better choices about health- and safety-related behaviors and products. Ideally, science produces information that is both accurate and objective or unbiased.

### Science Is Systematic

Studies following scientific protocols are more likely to result in accurate findings. For example, a key requirement in observational or descriptive studies is to make many observations. If we were interested in the effects of exercise at shopping malls, we would observe or interview ethnically diverse people, males and females, every day of the week, at all different times of the day, in different areas of the mall, and during all four seasons. We would keep careful records of what people said or did in order to arrive at accurate conclusions based on the evidence or data. When designing studies, scientists rely on representative samples, or sets of people reflecting characteristics of people about whom the scientists plan to draw conclusions. Scientific studies can be very expensive to complete and many studies include only small numbers of people. The chapter on cardiovascular disease references studies of fewer than 200 participants, but also refers to the Framingham heart disease study that has continued for two generations and is likely to add a third generation (Voelker, 1998). Science is more accurate than casual obervation because scientists follow systematic organized

---

**experiential learning** Learning through personal experience or activity rather than through reading or being formally taught by an instructor.

sets of rules. If findings are notable, they are published in professional journals and may be repeated or replicated so results can be compared. A meta-analysis compares results of several studies.

## Science Strives to Be Unbiased

A second scientific ideal is to be unbiased or objective. In reality everyone is biased, but scientists try to keep an open mind and reach conclusions based on what is discovered rather than on what they expected to discover. Being objective or unbiased is difficult. For example, in the 1960s scientists doing meta-analyses of many studies concluded that smoking cigarettes is harmful to health. If the scientists were smokers, it might be difficult for them to be unbiased, and this prejudice might taint their conclusions. It is also difficult to arrive at a conclusion of harm if organizations with a vested interest pay for the studies. For example, cigarette-producing companies sponsoring a study might find it difficult to accept and publicize the conclusion that smoking is harmful. We depend on science to be unbiased and rely on scientists to be truthful about what they discover. Fortunately, ethical principles guide new searches for knowledge and help keep scientists trustworthy. Students can use these same principles when evaluating research reports. The scientific method is not a perfect approach to increasing knowledge, but it is the best system devised so far.

## Review of Terms Used in Science

Theories, Models, and Generalization
"A theory is a set of interrelated concepts, definitions, and propositions that present a systematic view of events or situations by specifying relations among variables in order to explain and predict the events or situations" (Glanz, Rimer, & Lewis, 2002, p. 25).

**Theories** are important because they influence behavior. For example, at one time a widely accepted theory was that the earth was flat. Sailors feared sailing out of sight of land lest they fall off the edge of the world. The theory influenced behavior until some sailors demonstrated the earth could be circled, or circumnavigated. It was an experiment when people first sailed safely around the world returning to the same port from which they embarked. This experiment tested the theory of the flatness of the earth and eventually the theory was discarded.

A theory begins as a tentative idea or explanation usually based on observations. Health psychologists see persistent patterns of human behavior and develop ideas about why they occur. Observations become the bases for studies. Theories may begin as guesses, but may

**theory** In health psychology, a theory is a set of related statements or propositions from which hypotheses can be developed for research purposes; theories organize and explain observations.

end as organized sets of principles explaining phenomena. One theory we already know is Newton's theory of gravity.

The word **model** is also used when discussing theories in health psychology. Two examples of theories and models in health psychology are the theory of planned behavior and the health belief model. Both are discussed in the next chapter. They were developed to explain what motivates people to change health-related behaviors. Once health promotion specialists know what motivates people to change they can design programs to help people stop smoking or start exercising. For example, some theories include the prediction that attitudes precede behavior. Therefore, to change behaviors such as smoking, we must first change people's attitudes. Other theories suggest that serious threats or danger will change behaviors. That theory is often applied in childrearing: We all recall being punished for behaviors our caregivers did not like. Theories and models serve as frameworks for research, help organize and discuss scientific findings, and generate new searches for information.

One goal of theoretical sciences is to be able to generalize or make broad statements. When we generalize findings, we are saying those findings apply to many different people or in many different situations. Each study adds more knowledge about the world. Scientists use scientific methods to determine accuracy and usefulness of theories and models.

**Evaluating Theories and Models** Theories help make sense of the world, but a drawback of theories is limitations on our thinking. Even a theory or model based on scientific study can be wrong. This is why we are often urged to "think outside the box." We hope that research teams will eventually find new solutions to old problems through systematic scientific processes. Research outcomes may support existing theories or lead to new theories.

Scientists perform research to evaluate and to attempt to prove or disprove theories. One theory in health psychology research concerns the causes of obesity. Obesity is a major risk factor for a very destructive disease known as type II diabetes. Although some aspects of how people store fat on the body may be affected by genetic heritage, in general, obesity results when people consume more calories in food than they expend or use or burn by movement. The body stores the unused calories in the form of fat. Fat cells accumulate over the years, and eventually a person is said to be obese according to government standards for body mass index (BMI) (U.S. Departments of Agriculture and Health and Human Services, 2005). We could design experiments to test this theory of obesity by trying to reduce the amount of fat on people's bodies through limitations on their caloric intake and by encouragement of exercise to use up calories already stored in body fat. People pay a great deal of money to participate in such programs at gyms, spas, and diet centers. By having an accurate theory

> **model** In health psychology, a model is a set of statements explaining the relationship between factors or variables contributing to some phenomenon. For example, a model may include principles constructed to explain the human behavior of regular aerobic exercise or the behavior of choosing to be vaccinated against a disease. An example is the health belief model. A model is less formal than a theory.

about causes of obesity, health scientists and physicians can help people live longer and healthier lives by preventing diabetes that results from obesity. An accurate theory of obesity makes it possible to test the results of behavior change.

Variables

A **variable** is any factor used in research that can diverge or take on more than one form. Being human is not a variable, because there is no variation—a human being is a human being. Characteristics of humans such as gender, education, socioeconomic status, eating patterns, exercise patterns, mental health, and stress levels are all variable characteristics. One commonly used variable is age. We refer to infants being 1 hour old, adults being 90 years old, or rocks being millions of years old, and we make predictions or observations based on these ages. Scientists precisely define the variables used in their studies. **Operationalization** refers to the process of describing a variable by stating precisely how it will be measured in a study. For example, an investigator may operationalize age as the number of years a person has lived based on his or her last birthday.

The **independent variable (IV)** is the causal factor in research. It is the variable with the potential of influencing or causing changes in other variables, known as **dependent variables**. In the obesity example, food consumption and lack of exercise are independent variables while obesity is the dependent variable.

Hypotheses

A **hypothesis** (pl: hypotheses) is a prediction about the relationship between or among variables, and experiments can be used to test hypotheses. A hypothesis in health psychology

**variable** Any factor used in research that can diverge or take on more than one form, such as age or gender.

**operationalization** The process of defining a variable by stating precisely how it will be measured in a study.

**independent variable (IV)** The variable that is viewed as a cause affecting another variable within a hypothesis. For example, in the hypothesis that alcohol use by drivers increases the likelihood of automobile wrecks, the independent variable is alcohol use.

**dependent variable** The variable that is viewed as the probable result of the independent variable. For example, in the hypothesis that auto wrecks often occur because the person driving the car has been drinking alcohol, the dependent variable is automobile wrecks.

**hypothesis** A prediction about a relationship between variables. If the hypothesis is that when people believe they have a serious disease, they will usually seek medical treatment for the disease, the independent variable is the belief, the dependent variable is the behavior, and the hypothesis is the prediction about the effect of the independent variable on the dependent variable.

could be "A teenager is more likely to smoke cigarettes if one or more of the teen's friends smoke cigarettes." If this hypothesis is verified, then a next step might be to devise a health promotion intervention to prevent teens from starting to smoke cigarettes that takes peer infuence into account.

### Data

**Data** are bits of information collected about variables. A datum may provide evidence enabling scientists to accept or reject hypotheses. If the majority of teenage smokers never saw anyone else smoke before they started smoking, then we would doubt the original hypothesis about that independent variable contributing to cigarette smoking.

### Replication

**Replication** refers to the practice of repeating scientific studies in an attempt to obtain the same results. The methods used in experiments and other types of studies are recorded and described in professional scientific journals so other interested scientists can repeat, or replicate, the study. Replication increases the chance that the results are accurate.

## Research Methods and Science in Health Psychology

Many health psychologists work within different venues, including research, clinical work, and public health. Research areas include psychosocial models of health, behavioral theories of health promotion, disease prevention, personality theory, biobehavioral effects on health, and psychoneuroimmunology (Frank, Wallander, & Baum, 2004). This chapter provides a brief overview of empirical research methods that serve as the basis of knowledge in health psychology. Due to advances in communication, findings are shared, questioned, and corroborated or contradicted by other health psychologists throughout the world. This textbook includes examples of research done by health psychologists, but accumulation of knowledge in a scientific field does not end when a textbook is published. Students must rely on their professors to keep up to date with new empirical findings and to share them in class.

Research is a massive subject with many books dedicated to scientific methods used in social sciences including health psychology (Babbie, 2004; Howell, 2002; Cozby, 2007). This chapter assumes that students know about research methods used in psychology, so this

---

**data** Information assembled about variables. The word data is plural, and the word datum is singular. For example, the student assembled or amassed data about the variables relating to her class research project.

**replication** The practice of repeating scientific studies to affirm accuracy of study results.

chapter provides only a brief review. After reading this chapter, students will have the knowledge and skills to evaluate health psychology research, and even to design studies about health topics.

## Qualitative and Quantitative Research Methods

Two general approaches used in health psychology are **quantitative** and **qualitative research methods** (Cottrell & McKenzie, 2005; Murray, 2004). Quantitative methods include experiments and observational, correlational, or descriptive studies. Qualitative methods are often used to collect data on biopsychosocial phenomena for which quantitative measures are not appropriate (French, Yardley, & Sutton, 2004). Some scholars consider quantitative methods to be more systematic and qualitative methods to be more flexible and reflective. This chapter focuses mainly on quantitative methods, but students should also understand purposes, methods, and outcomes of qualitative research.

### Qualitative Methods

Qualitative methods include the study of subjective health-related experiences such as people's reactions to being diagnosed with heart disease or cancer. Research methods include interviews, focus-group discussions, observation (including participant observation), analysis of medical notes and patient diaries, and audio- and video-recording. Qualitative methods often reveal previously unknown motivations and attitudes of people struggling with health problems such as obesity or excessive alcohol use. This type of research can lead to new ideas about effective ways to change behavior. Psychologists engaged in critical health psychology prefer qualitative research methods and such methods often offer alternative approaches to the theories and methods found in most health psychology textbooks (Fox & Prilleltensky, 1997).

For example, a health psychologist might assert that some health conditions mainly reflect and result from social inequalities, including discrimination against and exploitation of particular groups of people, rather than from individual behaviors. In contrast, federal policy may emphasize individual choices while ignoring the role of social inequities in the causes of health problems (Murray, 2004). Critical health psychologists with this perspective may urge colleagues to promote health through social change rather than by focusing on changing individual behaviors.

**quantitative research methods** Types of research used to assemble numerical data about a variable; one example of a quantitative variable is age.

**qualitative research methods** Types of research used to assemble data on measures that are not numerical such as people's gender, their perception about their health risks, or factors affecting that perception.

Quantitative Methods

Quantitative methods include experiments and observational studies. The goal of experiments is to test theories about causes of phenomena such as stress, heart disease, traffic accidents, cancer, or substance abuse. A testable theory about stress might posit that thinking about college-entrance exams causes stress levels to rise among most high school students.

A second general quantitative approach is observational or descriptive research. Descriptive studies are systematic, but less focused on discovering causal factors than on finding conditions or situations that contribute to outcomes such as obesity, depression, stress, or lung cancer. Quantitative research methods usually rely on large numbers of participants and statistical analyses.

## Using the Experimental Research Method to Determine Cause and Effect

Determining causality, or the cause of some phenomenon, is a complex, controversial, and difficult task. Experiments test hypotheses against observations in the search for causality. The design of experiments is difficult because researchers must control all variables other than the independent variable, that could influence results in a study. If a goal is to say that Factor A causes Factor B, then the researchers must control conditions other than Factor A that may affect Factor B. The presence of many variables might change research results. Gender and age are examples of two important variables. Scientists cannot generalize study results to all people if only females are included in an experiment. Neither should we generalize findings if all subjects were 22-year-old college students.

## The Process of Setting Up an Experimental Research Study

1. Review the Literature and Write a Hypothesis

Imagine health psychology students are assigned a small research project just for the experience. College students often want to know how to lose the weight they gained since leaving high school. They could design an experiment to discover what helps or causes college students to lose weight. There is not much time or money to complete the study, so we limit the experiment to 12 subjects or participants and 6 weeks of time. With such strict limitations we know we will not be able to generalize study results to all people or even to all college students. We review applicable research reported in health psychology journals. Because our study is about college students, we examine journals that include college students in health-related studies. In the *Journal of American College Health* we read about an experiment using academic incentives to increase participation in physical activity programs for weight loss (DeVahl, King, & Williamson, 2005). That study found that students receiving academic rewards for exercising lost more body fat than students who were not offered academic incentives. This article gives us ideas about experiments to reduce body fat gained since high school. The hypothesis states a cause and effect relationship between variables: "College students offered an incentive will lose more fat than students who are not offered an incentive."

2. Identify, Define, and Operationalize Variables

We predict that rewards or incentives will cause or contribute to fat loss. The incentive or reward is the independent variable. The dependent variable is fat loss. The downward change or loss of fat-weight produced by the experiment depends on the independent variable, a reward. To operationalize variables, we specify how we will measure variables. A reward or an incentive is defined as something that incites to action. In this experiment the reward must be something college students desire. Most students want more time. We could operationalize the incentive (IV) as help with school work. We are not going to cheat and do their work, but we will save students time on routine school tasks so they have time to exercise for fat loss. For example, we will do time-consuming chores for them such as photocopying or returning books to the library.

The dependent variable, fat, is defined as adipose tissue on the body. When people gain fat, their girth or waist measurement usually increases, so we operationalize the dependent variable, fat loss, as a decrease in the distance around the waist measured in inches.

3. Obtain Approval for the Research

We must next complete paperwork for permission from the college institutional review board (IRB) to begin the research. We describe the experiment and include a copy of the informed consent form for participants to sign. Each subject or participant must read and understand the risks and benefits of participating in the study. They are also told they may withdraw from the research at any time, although we hope they will not. After receiving IRB approval we move on to the next step.

4. Recruit Participants or Subjects

We recruit 12 students to be subjects. For experiments we need at least 2 groups. The experimental group is the set of people who will be affected by the independent variable, the incentive. The control group is the set of people who will not be exposed to the independent variable. People in the control group and the experimental group will be similar except for the independent variable. For example, their ages and genders will be the same and they will all be college students. This is because age and gender might affect the outcome of the study.

5. Randomize Membership in the Control and Experimental Groups

Half of the participants are members of the experimental group, and they will receive help with school tasks so they have more time for exercising. Members of the control group will not receive any help. Random allocation of participants in experiments is central to accuracy and gives experiments greater creditability (French, Yardly, & Sutton, 2004, p. 333). After recruiting 12 college students, we designate who will be in the experimental and control groups. Each student recruited for the study must have an equal chance of being in either group.

We write their names on identical pieces of paper, put the names in a paper bag, and then draw names without peeking inside the bag. The first 6 names drawn will be in the experimental group and the remaining 6 people are in the control group. All 12 had an equal chance of being in either group. We can now conduct the experiment to determine if the incentive of "saving time by doing menial tasks" for the 6 students in the experimental group causes them to lose more fat from around their waists than the 6 students in the control group.

## Experimental Research Difficulties: Self-Selection and the Placebo Effect

### Self-Selection Bias

People who agree to participate in studies may be different in significant ways from people who refuse to participate. This can be a source of error in research. **Self-selection bias** limits generalizing research results, because what is found may not be true of all people, but only for the kind of people who agree to participate. For example, health intervention studies frequently include people such as smokers who want to quit or patients who want to reduce risks of another heart attack. People interested in improving their health may be significantly different from people who decline to participate. This fact limits the ability of scientists to generalize from a study.

### The Placebo Effect

A second problem in experimental research is the **placebo effect**. A **placebo** is a treatment that is inactive, e.g., a sugar pill. The placebo effect is especially problematic when the study

**self-selection bias** When participants decide to opt into a social science study as a respondent or are allowed to choose between being in the experimental group or the control group, this may affect the accuracy of research results. Making the choice risks the inclusion of an important bias or prejudice that might invalidate study results. Random selection of participants makes study results more likely to be accurate.

**placebo effect** An outcome or result attributed to a person's belief. For example, physicians gave patients sugar pills to encourage their recovery from an illness. If the patient believed the placebo would help them, it usually did. The placebo effect is a difficulty in experimental research.

**placebo** A treatment or substance believed to be ineffective by researchers that may contribute to positive changes in research participants due to their beliefs about its effectiveness. The placebo effect must be taken into account when designing experimental research.

is evaluating the effectiveness of a treatment or intervention. Histories of medicine cite cases when healing occurred in spite of the fact that treatments later proved to be useless or even harmful. Hoping for therapeutic gain, some physicians once gave sugar pills to please patients and improve healing, although the practice is now considered unethical (Thompson, 2005). The mind is very powerful, and placebo effects reveal the close connection between the mind and the body (Williams & Martin, 2002). For example, when people in pain are given inactive pills but are told the pills will reduce their pain, many people report they have less pain (see **Figure 2.1**).

The placebo effect demonstrates the fact that when people believe something to be true, it may have treatment effects even when there is no known scientific connection between the treatment and effect (Brannon & Feist, 1997). The placebo effect reflects beliefs of the user, and beliefs influence treatment outcomes (Brody, 2000a & 200b). Clinical trials for medical treatments and experiments in health psychology are affected by the placebo effect. The effect is any improvement occurring after treatment for which there is no scientific explanation. The placebo effect is an interesting phenomenon occurring in medicine, pharmacology, health psychology, and psychiatric research. The effect even occurs in cases of sham surgery (Moerman & Wayne, 2002). Treatments for ulcers, pain, colds, headaches, and asthma have generated the placebo effect (Turner, Deyo, Loeser, Von Korff, & Fordyce, 1994).

This may be why what we call a home remedy is often effective or successful. Some home remedies may have true medicinal value, but it is more likely the power of suggestion that makes the remedy effective. Studies show that placebo effects are related to patient characteristics, physical factors, and patient-physician relationships (Bensing & Verhaak, 2004). One explanation is that when people expect success from a treatment, they are more likely to follow their physician's suggestions, thus speeding their recovery. Further, if we believe we will recover from an illness, the belief may improve our immune system to resist a disease. Social support from family and friends may also help speed healing, even if recovery reflects the natural history of an illness (Sobel, 1990).

**Figure 2.1**

This is an example of the placebo effect that occurred during a clinical trial to test the effectiveness of medication.

*Source:* Edlin, G., & Golanty, E. (2007). *Health and wellness* (9th ed.). Sudbury, MA: Jones and Bartlett Publishers.

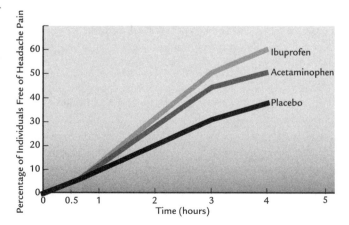

In clinical studies, members of the experimental group receive an active medication while control group members receive a placebo or inactive substance that looks, tastes, and feels exactly like the medication. Placebos may even have side effects similar to active medications. In experiments, the placebo effect is any improvement that occurs in control group members. Both real and inert substances usually have a beneficial effect, but the effect of the experimental treatment must be greater than the effect of the placebo before a medication is judged to be beneficial. The medication must outperform the placebo.

Double-Blind Studies

One way to counteract the placebo effect is the single-blind experimental design, in which subjects do not know if they are in the experimental or the control group. Scientists realized that they may also influence study outcomes due to their inside knowledge about which subjects are in the experimental group. **Double-blind studies** address this problem. In a double-blind experiment, neither participants nor researchers know who receives the placebo and who receives the treatment until after the experiment is complete. The ideal experimental model is a placebo-controlled, double-blind study.

There are other problems when doing experimental research. The results of experiments implemented in laboratory conditions may be different from what happens in real-world situations. Ethical concerns about doing harm also limit the use of experiments. Valid experimental results are more likely when a) they are based on a precise hypothesis, b) subjects or participants are similar with regard to important variables at the onset of the experiment, c) subjects are randomly assigned to experimental or control group, and d) both subjects and researchers are blind as to which subjects belong to the experimental and control groups. These conditions may not be possible, because of limited funding, limited participation, or ethical concerns. An alternative research method is a descriptive study.

## Using Descriptive or Correlational Studies to Discover Relationships Between Variables

The goal of observational research designs is to discover what variables contribute to outcomes or effects. In these types of studies, scientists draw conclusions about relationships between variables, but they cannot say one variable causes another. **Correlational studies**

---

**double-blind study** A study designed to eliminate the expectations of participants in a study and the biases of those conducting the study. In single-blind research designs, the participants do not know if they are receiving the treatment or a placebo but the providers of the treatment do know. In a double-blind study, neither participants nor scientists know who is in the experimental group and who is in the control group.

**correlational study** A research effort to discover relationships between variables.

are often used in cases where experiments would violate laws protecting human subjects. For example, it is possible to design an experiment to demonstrate smoking contributes to lung cancer or osteoporosis, but encouraging people to adopt behaviors that may be harmful would be unethical and no IRB would allow it. In **observational studies**, scientists are not controlling or manipulating variables; rather, they look for the existence of relationships between variables and the size and direction of those relationships. Examples of observational studies are surveys such as questionnaires and interviews: Perhaps you participated in a descriptive study when someone stopped you at the mall and asked you to answer a few questions.

Scientists using these research methods may decide to describe findings in terms of independence and dependence. Dependence and independence are a consequence of the time when one factor occurred in relation to the other. Usually only variables coming first can be independent. A variable cannot be independent if its occurrence follows the other variable in time. One example of the importance of the order of variables is lung cancer. If lung cancer occurred before people smoked cigarettes, then cigarette smoking could not be an independent risk factor for cases of lung cancer. In fact, some people who have never been exposed to cigarette smoke do develop tumors in their lungs, so we know cigarette smoke is not the *only* cause of lung cancer. On the other hand, people who smoke cigarettes are more likely to develop lung cancer than people who do not smoke. Scientists can accurately say that cigarette smoking is a likely contributor to many lung cancers.

Another health-related example is osteoporosis. Osteoporosis is a weakening of bones caused by reduced bone density and generally occurs in older people. We might conclude that osteoporosis is related to aging, but being old does not cause osteoporosis, because there are many old people who do not have osteoporosis and there are young people who do have osteoporosis. Scientists wanted to know if lifestyle factors contributed to osteoporosis. They compared lifestyles of people with osteoporosis to lifestyles of people without osteoporosis, and discovered that people who never exercised were more likely to develop osteoporosis than people who did exercise. We cannot demonstrate that lack of exercise causes osteoporosis, because an experiment would be unethical, but we can say lack of exercise contributes to some cases of osteoporosis or that lack of exercise is a risk factor for osteoporosis.

Sometimes scientists pay people to participate in experiments, but it would still be against the law in the United States to do a study if it was likely that subjects or participants would be harmed. Years ago, people in prisons and mental hospitals were placed in studies dangerous to their health and well-being. This is no longer allowed. Many people also believe that

---

**observational study**  A study in which no variables are manipulated as they are in experiments; the researcher is simply observing what occurs, such as watching a group of children to see how they share toys. When people know they are being observed, they may change their behavior.

animals should not be harmed in experimental studies. As laws are currently written, animal studies are permitted if the animals are treated as compassionately or humanely as possible.

## Samples of Participants, Respondents, or Subjects

It is impossible to study everyone in the world, so scientists study **samples** or sets of people who are representative of others. We understand the concept of sampling because we use it in food tasting. After eating one slice of cake we know how the whole cake will taste, even though all we took was a small sample. Statisticians know about accurate sampling techniques. In reports, scientists describe their sampling techniques to explain why the results of their study can be generalized to a larger population. Sample size and the way samples are drawn are two important pieces of information about a study.

Sample Size, Representative, and Random Samples
The number of people included in a study is important. Generally, a study based on many people is more generalizable than when conclusions are based on only a few people. There are mathematical formulas to help determine appropriate sample size. How representative a sample is also affects the credibility of a study. Samples must represent the type of people about which conclusions are drawn. There are statistical models to ensure that samples are sufficiently large and representative.

Samples should be **random samples**, that is, groups of people drawn randomly from a population. In the example of an experiment, membership in control and experimental groups was based on random assignment. Each person was equally likely to be chosen for either group. Randomness is often important in observational research, too. For example, if we want to draw conclusions about all students on our campus, it will be necessary to include a random sample of all students. We want a large, representative sample drawn randomly from the entire student body in order to ensure that most types of students are included. We could assign every student a unique number and then use a table of random numbers to help select study participants. We may first divide or stratify a list of students into sets based on number of hours passed to ensure we have freshmen, sophomores, juniors, and seniors in the sample, if the characteristic of class designation is important for

**sample** A small quantity of some phenomenon taken to understand the nature of the total phenomenon. For example, a scientist may interview a sample of a hundred cancer patients about the level of their optimism to survive the disease and draw conclusions about all cancer patients.

**random sample** The process of taking a sample in such a way that each member or part has an equal chance of being selected. For example, scientists might use a table of random numbers to select 1,000 students from among the 10,000 students in the sophomore class to be included in their study.

study results. Random selection can be expensive and time consuming, but it generally improves study design.

Non-Random Samples

Some studies are based on samples that are not representative of all the people about whom we want to draw conclusions. Some **non-random samples** are based on convenience. For example, if we are writing articles for a school newspaper, we might ask everyone in our carpool what she or he thinks about an event. This is a small, non-representative, non-random sample of people on campus. It is simply a convenient set of people, and the opinions given probably do not accurately reflect or represent the opinions of all students. (The opinions *may* be representative of some other group, e.g., "people I know.") Another example of a convenience sample is people standing in line to get into a new club or movie.

In **snowball samples**, we gather information from one person, who in turn refers us to others who had similar experiences or have similar characteristics. Snowball samples are not representative, because each person is connected to the previous and succeeding people, and experiences and opinions are limited by that fact.

Revisiting the Problem of Self-Selection

Self-selection is also a problem in observational research. People willing to participate in studies may not represent all people. The people who agree to fill out a survey or be interviewed may be significantly different from people who refuse to complete a survey. For example, research participants tend to be better educated and younger than the general population. These differences may affect accuracy or generalizability of conclusions. Scientists working in national health centers such as the Centers for Disease Control (CDC) often use a technique called random digit dialing to decide what homes to call when they are doing a survey. They hope to be able to generalize to all the people in the United States, but do not have the time or money to call all people in the country. Consequently they decide on a sample size and a computer randomly selects phone numbers. If someone does not answer, the next number on the list is called. CDC researchers can divide the country into geographic regions so they are more likely to have a representative sample of people from different parts of the country. Think about a survey about skin cancer. It would be important to have respondents from all geographic regions, because the amount of exposure to the sun is different in northern and southern regions of the country. It would also be

**non-random sample** The process of taking a sample in such a way that certain members or parts are more likely to be chosen thus biasing the conclusions of a study.

**snowball sample** A non-random sampling process that relies on participants to recommend others they know to be included in a study, for example, interviewing people with HIV/AIDS and then asking for names of other patients to be included in the study. This study may be biased because each participant knows the other.

important to distinguish between people who spend many hours outdoors and people who spend few hours outdoors, so the survey should ask about that. This structuring makes samples more representative for the purpose of generalization. Of course, by using telephones, CDC researchers miss the people who do not have phones or who are not at home when the call is made or who refuse to answer questions.

There are specific situations in which descriptive studies cover most people we want to generalize about when reporting study results. For example, many college administrators and faculty members want to know what students think about the courses they take. At the end of semesters, students in every class on campus are usually asked to complete evaluations of courses and teaching. Most students conscientiously fill out these forms. Scores generated probably accurately reflect class opinions. These surveys are important because they affect salaries and promotion of faculty members and because professors may change the way a course is taught based on student opinion (**Figure 2.2**).

## Questionnaires, Surveys, Interviews, and Scales

Designing Questions for Interviews and Surveys

Scientists take care when wording questions for interviews and questionnaires. A **loaded question** is one that leads to particular answers rather than giving respondents the opportunity to answer freely. Two examples of ridiculously loaded questions are "You didn't eat any fried foods today, did you?" and "You exercised every day this past week, didn't you?" We can pretest questions on a few people to see if the question is understandable and will provide answers that meet the purposes of the study.

Scales

Many health psychologists develop and use sets of questions that are combined to represent a complex concept. These sets of questions are called **scales**. For example, in studying eating disorders, researchers devised a series of questions incorporating various aspects of anorexia nervosa. Researchers found that people with anorexia nervosa answer questions in typical ways, and the scale could be used to identify other people with anorexia. Another

**loaded question** A question in an interview or survey that is phrased in such a way as to make a certain answer more likely. For example, asking "How often do you eat at fast food restaurants?" rather than asking, "Please give the names of the last three restaurants from which you bought a meal."

**scale** A measurement device. In psychology it often is a series of questions by which the combined answers represent a complex concept. For example, a life-events survey may measure major stressors. A stress inventory may assess sources and the impact of stressful events in people's lives. Mood, fatigue, self-efficacy, helplessness, and other social science factors may be measured by validated sets of questions or scales.

**Figure 2.2**
At the end of each semester college students are asked to evaluate courses and teaching. Questionnaire answers are collected, quantified, and reported for every course.

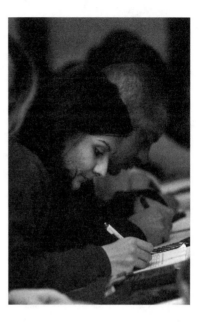

multifaceted or complex concept is body image. Research might include a scale or set of questions to discover ways people think about their own body shape. We recognize scales when we are asked about the extent to which we agree or disagree with statements. There are usually five to seven response categories or levels of agreement. Answers may be scored and added to arrive at composite scores. Scales are tested over and over again to improve their reliability and accuracy. Once validated, scales can be used by other scientists interested in the same kinds of topics. There are scales to measure many variables, including stress and hostility.

Reliability and Validity

**Reliability** and **validity** are possible characteristics of questionnaires, interviews, and scales. When sets of questions and scales are reliable, it means they provide consistent, stable results time and time again. For example, questions about people's ages are reliable if they resulted in the same answer today that they did last month (unless respondents have a birthday over that time period). Some questions are famously unreliable. For example, asking people

reliability The quality of getting consistent results from a set of questions or observations. For example, a stress scale is reliable if it consistently identifies or separates highly stressed people from less-stressed people and predicts who will get sick and who will not.

validity The accuracy of a test or measurement. For example, does the question or measurement accurately assess obesity or stress or anger?

about their blood pressure (BP) often produces different answers. One day people say their pressure is 190/40 and next month report it is 140/90. BP numbers are confusing and difficult to remember, so answers to that question are not reliable. To add to the confusion, a person's blood pressure can vary depending on the time of day, how recently he or she smoked or exercised, whether the person is seated or standing, and even whether the technician is wearing a white uniform.

Validity refers to accuracy. For questions and scales to be valid, they must be designed to obtain precisely accurate answers. A question is valid if it provides a measurement of what it is designed to measure. For example, which question is more likely to result in an accurate answer: "What was your weight in pounds when you weighed yourself this morning?" or "How much do you weigh?" The first question is more likely to be accurate, but not everyone weighs daily. Now think about questions designed to get an accurate answer about age. Is it better to ask "What year were you born?" and do the calculations yourself, or to ask, "How old are you?" The two ways may be equally valid or they may not. This brings us to the discussion about other sources of error in interviews and surveys.

Other Sources of Error

Surveys and scales are pretested repeatedly before being judged reliable and valid. Scientists are careful about words and the order in which questions are asked. As discussed earlier, it is unethical and dishonest to devise questions to lead to specific answers to support one's own opinions. A more likely source of error is respondents themselves. This is why pretesting questions is important. Respondents may forget information or be embarrassed. Some people make up answers to avoid saying "I don't remember" or "I don't know." Other times people are ashamed of what they did, so they give socially desirable answers. For example, people on weight-loss plans might be reluctant to report to a nutrition researcher that they ate an entire chocolate cake the previous day. This is why assuring people their answers are **confidential** or **anonymous** may improve accuracy.

Privacy Issues: Confidentiality and Anonymity

Researchers want accurate responses to questions, and promising privacy for respondents encourages greater accuracy. When interviews and questionnaires are said to be confidential, it means no one outside of the research team will know what people said in answer to questions. The principal investigator (PI) of the study is responsible for keeping records confidential, but anyone who works on the study may have access to names and answers. An

**confidentiality** A promise made to participants in research that their names and answers or information will be protected from people outside of the research staff.

**anonymous** An assurance given to research participants that any data collected will not be attributed to them. Participants filling out a survey form are assured they are anonymous and no one will ever know who filled out the form.

anonymous questionnaire is one in which no one knows how any one person answered. Anonymous surveys are more likely to elicit honest answers than confidential surveys. Of course, in interviews researchers conducting the interviews know how a person answered the questions, so only confidentiality can be promised.

## Correlations or Relationships Between Variables

In experimental research, the goal is to discover if one variable causes another. In descriptive research, the aim is to learn if variables are related. Using well-developed statistical techniques, researchers can also assess the strength of relationships between variables. For example, scientists report a strong, positive relationship between smoking and lung cancer. This can be said because people who smoke are much more likely to develop lung cancer than people who do not smoke. This is an important finding. Knowing this **correlation** encourages citizens, educators, scientists, and leaders of government agencies to work to prevent lung cancer by preventing smoking. This means some people could prevent lung cancer by avoiding cigarette smoking or stopping smoking. Lung cancer shortens life, interferes with productivity, and is difficult to treat. For these reasons federal, state, and city governments pass laws to try to prevent teenagers from starting to smoke and to keep smoke out of worksites, elevators, restaurants, and other public places.

### Strong and Weak Correlations

In observational studies, scientists are interested in uncovering what variables are correlated or related to each other. For example, two related variables are absence of exercise and obesity. It can be said there is a strong correlation between the two variables: The less people exercise, the more likely they are to be obese. It means there is a high degree of relationship between the two variables. Statistical analyses can tell researchers how closely two variables are related. A statistical finding of a zero (0) relationship means there is no correlation between the two variables. A statistical finding of plus or minus one (1) means there is a perfect or complete relationship between two variables. Correlations fall somewhere between +1 and 0 or 0 and –1. An example of a strong relationship between two variables is 0.85. An example of a weak relationship between two variables is 0.25. The correlation between smoking and lung cancer is so strong that scientists concluded that smoking is a significant risk factor for lung cancer.

### Interpreting Correlations

Variables can be related or correlated in the same or in opposite directions. For example, smoking and lung cancer have a strong positive relationship. This means that when rates

**correlation** The degree of relationship between variables. Correlations can be positive or negative. For example, the more cigarettes people smoke the more likely they are to develop lung cancer. There is a positive correlation between smoking and lung cancer.

of smoking increase then rates of lung cancer increase, or when smoking rates go down, lung cancer rates also go down. There is a strong positive relationship between the two variables. Variables can also be negatively correlated, that is, an increase in one is related to a decrease in the other variable. The two variables are highly correlated but move in the opposite direction from each other, so it is said they are negatively correlated. An example of a strong negative correlation occurs between the frequent use of sunscreen and development of skin cancer. These two variables are strongly related, but the relationship moves in opposite directions. The *more* often people use sunscreen, the *less* likely they are to develop skin cancer.

Correlations, or relationships between variables, do not demonstrate that one variable causes another as in experiments, but observational research shows relationships between variables. Scientists can say cigarette smoking probably causes lung cancer, because the relationship between the two variables is so powerful from a statistical perspective. See **Figure 2.3** to decide if there is a correlation between stress levels and aerobic exercise.

Intervening Variables

Even when there is a strong relationship between variables, scientists still must consider other explanations, because an intervening variable may explain correlations in observational research. In some cases, a strong relationship between two variables is discovered, but the correlation does not make sense from a scientific viewpoint. Many research textbooks use as an example of an intervening variable the positive correlation between the appearance of storks in northern Europe and the birth of babies. The common or intervening variable in this case is the arrival of spring. Storks go to certain locations to nest in the spring, and many babies are born in the spring. Another example of an intervening variable is the strong negative relationship between two variables: the number of peanut butter sandwiches eaten each week and the development of cancer. Among most segments of the population in the United States, when people's peanut-butter-sandwich consumption is high, their cancer rates are low. This is because there is an intervening factor common to both variables. In this case, the

**Figure 2.3**
Interpret the correlation. Is there a relationship between stress and exercise? If yes, is it a negative or positive relationship? Describe the relationship. Does this mean exercise affects stress levels, or stress affects exercise, or neither?

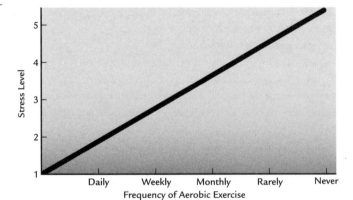

## Think About It!

### The Process of Advancing Knowledge in Health Psychology

*1. Review existing research literature.*
The first step in any research project is to review scientific literature about what is already known about the topic.

a. Upon completion of studies health psychologists present papers and write articles describing their methods and conclusions.

b. In most health psychology journals there is assurance that articles are worthwhile because they are reviewed by other knowledgeable health psychologists before being accepted for publication. Scientists send copies of their research report to journal editors who then send them out for blind review by other knowledgeable health psychologists. Reviewers recommend 1) the article be accepted for publication, 2) the article be accepted if revised, or 3) the article should not be published. Books go through a similar review or "vetting" process carried out by the publisher's editors and experts in a field of study. Getting scientific articles published in health psychology journals is a highly competitive endeavor.

c. If you were a health psychologist who decided to research the topic of alcohol consumption by college students, you could go into a "search engine" supported by library services and enter the topic "alcohol use by college students" to find pertinent journal articles. After reading several articles and books, you will have an idea of the knowledge already available in the area of interest and can then decide what you want to study that would add to existing knowledge. If you decide to replicate an existing study, the research design is already described for you to repeat. Otherwise, the next step is to design the study.

*2. Design, implement, and evaluate the study.*
There are college courses devoted entirely to research methods in specific fields. When you review research literature you read about a variety of ways to test hypotheses. You decide on an experimental method or a descriptive or observational method and design your study so your conclusions will survive the scrutiny of other scientists who also know about your topic.

*3. Share research findings.*
As a scientist your next step is to share your research findings with your peers at scientific meetings or conferences. By doing this, other scientists interested in your topic can listen to you describe your study, ask you questions, and make suggestions for further research. They may tell you they did a similar study and their findings are very different from yours. This will result in a lively discussion. Other researchers may make suggestions about ways to improve your work or ask you questions you failed to explain. All of this helps advance your work.

*(continues)*

## Think About It!

**4. *Submit an article to a reputable journal for publication.***
If you believe your research findings are worth sharing then you can submit your article to a peer-reviewed or refereed journal for publication. You describe your study sufficiently for replication. Remember also that one of the goals of science is to generalize findings. That means you hope to be able to say that under most circumstances the findings will hold true.

**5. *Choosing research methods: ethical and practical issues.***
Ethics in research is an important issue for scientists. There are significant ethical and legal decisions researchers must make. Federal laws protect human and animal research subjects. Most college campuses have an Institutional Review Board (IRB) or a Committee for Protection of Human and Animal Subjects. Committee members are experienced researchers who periodically meet and decide if other scientists on campus should be allowed to carry out proposed studies. The proposed research is described using a specific format designed to protect study participants. Included is a consent form that must be understood and signed by each participant or subject. When children are subjects in proposed studies, the parents or caregivers of children must read and decide whether to sign the consent forms. Respondents, or subjects, in research have the right to know all the risks that are involved in their participation. If you are ever asked to be in a study, read the informed consent form very carefully. The purpose of laws and forms is to protect you from harm.

The choice of research methods is affected by practical considerations including the amount of time available and the economic costs of a proposed study. For example, if you want to generalize to all people in the United States then you should probably study more than 100,000 people, ensuring the participants are representative of all people in the country. This would be very costly and time consuming. Most scientific studies do not include thousands of respondents or subjects. Scientists often choose what is possible and practical rather than spending their entire life doing one study. Research principles exist to guide scientists when deciding how many people should be included in studies and how long studies should last.

intervening variable is age. Age explains the strong negative relationship between peanut butter consumption and cancer. Young people and children are the age group least likely to be diagnosed with cancer and most likely to eat peanut butter sandwiches. When age increases, cancer increases. But the relationship between cancer and peanut butter sandwiches does not make scientific sense. There is no known ingredient in peanut butter related to cancer suppression. Scientists consider the possibility of intervening variables before drawing conclusions about relationships.

# Epidemiology and Other Health Sciences

**Epidemiology** is a branch of medicine that studies the occurrence, cause, and control of diseases. This word is similar to the word **epidemic**, which is an outbreak of a health problem within a geographic area. Because there is so much trade and travel among countries, many diseases become global or worldwide. For example, HIV/AIDS is said to be a worldwide epidemic, as was influenza in the early 20th century. Other diseases may become widespread enough to be considered global epidemics.

Epidemiologists can do experimental research, but more often they use observational research methods on diseases that have developed in specific geographic regions of a country or the world. From epidemiology come subfields such as risk factor analysis and health risk reduction. Health psychology research often includes terms, methods, and examples developed in epidemiology.

## The Terminology of Epidemiology and Other Health Sciences

This textbook uses some terms and concepts from epidemiology, so this chapter presents relevant definitions. The term **prevalence** refers to disease rates or the number of occurrences of a disease within a designated time period within a population. Prevalence is often expressed as a ratio, such as the number of cases of a disease per the number of people in the population at risk for the disease. For example, the prevalence of lung cancer can be stated as the number of cancer cases per 100,000 people in the United States.

The term **incidence** refers to the number of times an event occurs within a given period of time, usually a year. The incidence of flu is the number of new cases of that disease in a population during the year a count was made. Health scientists are very interested when prevalence and incidence begin to increase.

**epidemiology** A branch of medicine that studies the occurrence, cause, and control of diseases.

**epidemic** An outbreak of a specific health problem affecting a large number of people within a geographic area.

**prevalence** Disease rate, or the number of occurrences of a disease within a designated time period within a population. Prevalence is often expressed as a percentage. For example, a study may find that 10% of people who use tanning beds develop skin cancer.

**incidence** A measure of frequency, or the number of times a new event occurs within a given period of time, usually a year. For example, a study might find that the incidence of new cases of the sexually transmitted disease of genital warts or HPV is over 5 million each year.

**Morbidity** tells us about the extent of a disease in a population. It is the ratio of persons who are ill compared to those who are well within a geographic area. The word *mortality* refers to deaths, and the **mortality rate** is the number of deaths compared to the number of people in an area. For example, scientists might be interested in morbidity and mortality rates due to AIDS per 100,000 people in the United States, or per 100,000 people in the 30–40-year-old age group, or per 100,000 people residing in the state of Alabama.

To summarize the usefulness of these four terms, we can say that prevalence tells us how common a disease is at any given time; incidence tells us about new cases of a disease in a population; morbidity tells us about the extent of an illness or disability; and mortality tells us about the number of deaths due to the disease. A serious disease is one that is common or prevalent, there are many new cases appearing each year (incidence), many people in a population have the disease (morbidity), and many people are dying from it (mortality).

## Special Types of Studies in Health Sciences

Understanding the types of research used in the health sciences helps in evaluating research reports. Students should also be aware of the advantages and disadvantages of each type of study. When searching for likely contributors to accidents or illness, health scientists often turn to specific types of observational research methods that take into account issues such as how long the research must continue before conclusions can be reached.

### Longitudinal Studies and Cross-Sectional Studies

Health scientists must decide if they want to extend research over the normal lifetime of participants (about 75 to 80 years) or if the study is to be completed in less time. The amount of time and money available for research often influences decisions about whether or not a study will be longitudinal or cross-sectional. A **longitudinal study** includes the same respondents and continues over a long period of time. A **cross-sectional study** includes par-

---

**morbidity** A proportion of illness or the ratio of persons who are ill compared to others within a geographic area. For example, a study may find that at any given time about 33% of the population is ill.

**mortality rate** Frequency of death or the death rate associated with a health problem or geographic area; for example, a study might find that 10 out of every 1,000 people die of heart disease.

**longitudinal study** A research design that studies the same respondents over a long period of time.

**cross-sectional study** A research design that studies participants representing all age sets and occurs over a short period of time.

ticipants representing all age sets and occurs over a shorter period of time. Study participants in longitudinal research are interviewed periodically, asked to fill out forms, and have physical examinations. One example is the National Women's Health Initiative which began in 1991 and studies post-menopausal women. Data include 7.5 million completed forms and information from 1 million clinic visits. Another example of longitudinal research is the Framingham heart study, which has continued for many decades and now includes three generations of families. Look at **Figure 2.4** and think about a correlation between hostility and heart attacks.

Scientists using a cross-sectional research approach may interview and examine samples of people in selected age sets. For example, a study might include participants ranging in age from 10 to 49 years. The people are all studied at the same time, but information is drawn from people of age cohorts such as 10–19, 20–29, 30–39, and 40–49 years. The advantage of cross-sectional research is that it can be accomplished in a much shorter time than longitudinal research. Scientists are assuming the 20–29-year-olds of today will eventually be very similar to the 80–89-year-olds of today.

Retrospective and Prospective Studies

When evaluating research reports, students should also consider the timing of questions in terms of respondents' lives and memories. What information would be more accurate? A researcher is trying to choose between asking people what happened in their lives 20 years ago, or asking people what happened yesterday. In most cases, the more recent the condition or event being studied, the more likely people are to clearly remember what occurred. For example, in a recent national health study, adult participants were asked if during their infancy their caregivers used talcum powder on them when changing their diapers. There is some research indicating that the use of talcum powder may be a risk factor for cancer of the reproductive tract. It is very difficult for most people to give an accurate answer to that

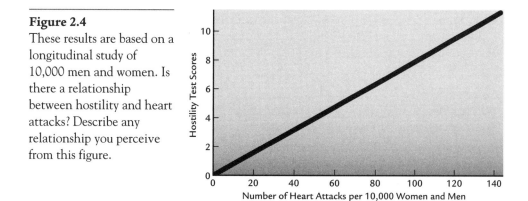

**Figure 2.4**
These results are based on a longitudinal study of 10,000 men and women. Is there a relationship between hostility and heart attacks? Describe any relationship you perceive from this figure.

question, yet answers affect research conclusions and reports. This is an example of **retrospective** observational research. Respondents are being asked about something that happened far in the past. Generally the further away in time in respondents' lives, the less likely the research data will be accurate.

The idea of remembering things that occurred a long time ago is not absurd. For example, mental health therapists often ask about events in their patients' childhoods. Some therapists use hypnosis to help patients recall past experiences. What other options are available to study the talcum powder–cancer connection? Experimental research would be unethical because talcum powder may cause harm. **Prospective studies** might be a choice, because they occur when people are actually having experiences of scientific interest. Researchers could advertise for parents of newborns to participate in a study and then follow those infants all their lives. In order to make comparisons, researchers would include parents who choose to use talcum powder and those who do not. This would be an observational, prospective study but given the suspected link between talc and cancer, this study is unethical and an IRB probably wouldn't approve it. It would take many years to finish. For these reasons many researchers use animals for testing such as mice and rats. Many products, such as artificial sweeteners, were first tested on rats to see if illnesses developed down through several rat generations. The problem, of course, is that people may not be like rats in variables important to research findings.

## Developing Skills for Analyzing and Evaluating a Scientific Study

This chapter began with the idea that everyone should develop the knowledge and skills to evaluate scientific studies because new research findings continue to emerge. People may even change their behavior due to scientific findings and later read that the study was flawed. Articles in newspapers and magazines are usually so brief no one can really determine the accuracy of studies. Fortunately, journalists sometimes give a reference to scientific reports so we can look them up. Scientific journals are also limited in text space, but if we have questions after we read a description of a study, we can contact the lead author for more information. Studies described in peer-reviewed scientific journals follow a prescribed format and are judged worthy of publication by experts prior to publication. We should pay close attention to all aspects of published studies.

**retrospective study** A longitudinal research design that asks participants or subjects to tell about what happened in their past or looking backward.

**prospective study** A longitudinal research design that looks to the future by following subjects forward from a starting point, for example, a study of the children of women who drank alcohol during pregnancy.

## Think About It!

### Would You Buy This Medication?

Evaluate this study based on the data. Would you use the medication? Would you advise a friend or relative to use this medication?

---

**Clinical Study Results***

A. Less elbow pain during exercise for 80% of participants

B. Improved ability to move elbows without pain for 75% of participants

C. Improved ability to carry out daily activities requiring the use of arms in 65% of participants

---

*Results shown are from a randomized, double blind, placebo-controlled study of 25 participants of various ages completed in 1945 by XYZ pharmaceutical company, the proud producers of this product.

## Who Provided Financial Support for the Study?

**Objectivity**, or the absence of bias, is an important goal of science. Scientific findings should be based on well-designed, meticulously implemented, accurate, unbiased studies. Sometimes financial support comes from organizations or groups that could benefit from the findings. Having this information reminds us to be very careful in our scrutiny of study methods and findings. For example, if a trade group, such as the National Dairy Council, supported a study, and study results might increase their profitability, then we should examine that study carefully before accepting conclusions. Information about how research was financially supported is usually found at the bottom of the first page of journal articles.

## How Many People Participated in the Study?

This is an important question to ask when evaluating research. In most cases, the more people involved, the more likely the findings can be generalized. The ideal is large samples randomly drawn from the general population. The reality is that many studies are very limited in fiscal support and may include relatively few people drawn from one geographic region. After students read a few studies referenced at the end of each chapter in this textbook, they will begin to understand that some findings are based on relatively few people. For

---

**objectivity** A goal of scientists to avoid prejudice or their own biases in research.

example, many studies are based on freshmen and sophomores in college psychology classes. Should scientists generalize to all college students from such a limited sample? Due to lack of research funding, many studies are based on convenience samples. Information about the sample will also be included near the beginning of most articles or in the research method section of the article.

## How Were Subjects or Participants Recruited?

This information is usually reported in the methods section of published studies. In the United States, no one should be forced to participate in a study. It is often difficult to get people to take their time to participate. This is why college students often make up study samples. In some cases, it is possible to offer an **honorarium** to respondents who agree to be study subjects and participate in research. Honorariums are rewards recognizing participation. These can be included in a request for grant money to support the study. For example, a study of family health practices included $35 to be given to each of 60 participant families. The researchers thought families could use this money to go out to eat together after completing the study questions (Snooks & Hall, 2002). It is ideal when participants are true volunteers and participate for the benefit of scientific knowledge.

## Were Comparison Groups Used?

If the researcher used an experimental model, then read carefully about how participants were recruited and divided into control and experimental groups. This should be done on a random basis, and, ideally, in a double-blind way, so neither subjects nor researchers know who is in the experimental group and who is in the control group.

## Were the Measures Reliable and Valid?

Research instruments, especially scales, should go through an elaborate process to be affirmed both valid and reliable. Scientists often use questionnaires or scales validated by other scientists, and references to those studies will be given for further information.

## Were the Conclusions Based on the Findings?

Are the findings and conclusions compelling? This may seem like an odd question, but thinking about possible conclusions is important. After reading about a study and its find-

**honorarium** A reward in recognition of participation in a study; For example, participants in the Women's Health Study were given pencils and emery boards after filling out forms.

ings, but before reading the author's conclusions and implications, ask yourselves what conclusions you would draw from the findings. Then read the author's conclusions to see if they are the same as yours .

## What Are the Limitations of the Study?

There are no perfect studies. Authors of research articles are expected to explain the limitations of their studies. For example, ethical concerns are very important for the protection of human and animal subjects, but may limit the ability of scientists to generalize to entire populations. These limitations also control the range of research methods available to scientists.

## Summary

Health psychology is a science, and its findings are based on scientific research methods. An advantage of using scientific methods is greater accuracy. New findings are reported and challenged at professional conferences, through journal articles, and in textbooks. Many health psychologists develop theories and models to organize their research. Ethical concerns, laws to do no harm, and practical issues such as money and time often limit the breadth and depth of studies.

Two important approaches in health psychology are experimental research methods and observational research methods. Experimental studies may result in explanations or causes of phenomena and begin with a hypothesis about relationships between variables. The proposed cause is the independent variable, while an effect or result is the dependent variable. Variables are operationalized by specifying the precise way each will be measured. To ensure greater accuracy, research participants are randomly assigned to either the experimental group or the control group. Only experimental group members will be exposed to the independent variable. Members of the control group may be exposed to a placebo. Scientists use double-blind experimental models to control for the placebo effect. Using subjects or respondents who self-select into a study may affect research outcomes.

An alternative approach to experimental research is the observational or descriptive study. A major goal of observational research is to discover relationships between variables. An important consideration in designing observational research studies is the number of people or events to be included. One goal of science is to generalize findings to large numbers of people. This is more likely when the sample, or set of research participants, accurately reflects the general population. Observational research often involves questions for study participants, either through interviews or questionnaires. Validity refers to the accuracy of information gathered through questions. Reliable questions will be answered in the same way regardless of how much time has passed between interviews.

Relationships or correlations between variables can take a variety of forms. They can be strong or weak, positive or negative. An important part of the science of observational studies is interpretation of data. Observational research is especially characteristic of a special branch of medical science called epidemiology. Health psychologists use many terms from epidemiology, such as *prevalence, incidence, mortality,* and *morbidity* to describe findings. In the health sciences, research designs can be longitudinal or cross-sectional. Prospective studies follow participants forward through time, while retrospective study designs include questions about past experiences. When reading reports of research, students should consider sample size, how subjects were recruited, and any funding received from sponsoring organizations. After thoroughly describing the methods and findings of their studies, scientists should clearly explain why they reached their final conclusions and explain any limitations on their research findings.

## Review Questions

1. What is beneficial about using a scientific approach to gain knowledge about the world?

2. List and briefly describe the most important aspects of steps scientists go through to verify their ideas and theories.

3. What are the benefits and risks of developing theories and models?

4. Define and give an example of a theory, a model, a variable, a hypothesis, data, and replication.

5. Clarify differences between qualitative and quantitative research methods in health psychology and give one example of each.

6. What is the purpose of experimental research methods?

7. Briefly describe the task of institutional review boards or committees for the protection of human subjects on a college campus.

8. Explain how to randomize membership into experimental and control groups. Why is this important?

9. What is the placebo effect and why is it important to control for it in research?

10. What are the limitations of the experimental research method?

11. Describe important factors health psychologists should be aware of when planning observational research.

12. List and then explain three significant points about designing questionnaires.

13. What kind of assurance given to respondents about the information they provide is most likely to result in valid answers to questions?

14. How do health psychologists arrive at conclusions about relationships among variables?

15. Distinguish, or explain the differences, between longitudinal and cross-sectional studies, and between retrospective and prospective studies. For each set, choose the type most likely to result in accurate results and briefly explain why accuracy is more likely.

16. Compare experimental and observational research methods in terms of their goal or purpose.

17. List five important questions you would want answered before accepting the results of research reported in a health psychology journal.

18. Design a health psychology research study on a topic of interest.

## Student Activity

Evaluate the following fictitious report in relation to what was learned in this chapter.

ASTOUNDING FINDINGS IN RECENT PILL STUDY

Dr. Mary Mason and Dr. Gary Grayson, faculty members of the University of Texas School of Medicine, recently reported findings from their study of the effectiveness of color-coding pills to increase patient adherence to medical regimens. Following their study, the researchers concluded that color-coding pills increases the likelihood that pills will be swallowed. The study was based on a sample of 1,000 undergraduate college students who agreed to participate. The institutional review board approved the experiment. For participation, students received an award of season tickets to Sea World. On a random basis, 500 students were placed in the experimental group and 500 students were put in a comparison group. The students in the experimental group received color-coded vitamin pills with a different color for each day of the week. For example, the Monday pill was blue, the Tuesday pill was green, the Wednesday pill was yellow, etc. The control group received the same vitamin pills labeled for days of the week, but all pills were colored gray. Graduate students who were blind to the research hypotheses distributed pills on a weekly basis. At the end of 6 weeks the researchers asked for all the pills not consumed to be returned. The number of remaining colored pills was only half of the number of the remaining gray pills. Drs. Mason and Grayson concluded that color-coding pills by day of the week makes people more likely to take their pills. ABCDEF Pharmaceuticals provided funding for the study.

## References

Babbie, E. (2004). *The practice of social research* (10th ed.). Belmont, CA: Thomson/Wadsworth.

Bensing, J. M., & Verhaak, P. F. M. (2004). The medical encounter as a powerful placebo. In Kaptein, A. & Weinman, J. (Eds.), *Health psychology* (pp. 261–287). Malden, MA: Blackwell.

Brannon, L., & Feist, J. (1997). *Conducting health research*. NY: Brooks/Cole.

Brody, H. (2000a). Mind over medicine. *Psychology Today*, July/August 60–67.

Brody, H. (2000b). *The placebo response*. New York: HarperCollins.

Cottrell, R. & McKenzie, J. F. (2005). *Health promotion and education research methods*. Sudbury, MA: Jones and Bartlett Publishers.

Cozby, P. C. (2007). *Methods in behavioral research* (9th ed.). Mountain View, CA: Mayfield Publishing Company.

DeVahl, J., King, R., & Williamson, J. W. (2005). Academic incentives for students can increase participation in and effectiveness of a physical activity program. *Journal of American College Health, 53,* 295–298.

Fox, D., & Prilletensky, I. (1997). *Critical psychology: An introduction.* London: Sage.

Frank, R. G., Wallander, J. L., & Baum, A. (2004). Introduction to Volume 3: Models and Perspectives in Health Psychology, pp. 3–5. In *Handbook of Clinical Health Psychology, Vol. 3.* Washington, DC: American Psychological Association.

French, D. P., Yardley, L., & Sutton, S. (2004). Research methods in health psychology, pp. 326–359. In *The Sage Handbook of Health Psychology.* London: Sage Publications Ltd.

Glanz, K., Rimer, B. K., & Lewis, F. M. (2002). Theory, research, and practice in health behavior and health education. In K. Glanz, B. K. Rimer, & F. M. Lewis (Eds.), *Health behavior and health education: Theory, research, and practice* (3rd ed., pp. 22–39). San Francisco: Jossey-Bass.

Howell, D. C. (2002). *Statistical methods for psychology* (5th ed.). Pacific Grove, CA: Duxbury/ Thomson Learning.

Moerman, D. E., & Wayne, B. J. (2002). Deconstructing the placebo effect and finding the meaning response. *Annals of Internal Medicine, 136*(6), 471–476.

Murray, M. (Ed.) (2004). *Critical health psychology.* New York: Palgrave MacMillan.

Snooks, M. K., & Hall, S. K. (2002). Body image and self-esteem in three ethnic groups. *Health Care for Women International, 23*(5), 460–466.

Sobel, D. S. (1990). The placebo effect: Using the body's own healing mechanisms. In R. Ornstein & C. Swencionis (Eds.), *The healing brain: A scientific reader* (pp. 63–74). New York: Guilford.

Thompson, W. G. (2005). *The placebo effect and health: Combining science and compassionate care.* Amherst, MA: Prometheus Books.

Turner, J. A., Deyo, R. A., Loerser, J. D., Von Korff, M., & Fordyce, W. E. (1994). The importance of placebo effects in pain treatment and research. *Journal of the American Medical Association, 271,* 1609–1614.

United States Departments of Agriculture and Health and Human Services (2005). *Dietary guidelines for Americans* (6th ed.). Washington, DC: U.S. Government Printing Office.

Voelker, R. (1998). A "family heirloom" turns 50. *Journal of the American Medical Associaton, 279,* 1241–1245.

Williams, M. A., & Martin, M. Y. (2002). Symptoms, signs, and ill-defined conditions. In S. B. Johnson, N. W. Perry, Jr., & R. H. Rozensky (Eds.), *Handbook of clinical health psychology,* Vol. 1 (pp. 9–28). Washington, DC: The American Psychological Association.

Women's Health Initiative (WHI). (1991). Women's Health Initiative scientific resources Web site. Retrieved August 6, 2008 from http://www.nhlbi.nih.gov\whi.

# Chapter 3

# Changing Behavior to Improve Health

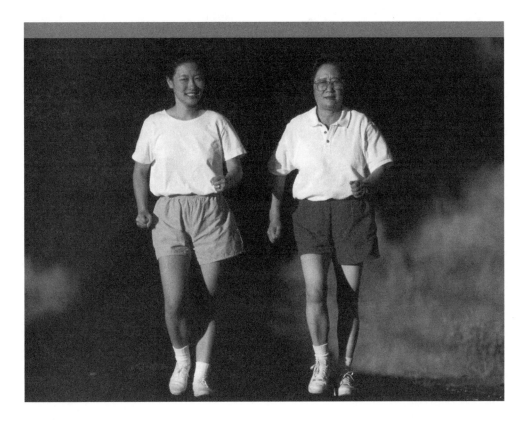

## Learning Objectives

After studying this chapter students will have the knowledge and skills to be able to:

1. Explain why there is a major emphasis today on changing health-related behaviors.

2. Enumerate the benefits of developing models for changing health-related behaviors.

3. Differentiate between types of health-related recommendations and three kinds of prevention.

4. Compare and contrast the health belief model and the theories of reasoned action and planned behavior.

5. Explain how changing health behavior is affected by self-efficacy and the three-pronged idea of reciprocal determinism.

6. List and briefly explain the stages of the transtheoretical model or the precaution-adoption process. Give one

55

example of each stage based on a change different from those used in this chapter.

7. Define optimistic bias, and explain how it affects health-related behavior and recovery from illness.

8. Define the concept of relapse, and evaluate methods of relapse prevention

likely to help people maintain changes in health-related behaviors.

9. Explain adherence. Describe and evaluate the ways it can be measured.

10. Identify and describe factors that affect adherence to medical recommendations.

## Introduction

Many researchers in health psychology focus on health promotion and illness prevention. Two intriguing questions shape the development of theories and much of the research. When the focus is prevention of illness or accidents, the question is, How can people be encouraged to behave in ways protective of health and safety? A second question centers on ways to convince people to stop behaviors harming their health and asks, What kinds of interventions persuade people to change existing behaviors dangerous to health and safety? Interventions or programs for behavior modification are based on theories and models. Health psychologists and health promotion specialists implement and evaluate interventions for effectiveness. This chapter summarizes several theories used in health psychology. The chapter also includes a discussion of the important concept of **adherence**, which refers to the likelihood that people will follow medical directives and stick to the behavior changes they made.

Health-related behaviors often become habitual. This makes them more difficult to change. Habits are deep-seated, well-practiced, repetitive ways of acting. Beginning in childhood, we develop habits affecting our health and safety. Childhood behaviors such as toothbrushing are beneficial, while others, such as playing in the street, are very dangerous. Adolescence is the time when some people begin unhealthy behaviors such as smoking and abusing alcohol, while their peers reject tobacco and alcohol and continue to exercise and eat healthily. Students might want to use this chapter to think about their own health-related behaviors. For example, most college students exercise less than they did as high school students. Recent data indicate that the percentage of adults who engage in regular leisure-time physical activity is declining. In 2003, about 33% of adults exercised. That percentage dropped to 30% the following year (National Center for Health Statistics [NCHS], 2004). This means that less than one third of adults in the United States use leisure time to exercise. Successfully changing or modifying behavior is more important for health than ever before, because most premature deaths are caused by unhealthy and unsafe lifestyle practices. This was not always true.

**adherence** The degree to which a person follows a medical directive or continues with a behavior change.

## Historical Changes in Major Causes of Illness and Premature Death

The current emphasis on health-related behavior came about due to changes in core causes of premature death. Early in the 20th century, infectious diseases were the major causes of death. For example, in 1900 the leading causes of death included pneumonia/influenza, tuberculosis, diarrhea, and diphtheria (NCHS, 2005). Today, most of the leading causes of death are linked closely to lifestyle choices. Major causes of death, in descending order, are heart disease, cancer, stroke, chronic lower respiratory disease, accidents (unintended injuries), diabetes, pneumonia/flu, Alzheimer's disease, kidney disease, and suicide (NOVS, 2008). Illness, injury, and premature death result from choices people are making about their own behavior. Some common actions leading to premature deaths are physical inactivity, harmful eating patterns, tobacco use, unsafe sexual practices, the abuse of alcohol and other substances, and reckless or unsafe behaviors including driving while under the influence of alcohol. (See **Table 3.1** for risk factors for preventable death in the United States.)

TABLE 3.1   **Numbers of Preventable Deaths in the United States in 2000**

*Estimates are from data including actual numbers (firearm deaths) and calculated risks (tobacco deaths). More than 1 million deaths are caused by lifestyles and behaviors—all preventable deaths.*

| | Deaths | |
|---|---|---|
| Cause | Estimated no. | Percentage of total deaths |
| Tobacco | 435,000 | 18 |
| Diet/activity patterns | 365,000 | 15 |
| Alcohol | 85,000 | 3.5 |
| Microbial agents | 75,000 | 3.1 |
| Toxic agents | 55,000 | 2.3 |
| Motor vehicles | 43,000 | 1.8 |
| Firearms | 29,000 | 1.2 |
| Sexual behavior | 20,000 | 1 |
| Illicit use of drugs | 17,000 | <1 |
| Total | 1,124,000 | 47.4 |

*Source:* Edlin, G., & Golanty, E. (2007). *Health and wellness* (9th ed.). Sudbury, MA: Jones and Bartlett Publishers, LLC, and Mokdad et al. (2004). Actual causes of death in the United States, 2000. *Journal of the American Medical Association, 291,* 1231–1243.

## Biopsychosocial Origins of Health-Related Behaviors

Complex connections exist among biological, psychological, and sociocultural factors affecting health, safety, and life expectancy. Eating a high-fat diet raises cholesterol levels, increasing risk for cardiovascular disease. On the other hand, regular exercise elevates high-density lipoproteins (HDL), or good cholesterol, which reduces the risk of cardiovascular disease. Smoking and alcohol use increase blood pressure and contribute to cancer. Insulin-level problems leading to diabetes are increased by obesity, which can result from both high-fat diets and absence of regular exercise. Stress, a major psychosocial concept in health psychology, is also connected to lifestyle choices and premature death.

Stress has negative effects on the nervous and immune systems and sends chemical messages throughout the body (Danzer, 2001). Cruess, Schneiderman, Antoni, and Penedo (2004, p. 60) note, "There is strong evidence that psychosocial factors can influence the development and course of disease." Some heart attacks are directly associated with stressful situations. A tendency to respond to social and cultural situations with anger and hostility is associated with heart disease (Williams et al., 2000). Biobehavioral bases of disease processes include the findings that faster progression to AIDS is associated with higher cumulative stressful life events, with patients using denial as a coping mechanism, and with less satisfaction with patient social support (Leserman et al., 2000).

Physical environments also influence the adoption of both healthy and unhealthy behaviors. For example, you may live in a densely populated urban area where there are few safe places to exercise or in a rural area with few gyms. People with low incomes may live in areas where fresh food is more expensive and less available than cheaper fast food. Family and child-rearing practices are important social influences on health. Many boys are encouraged to exercise for sports participation and parents spend hours watching their games. Extensive encouragement in athletics continues to be less likely for girls (Zophy, 2000, pp. 46–47).

Some behaviors are based in the psychosocial processes of learning, such as being rewarded, ignored, or punished for some action (Sarafino, 2001). For example, parents and other caregivers tend to use rewards and punishment to change children's behaviors. Nicotine is highy addictive and smoking continues as a behavior as long as the smoker believes the rewards exceed the costs. From a psychological viewpoint, we become very attached to persistent behaviors such as smoking. Smoking a cigarette or chewing tobacco even becomes part of a person's personality and self-image. Changing the smoking habit feels wrong and unnatural.

## One Example of Gradual Change to a Healthy Behavior

We can better understand risky health-related behaviors if we think about how healthy behaviors begin. A common and beneficial health habit is daily brushing of teeth. Our caregivers and parents, with encouragement from the American Dental Association, convinced us when we were children that brushing our teeth was an important behavior. We were taught that regular brushing prevents decayed, painful, and unsightly teeth. Many adults still feel guilty if they go to bed without brushing their teeth. Think back to the ways your caregivers encouraged you to develop this habit when you were a child. You received positive attention and praise when you brushed. Elementary teachers often gave gold stars to students who report brushing their teeth. Later television advertising convinced you that brushing and using mouthwash would prevent bad breath, making you more popular among your peers. As an adult, you brush your teeth out of habit and to avoid painful and expensive dental visits involving drilling, filling, root canals, and gum surgery. A great deal of effort went into developing the teeth brushing habit. Regular exercise, nutritious eating patterns, adequate sleep, and wearing seat belts are other examples of habitual behaviors beneficial to health and safety.

## Types of Health-Related Recommendations

There are many health and safety adages or common sayings in our culture: "An apple a day keeps the doctor away." "It is better to be safe than sorry." You learned general health-related recommendations beginning in preschool or kindergarten. In high school you took a health class. Physical education teachers and coaches were additional sources of general health- and safety-related information including advice about exercise, strength training, and stretching. See the "Think About It!" feature for challenges we all face.

---

### Think About It!

#### Challenges: Can You Meet Them?

- To experience psychological adjustment and growth, set realistic goals, plan effective ways to achieve those goals, take actions that are based on reasonable judgments and decisions, and evaluate the consequences of your choices.

- To facilitate your psychological adjustment, learn ways to manage interpersonal conflicts constructively, without being aggressive. When such conflicts arise, decide when it is best to compromise or assert your position.

- To improve your self-esteem, avoid making negative statements about yourself. Identify and be realistic about your strengths and weaknesses; focus on your accomplishments and positive characteristics.

- To improve your psychological health, take steps to improve the quality of the other dimensions of health.

*Source:* Alters, S., & Schiff, W. (2009). *Essential concepts for healthy living* (5th ed.). Sudbury, MA: Jones and Barlett Publishers.

While growing up, you may have had regular checkups by physicians and dentists who gave you additional advice on ways to maintain your health. Interestingly, many people find it difficult to comply with this advice, even when paying for it. A surprisingly large percentage of people do not follow physicians' advice. For example, we know antibiotics are more effective when the entire dose is taken as prescribed, but some patients stop using antibiotics as soon as they start feeling better. Infections return and bacteria mutate, making the antibiotic ineffective in the future. This is the issue of adherence, which this chapter covers later.

## Prevention: Primary, Secondary, and Tertiary

Understanding the causes of diseases and injuries helps us to discover the best ways to prevent and treat them. When scientists talk about reducing health risks, they focus on three stages of prevention: primary, secondary, and tertiary. **Primary prevention** is any effort to completely avoid a health or safety problem. For example, regular exercise and avoiding tobacco smoke are primary prevention strategies with regard to cardiovascular disease. Practicing safer sex during every sexual encounter is a primary prevention strategy for avoiding HIV/AIDS, sexually transmitted diseases, and unwanted pregnancy.

**Secondary prevention** refers to screening so disease and injury are discovered at an early stage when chances are better for healing. Common screenings for heart disease are blood pressure, heart rate, and cholesterol levels. **Tertiary prevention** includes controlling complications of illness, improving patients' quality of life, and preventing death. Patients are often advised to involve friends and family members in their treatment and recovery process and to make every effort to maintain good mental and social health. Biology, emotions, and social relationships all play an important part in prevention of illness and accidents, in their development, and in recovery. Prevention of disease and death is an important goal of interventions to change health behaviors. Health-promotion interventions can be aimed at individuals, organizations such as schools and businesses, and whole communities or countries. For example, large populations are affected by laws requiring seat belts or forbidding smoking at worksites and in restaurants.

Developing interventions and ways to assist in making changes in health-related behavior is central to health psychology. Models and theories about behavior change include giving

primary prevention  Any effort to completely avoid a health or safety problem.

secondary prevention  Screening so disease and injury are discovered at an early stage, when chances are better for healing.

tertiary prevention  Controlling complications of illness, improving patients' quality of life, and preventing death.

information about benefits and risks of change, skills for making behavioral changes, and ways to increase self-efficacy and social support (Westmaas, Gil-Rivas, & Silver, 2007; Cruess et al., 2000).

## Models and Theories of Health Behavior Change

### Interventions for Behavior Modification

You remember efforts made by your parents and caregivers to modify your behaviors during childhood. For example, at mealtime, when you ate all your vegetables did you receive praise and a reward like a sweet dessert? This was an effort on the part of your caregivers to encourage vegetable-eating behavior, because they believed the vitamins in vegetables were good for you. You may already know a great deal about how to change your own behavior. Perhaps you recently changed your high school study habits to match college-level assignments.

**Behavior modification** describes interventions to start, stop, or change behaviors. Health psychologists first devise theories and models about behavioral change, and then health promotion specialists develop interventions based on theory. Modification of health-related behavior can move in two directions. Sometimes interventions are designed to encourage people to begin a healthy behavior, such as regular exercise. At other times interventions are intended to stop an unhealthy behavior, such as smoking. Some interventions for behavior change focus on shifting thought processes about the behavior before actually attempting to change the behavior itself (Sarafino, 2001). The **health belief model (HBM)** is one of the earliest theories about health-related behavior.

### The Health Belief Model

This theory of behavior change originated in the field of public health and focused on cognitions or thought processes people experience when considering making a behavioral change. The HBM assumes that humans are rational and will change health-related behaviors after following logical thinking patterns (Hochbaum, 1956; Becker, 1974; Rosenstock,

**behavior modification** Interventions to encourage behaviors such as exercise or extinguish behaviors such as smoking; for example, efforts to change or shape a behavior by reinforcing that behavior with rewards.

**health belief model (HBM)** One of the earliest explanations or theories of health-related behaviors; the model proposes that people will take action to protect their health if they believe they are susceptible to a serious threat, that taking action will be an effective deterrent to illness or injury, and that the barriers to taking action are worth being overcome.

1974). Two important parts of the model are people's beliefs about the seriousness of a health or safety risk and their perceived susceptibility to the risk. Perceived susceptibility refers to people's beliefs about the likelihood of their actually experiencing an illness or injury as a result of the health or safety risk in question. People weigh the seriousness, susceptibility, and benefits of changing a behavior against the difficulties involved in making a change; they consider the probability of their experiencing an illness or accident, how serious it would be if it did occur, and the likelihood that changing their behavior would eliminate or reduce the threat. They compare potential benefits to the difficulty of making changes. When comparing risks and benefits, people often become more knowledgeable about ways to reduce risks and about ways to change their behavior, and they can predict how effective they will be in making a change.

Health-promotion specialists planning interventions use the HBM to select important determinants of behavior and any environmental conditions that would be favorable to a behavior change (Bartholomew, Parcel, Kok, & Gottlieb, 2001). For example, many cancers are life threatening, so cancer poses a serious threat. In 1964, a report of the U.S. Surgeon General's Office labeled smoking as a risk factor for death from lung cancer. According to the HBM, smokers will consider the seriousness of lung cancer and their susceptibility to the disease. They will weigh the health benefits of stopping smoking against the difficulty of giving up their smoking habit. Some smokers decide the difficulties of stopping exceed any potential benefits, so they continue to smoke. Thousands of others weighed the risk and successfully quit (NCHS, 2004).

In 1984, Janz and Becker added to the model the idea that internal factors, such as having difficulty breathing, and external factors, such as being advised to quit by their personal physicians, also influence people's decision to change behaviors. Janz and Becker called these two factors **cues** and **motivators**. For example, smokers may develop persistent morning coughs that are internal factors that may encourage them to stop smoking. One day their children (external factor) come home from school saying they are afraid their parents are going to die from lung cancer due to smoking. These two types of factors, internal and external, may be sufficient to encourage smokers to stop.

The HBM has been applied to many types of behavior modification, including smoking, alcohol abuse, getting health checkups and immunizations, improving nutritional and ex-

**cue** Something that motivates or incites to action, a stimulus; billboard advertising, or a delicious odor may be a cue to eat or drink something.

**motivator** A factor that encourages an idea or a behavior; for example, the likelihood of improvement in their personal appearance and health may motivate people to exercise or stop smoking.

ercise behaviors, and participating in screenings for cancer and other illnesses (Hamilton, Cross, & Resnicow, 2000; Steptoe, Coherty, Kerry, Rink, & Hilton, 2000). Research using the HBM also indicates that dealing with the barriers to stopping a behavior is probably the most powerful component preventing change (Conner & McMillan, 2004). The health belief model was applied to exercise using the key concepts of susceptibility, severity, benefits, and barriers. McKenzie, Neiger, & Smeltzer (2005) described this scenario: a college student majoring in fitness and health completes a health risk appraisal in class. She realizes that due to her current lifestyle, her weight, and family history she is at increased risk for cardiovascular disease. She is now motivated to start an exercise program and uses herself as a project for class. The HBM has also been applied to efforts to encourage 1) young women to do monthly breast examinations and young men to screen themselves for testicular cancer, 2) condom use behaviors, 3) skills for refusal of cigarettes or alcohol by teens, and 4) parents' use of car restraint systems for infants.

Students thinking about changing their behavior can analyze 1) whether their current behavior (including their neglect of a recommended behavior) will make them susceptible to a serious health threat, 2) what obstacles or barriers are preventing them from changing their behavior, 3) how effective changing the behavior will be in preventing an illness or injury, 4) how motivated they are to change, and 5) what factors, external and internal, might encourage them to make a change in their behavior. See **Figure 3.1** for an illustration of how the health belief model can be applied to the behavior of monthly checks for testicular cancer.

## The Theories of Planned Behavior and Reasoned Action

According to the **theory of planned behavior (TpB)**, human action or behavior is influenced by 1) behavioral beliefs about the outcome of the behavior and the value of that outcome to the person, 2) normative beliefs about the expectations of others and the person's willingness to comply with others' expectations, and 3) control beliefs about what factors might influence the success of the behavioral change (Ajzen, 2007). This theory also assumes humans are logical and behavioral change follows cognitions or thoughts including attitudes and intentions. Ajzen's web site (2007) gives advice on how to construct a TpB questionnaire on any behavioral change topic.

**theory of planned behavior (TpB)** According to this theory, human behavior is influenced by three kinds of beliefs. In addition to their attitude toward a behavior and the attitudes of others, people are also influenced by their perceived behavioral control. When people have resources and opportunities, they are more likely to believe they can successfully change their behavior and intend to do so.

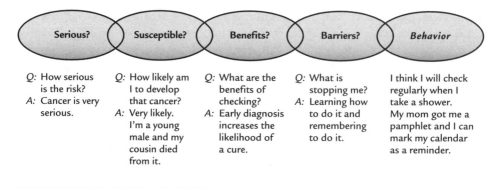

**Figure 3.1**   The chain of decision making based on the health belief model. The American Cancer Society (ACS) recommends monthly testicular self-examinations for young men. This behavior may reduce cancer risk (ACS, 2008).

The **theory of reasoned action (TRA)** is closely connected to attitude theory and measurement (Fishbein, 1967). In a 1975 book, Fishbein and Ajzen focused on the influence of beliefs, attitudes, and intentions on human behavior. Beliefs and attitudes about a behavior shape intentions, and the intention to act precedes the behavior change. A second part of the theory describes how social pressure, or what is called the subjective norm, influences actions. People are motivated to change their attitude and behave differently when they believe other people whose opinions they value want them to change. According to the TRA, when thinking about changing behavior, people also consider the likelihood of the goal being achieved if they try to change. Many variables affect planned behavior and reasoned action including past experiences, personality, age, gender, education, income, and religion. In a later publication, Ajzen and Madden (1986) modified the theory to include **perceived behavioral control**. This refers to the idea that people are more likely to change if they believe they are capable of doing so.

**theory of reasoned action (TRA)**  The theory that people take action if they believe a behavior change will achieve a desirable outcome and that other people whose opinion is important to them also believe the change is desirable (the subjective norm). Humans weigh their own negative attitudes about a change against the importance of the change to others and may develop the intention to act that is followed by the actual behavior.

**perceived behavioral control**  The idea that humans are more likely to intend to change their behavior if they believe they have the will and strength to do so.

For example, a woman believes that by having three alcoholic drinks every evening she is more relaxed, patient, and loving with her husband and children when they return home after work and school. One evening, both the children and husband tell her they dislike the fact that she smells like liquor and often embarrasses them in front of their friends. According to the theory of reasoned action, she is more likely to stop having drinks every evening if 1) her attitude toward her behavior becomes negative instead of positive, 2) she knows others disapprove of her behavior, and 3) she believes she has the self-control necessary to change. Based on this logic, she decides she can quit and plans her behavior change. Similarly, people are more likely to intend to quit smoking if the three elements exist: they think it would be better for their health (attitude), they think family and friends will appreciate their quitting (subjective norm), and they think they can control their smoking behavior (perceived behavioral control) (McKenzie, Neiger, & Smeltzer, 2005). These three factors contribute to the intention to stop smoking.

Research provides empirical support for TRA and TpB models in health-behavior change through the connection of intentions to behavior (Albarracin, Johnson, Fishbein, & Mullerleile, 2001). For example, students probably know that sexually transmitted diseases (STDs) infect millions of people each year (Centers for Disease Control [CDC], 2000, 2001). Researchers evaluated the TpB theory and found it useful in preventing diseases and infections through condom use (Bogart & Delahanty, 2004). See **Figure 3.2** for an application of the TpB.

## Social-Cognitive or Learning Theory, Self-Efficacy, and Reciprocal Determinism

**Self-efficacy** is a critical component of changing a problem behavior. "Perceived self-efficacy refers to belief in one's capabilities to organize and execute the course of action required to produce given attainments" (Bandura, 1997, p. 3). It is a cognitive determinant, because it refers to peoples' belief that they are capable of change (Bandura, 1986). Improving beliefs about self-efficacy makes it more likely people will change to healthier behaviors.

**Reciprocal determinism** refers to mutual interdependence and interplay among three types of interacting factors, including 1) social, cultural, and physical environments, 2)

**self-efficacy** A theory of human behavior that people are more likely to change if they believe they have control over their lives and can change. People act or change behavior if their thinking or cognitions include the idea that they are capable of overcoming the barriers that are currently preventing change.

**reciprocal determinism** A concept that human action is influenced by people's environments and also by personal beliefs such as self-efficacy, expectations, standards, and by other cognitions or perceptions, knowledge, and thinking.

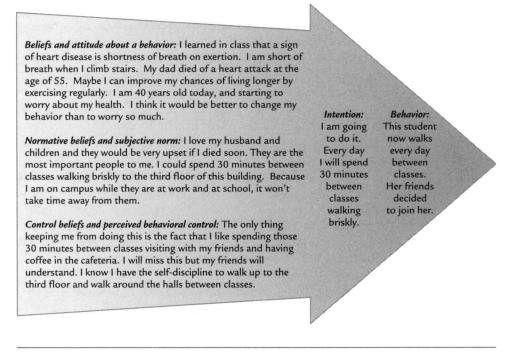

**Beliefs and attitude about a behavior:** I learned in class that a sign of heart disease is shortness of breath on exertion. I am short of breath when I climb stairs. My dad died of a heart attack at the age of 55. Maybe I can improve my chances of living longer by exercising regularly. I am 40 years old today, and starting to worry about my health. I think it would be better to change my behavior than to worry so much.

**Normative beliefs and subjective norm:** I love my husband and children and they would be very upset if I died soon. They are the most important people to me. I could spend 30 minutes between classes walking briskly to the third floor of this building. Because I am on campus while they are at work and at school, it won't take time away from them.

**Control beliefs and perceived behavioral control:** The only thing keeping me from doing this is the fact that I like spending those 30 minutes between classes visiting with my friends and having coffee in the cafeteria. I will miss this but my friends will understand. I know I have the self-discipline to walk up to the third floor and walk around the halls between classes.

**Intention:** I am going to do it. Every day I will spend 30 minutes between classes walking briskly.

**Behavior:** This student now walks every day between classes. Her friends decided to join her.

**Figure 3.2** The Theory of Planned Behavior can be applied to reduce the risk of cardiovascular disease by exercising on a regular basis.

psychological factors, such as thinking or cognitions, emotions, or affect, and 3) the action or behavior itself (Bandura, 1997, p. 6). The likelihood of changing any behavior requires analyzing the behavior, the social and physical environment where the behavior occurs and the person lives, and internal personal factors.

In studies, self-efficacy was positively related to dietary behavior change, exercise, and quitting smoking (Bogart & Delahanty, 2004). In other studies, self-efficacy had a positive effect on biological systems and health status, alcohol and drug abuse, athletic functioning, and improvement in cognitive functioning, such as making a better grade in a college course (Bandura, 1997). Students might think about ways to increase their own self-efficacy by applying this theory to make better grades. Self-efficacy is achieved by practicing behaviors such as studying alone and with other students. This may mean finding quiet locations without distractions (environment) to read this textbook and review class notes (personal). It may include staying well and getting adequate sleep (biological) so as to give complete attention to the subject matter in the course.

Developing self-efficacy may also include self-testing (personal) on important course concepts. Students can also decide to attend all classes (environment) and spend 3 hours studying for every hour spent in class (personal). Reorganizing one's life so that a particular behavior can be changed is central to self-efficacy and making successful changes.

## The Transtheoretical Model of Change

Another model frequently used in health psychology for health promotion interventions is the **stages of change model** (SOC). It focuses on stages or processes people go through in their efforts to change health-related behaviors. The **transtheoretical model of change** incorporates suggestions from other behavior change theories and emphasizes that behavior modification is a gradual, transitional process (Prochaska & DiClemente, 1984; Prochaska, DiClemente, & Norcross, 1992). Knowing about change processes and planning for each stage may help individuals whether they are working alone, in groups, or with health-promotion specialists.

The transtheoretical scheme provides a road map for navigating the process of behavior changes across six stages: 1) pre-contemplation, 2) contemplation about making a change, 3) preparation for the action of changing, 4) action or making the change, 5) maintenance of the change or about 6 months of adherence, and 6) termination of the problem behavior. People move through stages of change in a spiral fashion and may regress or return to an earlier stage and even to the beginning stage (Bogart & Delahanty, 2004).

Pre-contemplation refers to a stage in which people are risking their health by a behavior but are not thinking about making a change. In the past they may have tried to change but failed. They now believe it is unlikely they will ever be able to change, so they avoid thinking about it. People sometimes attribute their failures to factors outside of their own control

**stages of change model** Model that suggests that people go through a series of stages or phases when altering their behavior.

**transtheoretical model of change** A stage-of-change model of health-related behavior that applies several components of other theories describing the behavior change process. The stages include 1) pre-contemplation, which exists when a person is not even thinking about changing a behavior, 2) contemplation, which exists when a person thinks about making a change and weighs the pros and cons of the change, including their own attitudes and the attitudes of others, 3) the preparation stage, in which a person gets ready to implement the change he or she has been considering, 5) the action stage, in which people actually change their behavior, and 6) the maintenance stage, in which a person has successfully implemented the behavior change.

such as genetic or family background. When confronted about their behavior, some people feel helpless about making a change.

Contemplation or thinking about a change comes next. A specific event can trigger contemplation. One example is a smoker being told by a pediatrician that smoke contributes to his or her infant's ear infections. During contemplation, the parent evaluates the pros and cons of giving up smoking. When thinking about a change, it is better to emphasize the advantages while also recognizing the disadvantages. For example, the smoking parent worries about feeling deprived and resentful, which acts against change, but then the infant cries, runs a high fever, and must be taken back to the doctor with another painful ear infection. People may stay in the contemplation stage for many years. On the other hand, our imaginary smoker may decide the child's health is important and the benefits of quitting outweigh withdrawal discomforts. Fear of disease and death are psychosocial factors that often influence outcomes of contemplation.

During the preparation stage, people make plans for changing their behavior. Smokers decide on a quit date, they begin to reorganize their lives to avoid smoking, and think about ways to stop smoking. For example, some choose to cut back gradually by one cigarette each day each week, while others decide to quit all at once or "cold turkey." Many now choose to substitute nicotine patches or gum, and there are medications that can help reduce cravings.

It may be worthwhile for people planning a change to also consider the effects of social and physical environments on their behavior. Taking a different route to avoid driving by fast-food restaurants at noon may be part of changing eating behavior. Staying out of bars may help people avoid alcohol and cigarette smoke. When friendships are based around smoking, drinking, or eating together, a person can plan to meet friends where smoking, drinking, or eating fast food are not possible.

The action stage, the fourth step, is when the change actually begins. For a smoker this would be the quit day. For exercisers it is the day they actually begin to exercise. For dieters it is the day they make their lunch to avoid eating at a fast-food restaurant. When change appears to be established then a person enters the maintenance stage. There will be concerns about slipping or returning to old habits. It may help for people to plan what they will do if they slip. The sixth stage, **termination**, exists when people are no longer tempted to go back to the previous behavior and have great confidence that they changed their behavior permanently.

Health-promotion techniques can be planned specific to each stage. For example, when people are in pre-contemplation, consciousness raising and education are beneficial. Social support and building self-efficacy help when preparing for the action stage. The stages of

---

**termination**　The act of ending a behavior.

**The Transtheoretical Model or Stages of Change Process**

*5. Maintenance:*
Wow! In just one
year I lost 30 pounds
and I feel and look great!
I am sticking with this plan.

*4. Action:*
Here I am ordering food every day
with 30 fewer fat grams in each meal
than what I had been eating. I do get
hungry in the afternoon, so I take an apple
to eat at about 3:00 while I'm still at school.

*3. Preparation:*
I took a health class and remembered that fast food
places were inexpensive, but had lots of high-fat foods on
their menus. Maybe I could eat differently at lunch. The local
restaurant gave me a chart about the fat grams in their food,
and I am going to choose foods that are lower in fat.

*2. Contemplation:*
Mom just told me that my cousin Lisa has diabetes. She is the same age as I am.
I don't want to develop diabetes. Our uncle had to go to a dialysis center every week
because he had diabetes. The doctor told Lisa it was because she was obese and to cut
back on calories and start exercising. I'm about the same size as Lisa, so maybe I should
cut back too.

*1. Pre-contemplation:*
I love my life! Every day my boyfriend and I eat at fast food places on the main street across from campus.

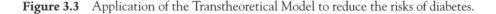

**Figure 3.3**   Application of the Transtheoretical Model to reduce the risks of diabetes.

change model can be applied to a variety of health- and safety-related behaviors including aerobic exercise, wearing seat belts, and avoiding foods high in fat. Web-based interventions can be used for behavior modification based on stages of change (Bock et al., 2004).

Critics of the transtheoretical model suggest the change process is difficult to evaluate, that changing behavior is more complex than represented in this model, and that each stage of behavior change requires new knowledge, skills, and resources (Ewart, 2004). It is also suggested that this model may be very useful in community-wide interventions (Leviton & Raczynski, 2004). See **Figure 3.3** for an example of applying the stages of change model to a health risk.

## The Precaution Adoption Process Model and Optimistic Bias

The **precaution adoption process model (PAPM)** broadened previous models and theories by including more stages and focusing on stages of belief having to do with readiness to adopt a behavior change (Weinstein, Rothman, & Sutton, 1998). The model assumes that people are hesitant to change and go through a complex thinking process before adopting a new behavior. In PAPM, the first stage is ignorance about the health risks of a behavior. For example, prior to 1964, many people were unaware of the health risks of tobacco use.

Weinstein writes that people in stage 2 may have a bias regarding their personal degree of risk. For example, they accept that smoking may be dangerous for many people but believe it is not as dangerous for themselves (Weinstein, 1982). Weinstein called this an **optimistic bias**. Optimism refers to a tendency to look for the most favorable side of any circumstance and focus only on favorable outcomes.

Weinstein's third stage, engagement, occurs when people actually consider making a change. Some decide (in stage 4) they can wait and change later if necessary. Other people go on to stages 5, 6, and 7. They decide to change, implement the change, and move into maintenance. Maintenance means the individual always carries out the health-related behavior; this usually requires conscious self-management for the rest of one's life. (For example, people with diabetes must always balance medication, food intake, and energy use, including exercise and stress.) Behavior changes also make demands on family members and friends.

Are you optimistic about your health? In an early study of his college students, Weinstein learned that the only health problem his students worried about was developing ulcers (1982). Are you worried about developing an ulcer? What are your fellow class members worried about? An optimistic bias sometimes leads people to underestimate the probability of their developing an illness or sustaining an injury as a result of their behavior. Optimistic people also underestimate the difficulty of making a health-behavior change. Many see themselves as invulnerable to sickness and death, and so they do not even think about changing a risky behavior. For example, you probably know smokers who say, "By the time

**precaution adoption process model (PAPM)**  Theory that emphasizes that people move backwards and forwards through stages of belief about their susceptibility to a health risk. In stage 1 people are unaware of their risk, and in stage 2 they are aware of a risk but, due to their optimistic outlook, they do not believe they are at risk. In stage 3 they accept their susceptibility and become more cautious. In stages 4 and 5 they either decide to act or decide not to do anything about the perceived risk. In stage 6 they have taken precautions about avoiding the risk. Stage 7 is maintenance of the precautionary steps.

**optimistic bias**  Part of the precaution adoption process model referring to a tendency on the part of people to be aware of a risk but not believe it applies to them.

I get cancer from smoking there will be a cure for it!" or, "There are millions of obese people who never develop diabetes, so why should I worry?" One concern in health promotion is that optimism discourages people from taking a variety of protective actions, such as having mammograms for early diagnosis of breast cancer or using condoms to avoid diseases and pregnancy. Due to optimistic bias, parents may believe their children do not need seat belts or child-restraint devices (Bartholomew, Parcel, Kok, & Gottlieb, 2001).

Students should be aware that optimism may also positively affect improvement in physical and mental health. Optimism is related to self-efficacy and feelings of being in control of one's life (Smith & Ruiz, 2004, pp. 170–172). For example, Taylor, Kemeny, Reed, Bower, and Gruenewald (2000) studied the relation of optimistic beliefs about the future among men infected with HIV. Based on the study, the authors suggest that psychological resources influence positive mental states by improvement in perceptions of self-worth, beliefs in personal control, and by encouraging better health habits and social relationships. They concluded that patients who find meaning in an illness, have a belief in personal control, and are optimistic about outcomes will better adapt to stressful events. Optimism protected physical health.

## Relapse Prevention

Another important concept in behavior change theory is **relapse prevention**. People may relapse or return to their former risky behavior. Different terms for this issue include nonadherence, lapsing, or relapsing. Relapse occurs whether people are stopping an unhealthful behavior such as smoking, or starting a healthful behavior such as exercising. Cigarette smoking, excessive alcohol use, avoiding exercise, and poor eating practices are well-practiced, persistent behaviors or lifestyle patterns, and changing long-standing behaviors is difficult. One approach to take when planning a behavior change is to expect relapses to occur just as they would during any process of learning and practicing a new skill. Being aware of the possibility of a relapse makes it possible for people to plan to avoid risky situations.

A lapse or reversion to previous behavior patterns is an opportunity to learn more about oneself by analyzing why it occurred (Marlatt & Gordon, 1985). Using this viewpoint, a relapse is not a failure, but is similar to taking the wrong turn on a road, discovering the error, taking another look at the map, and getting back on the right road. Following a relapse, people can analyze the causes of the relapse and avoid similar situations in the future (Marlatt & Witkiewitz, 2004).

Setting challenging but feasible goals for one's own behavior and meeting regularly with others to review specific goals may be beneficial (Strecher, Seijts, Kok, et al., 1995). This is one reason why group settings are effective in behavior change. Groups typically have experienced

---

**relapse prevention** Efforts to avoid a lapse or reversion to previous unhealthy behavior.

leaders who have already made a difficult change, and groups include other people ready to change. Social support from family, friends, and coworkers is also beneficial to behavior change.

Central to relapse prevention is planning and developing methods of coping in situations that pressure people to return to a behavior they want to stop (Dimeff & Marlatt, 1998). Relapse can be caused by psychological factors, such as feeling lonely, bored, angry, or stressed. Some formal interventions include relapse prevention training, such as identifying and avoiding high-risk situations (Smith & Ruiz, 2004). Relapse also occurs for social or cultural reasons. Many unhealthy products are highly advertised, and advertisements send powerful messages to revert to unhealthy practices. Even public health announcements may help people remain resistant. To avoid relapse, participants in formal group programs are taught to plan ahead what they will do when tempted to return to the unhealthy behavior. Some programs provide hotlines and relaxation tapes for this purpose. When the behavior is addiction to alcohol, members of Alcoholics Anonymous (AA) have sponsors or other members they can call. AA meetings are widely available and reinforce the behavior of abstaining from alcohol. Many smoking cessation programs also involve partnerships to prevent relapse (Brandon, Meade, Herzog, Chirikos, Webb, & Cantor, 2004). To quit and stay quit of smoking usually takes at least 6 months. People achieve the stage of termination when they have mastered the behavior and are no longer likely to relapse.

Dropping out of behavior change programs occurs because health-related behavior change is difficult. Therapists and health promotion specialists are advised to lead drop-out prevention sessions early in intervention programs. Stage-matched programs can be designed for participants in programs at clinics, schools, hospitals, worksites, or recreational facilities (Bartholomew, Parcel, Kok, & Gottlieb, 2001).

## Health Behavior Interventions at the Sociocultural Level

The theories and models of health-behavior change typically focus on an individual level of behavior change, but interventions may also be used to change the behaviors of many people at the same time. These are known as **community-based interventions**. Change is accomplished through changing the sociocultural environment. Behavioral-change interventions at the group or community level are now included in health psychology discussions (Leviton & Raczynski, 2004). Examples of cultural-level changes are sometimes described as public-service or health-promotion interventions.

**community-based intervention**  A health-behavior-change program that focuses on an entire community of people rather than on one person or a small group. One example is townspeople deciding to develop and implement a campaign to prevent smoking by their young people.

Health-behavior change can be carried out at a national, state, county, or local level through changes in laws. For example, the Environmental Protection Agency enforces legal limitations on air, water, and ground pollution to protect human health. Other examples are city and state laws banning smoking in public places. Most states have legal restrictions on age requirements for the purchase of cigarettes. Studies show that increasing taxes on alcohol and tobacco products makes their purchase less likely. Other examples are distributing free condoms and needles to prevent the spread of HIV/AIDS. A major difference in these types of interventions is that individuals may not have sought help in making a change and are included only because of their membership in a community or organization. Some people resent being forced to change by government, workplaces, or school system rules.

From a national viewpoint, one of the most ambitious health promotion efforts is the Healthy People objectives (U.S. Department of Health and Human Services [USDHHS], 2007). This national plan challenges individuals, communities, and professionals to take specific steps to improve both the quality and years of healthy life and to eliminate health disparities among population groupings within the United States. The initiative began in 1979 with a surgeon general's report on health promotion and disease prevention. It is a management-by-objectives planning process, currently includes 28 focus areas, and establishes baselines and target objectives. Focus areas include physical fitness, nutrition and overweight, tobacco use, prevention of injury and violence, and substance abuse.

From a community-intervention viewpoint there are several examples of health promotion in schools, churches, ethnic groups, and workplaces. To be effective, a population-based approach should include planning, implementation, and evaluation (Leviton & Raczynski, 2004). The Uniontown Community Health Project was implemented as part of the Women's Health Initiative programs (Raczynski et al., 2001). This program focused on exercise, nutrition, and smoking cessation. Community health advisors provided risk-reduction classes and interpersonal counseling and used social marketing strategies to reduce risks of cancer and cardiovascular disease. Health-behavior improvements were made in food preparation, exercise, and decreases in smoking prevalence. Advantages of behavior change in community settings include reaching people ordinarily not seen in other settings and the ability to modify interventions to conditions specific to target communities. Students may enjoy reading about the population-based approach known as the Rapid Early Action for Coronary Treatment (REACT) intervention based on social cognitive theory and the self-regulatory model of health and illness behavior (Raczynski et al., 1999; Luepker et al., 2000). Another example is the AIDS Community Demonstration Projects (Higgins et al., 1996).

## Self-Directed Behavior Change

Watson and Tharp (1997) believe that people can change themselves. Their book describing this process is now in its seventh edition. Changeable behaviors include feelings and thoughts as well as actions. The authors provide a wide range of examples, including improving athletic performance and study habits, eliminating teeth grinding, smoking cessation, and controlling Type A behavior. The authors use information from theories discussed earlier, including goal setting or targeting behaviors to change, using cues and antecedents, observing and recording one's behavior, and changing gradually. Self-efficacy beliefs, optimism, conditioning, reinforcement, and changing cognitions, behaviors, and feelings are all part of the self-directed behavior change intervention. Learning behaviors from observation of others (modeling) and conditioning are believed to be beneficial, but punishment is not helpful. The authors also discuss relapse prevention and distinguish between unintended slips and mistakes, which they view as failures in planning. References to self-directed behavior change can be found in professional journals, including *Health Psychology, Clinical Psychology Review, Behavior Therapy*, and the *Journal of Consulting Psychology*. Related to issues involved in behavior change is the difficulty of adhering to health-related recommendations.

## Adherence to Health-Related Recommendations

Do you make New Year's Day resolutions about starting a new behavior but fail to follow through in spite of your best intentions? Have you ever sought a doctor's advice but then ignored it? What you did is called non-adherence. Adherence in behavior modification programs is an important issue, because most health behavior changes should be permanent. Adherence is related to the problem of relapse discussed earlier. Constant self-management of behavior is another phrase applied to the issue of adherence.

### The Concept of Adherence

Adherence refers to the practice of following recommendations made by medical professionals or the advice of other health experts. Adherence is sometimes referred to using the terms *compliance* and *cooperation*. Some psychologists prefer the term cooperation, because compliance implies reluctant or grudging conformity to health-related suggestions. Adherence is a difficult issue in behavior modification and health care. Many people are unwilling to follow through on professional recommendations to improve their health or even to save their own lives.

Biological, psychological, and sociocultural factors contribute to failures in adherence. For example, after seeing a physician about an illness or injury, many people never get their prescriptions filled. One example of a biological determinant is fear the medicine will cause stomachaches. A psychological reason might be resistance to the idea that they actually need to take a medicine, and sociocultural reasons may include economic concerns about the cost of the medicine or the time it will take to get the prescription filled or that their spouse would not approve. Sometimes doctors give samples of medications to address these problems. Many people get prescriptions filled, but never finish the dose. Measuring adherence is a complicated process in medicine and health psychology.

### Assessing Adherence

All techniques for measuring adherence have advantages and disadvantages. None are foolproof with regard to reliability and accuracy. Medical practitioners tend to overestimate patient adherence to their recommendations. Many physicians simply assume patients will follow their instructions. When they do not hear from patients, they assume their treatment recommendation was followed and was effective. Patients give many and varied reasons for not following through with medical instructions.

### Measurement

Measuring the amount of remaining medication is one way to monitor patient cooperation. Counting remaining pills and weighing liquid medications left in bottles are used when studying the effectiveness of drugs. These efforts require constant vigilance in closely controlled situations. For example, in hospitals, the people who distribute medications are told to stay at the bedside until patients swallow their medication. There is less control in home situations. Other techniques are pharmacy database reviews, computer-based monitoring, and home nursing visits to ensure medication is taken and bandages are changed.

### Biological and Chemical Monitoring

Measurement of adherence may include assessing the effect of the recommended process or medication to be sure suggestions were followed. Some examples are weighing for weight loss or gain, taking blood pressure and heart rate, and analyses of blood and body wastes. Some smoking cessation programs monitor adherence by analyzing exhaled breath. Repeated assessment is difficult if patients refuse to keep monitoring appointments.

### Patient Self-Reports

It may seem straightforward to ask patients or participants if they followed recommendations, but many times self-reports are inaccurate. For example, many weight loss programs require patients to write down everything they eat each week. People are embarrassed when they eat an entire package of cookies, so they simply omit writing about it. The same behavior occurs with regard to reporting exercise adherence, because people want to please their trainers or coaches. In cases of asthma attacks or chest pain, patients are more likely to use medication, but may not remember how many times an attack or pain occurred. One of the newest ways to measure adherence is computer-based monitoring and telehealth (Glueckauf, Nickelson, Whitton, & Loomis, 2004). Web-based interventions are accessible, low in cost, standardized, personalized, private, convenient, and may produce more accurate reporting of behavior (Westmaas, Gil-Rival, & Silver, 2007, p. 61).

## Adherence Rates

It is important for health specialists to know the rate of patient adherence in order to evaluate the effectiveness of counseling sessions, health-promotion programs, medical advice, or prescribed medications. Adherence is difficult to measure, but clinical studies give some indications (Rand & Weeks, 1998). Between 50% and 65% of outpatients do not adhere to their medication regimens (Schaub, Steiner, & Vetter, 1993; Melnikow & Kiefe, 1994). Many smokers relapse in the first 3 months after quitting. Several factors affect rates of relapse (Ockene, 2000). In alcohol addictions, relapse often occurs during the first two years (Nathan,

1986). In weight-loss programs, relapse is less likely if people can maintain the loss for a few years (McGuire, Wing, Klem, Lang, & Hill, 1999).

## Factors Affecting Adherence

Students might assume that cost would be a factor in adherence and predict that costs affect adherence. Only half of patients adhere even when a program is free. When symptoms of illness disappear, adherence drops. Controlling pain is often a motivator for patients to adhere to a behavior change, even to exercise programs designed to control back pain or arthritic pain. Negative side effects of medications such as nausea and vomiting reduce adherence, even in the presence of serious illnesses such as a cancer. The complexity of a treatment discourages compliance. For example, most people will do something once a day, but doing it three times a day requires more-organized reminder systems and is more difficult. Social support helps compliance; isolated people reportedly exhibit poorer adherence with behavior change regimens. Spouses or partners usually help with adherence.

## Improving Adherence

It is helpful if people are convinced they are responsible for their health and for maintaining a health-related behavior. Smoking cessation programs and taking insulin for diabetes illustrate this phenomenon. It is also beneficial to provide people with information about the necessity for behavior change. For example, most people will not conform to a medical recommendation just because a doctor said so, although parents of young children frequently use this kind of reasoning to change their children's behavior. People are more likely to adhere to suggestions by a fitness or diet consultant when the reasoning behind a recommendation is clearly stated. Simplifying recommendations is usually beneficial. Ways to reduce barriers to a behavior change are worth discussing to improve adherence. Cues to positive behaviors are also helpful. For example, putting running shoes in plain sight and cookies out of sight may encourage exercise and discourage snacking. Specially designed pill packages and calendars increase adherence for taking medications. Phone calls and postcards remind people of behavior modification classes and increase attendance and adherence. Some fitness trainers charge the same fee even when participants do not attend a workout session. Knowing this encourages participants to make every session or call in advance to cancel. Tailoring a regimen to one's lifestyle is also effective.

## Summary

This chapter surveyed several theories, models, and concepts involved in changing health-related behaviors. The health belief model suggests people will start or stop a behavior if it involves a serious threat to which they believe they are susceptible. The model proposes that individuals evaluate barriers to change relative to the benefits if a change is accomplished. The theory of reasoned action incorporates the concepts of intention, belief, attitude, and social pressure, or the subjective norm, as being influential for behavior change processes. Self-efficacy is another concept influencing outcomes of efforts to change behaviors. The behavior itself, along with the social and physical environment, all have reciprocal effects when humans try to change.

The transtheoretical model proposes that people go through a serious of steps or stages when changing their behavior. Relapse, or returning to the previous pattern of behavior, frequently occurs. Relapse may be less likely with advance planning and may be ameliorated by assuming a tolerant viewpoint about the relapse. Most people assume they will never fall victim to an illness or accident due to their behavior. This is an optimistic bias. Even college students worry very little about tragic outcomes of risky actions.

Adherence refers to the practice of following health-related recommendations and maintaining behavior changes. It is difficult to directly measure adherence. Research reports suggest adherence rates are very low for most health-related behaviors, including taking prescribed medications. Health-promotion interventions should always include plans for promoting adherence.

## Review Questions

1. Explain why there is a major emphasis today on changing health-related behaviors.

2. Enumerate the benefits of developing models for health-behavior change.

3. Differentiate between types of health-related recommendations and the three kinds of prevention.

4. Compare and contrast the health belief model and theories of reasoned action and planned behavior.

5. Explain how changing health behavior is affected by self-efficacy and the three-pronged idea of reciprocal determinism.

6. List and briefly explain the stages of the transtheoretical model or the precaution-adoption process. Give one example of each stage different from those mentioned in this chapter.

7. Define the concept of relapse and evaluate three methods of relapse prevention likely to help people maintain a change in health-related behaviors.

8. Define optimistic bias and explain how it affects health-related behavior and recovery from illness.

9. Explain adherence. Describe and evaluate ways it can be measured.

10. Identify and describe factors that affect adherence to medical recommendations.

11. Discuss ways to improve adherence.

## Student Activity

1. Choose a health-related behavior you would like to change over the first half of the semester. Devise plans based on the transtheoretical model, including dates for each step of this behavior change process.

1. Analyze and describe in writing:

   a. Factors affecting your self-efficacy about the likelihood of your making this change.

b. Ways your environment, including friends, family, and coworkers, may affect your success.

3. Over the next 6 weeks, keep daily records about your progress using concepts discussed in the chapter and in class. This will be added to your report as an appendix.

4. At the end of 6 weeks, write a report describing your efforts to make this change.

5. Analyze the reasons for your success or your lack of success in making this health-related behavior change.

6. Evaluate the model based on your own experiences.

# References

Ajzen, I., & Madden, T. J. (1986). Prediction of goal-directed behavior: Attitudes, intentions, and perceived behavioral control. *Journal of Experimental Social Psychology, 22,* 453–474.

Ajzen, I. (2007). Behavioral intentions based on the theory of planned behavior. Retrieved October 15, 2007 from http://www.people.umass.edu/aizen/research.html

Bandura, A. (1986). *Social foundations of thought and action: A social cognitive theory.* Englewood Cliffs, NJ: Prentice Hall.

Bandura, A. (1997). *Self-efficacy: The exercise of control.* NY: W. H. Freeman.

Bartholomew, L. K., Parcel, G. S., Kok, G., & Gottlieb, N. H. (2001). *Intervention mapping: Designing theory and evidence-based health promotion programs.* Mountain View, CA: Mayfield Publishing Company.

Becker, M. H. (Ed.). (1974). *The health belief model and personal health behavior.* San Francisco: Society for Public Health Education.

Bock, B. D., Graham, A. L., Sciamanna, C. N., Krishnamoorthy, J., Whiteley, J. Carmona-Barros, R. N., et al. (2004). Smoking cessation treatment on the Internet: Content, quality, and usability. *Nicotine and Tobacco Research, 6,* 207–219.

Bogart, L. M., & Delahanty, D. L. (2004). Psychosocial models. In R. C. Frank, A. Baum, & J. L. Wallander (Eds.), *Handbook of clinical health psychology* (pp. 201–248). Washington, DC: American Psychological Association.

Brandon, T. H., Meade, C. D., Herzog, T. A., Chirikos, T. N., Webb, M. S., & Cantor, A. B. (2004). Efficacy and cost-effectiveness of a minimal intervention to prevent smoking relapse: Dismantling the effects of amount of content versus contact. *Journal of Consulting and Clinical Psychology, 72,* 797–808.

Centers for Disease Control and Prevention, (2000). *Sexually transmitted disease surveillance, 1999.* Atlanta, GA: Department of Health and Human Services, Division of STD Prevention.

Centers for Disease Control and Prevention. (2001). *HIV/AIDS surveillance report, 12*(2), 1–48.

Conner, M., & McMillan, B. (2004). Health belief model. In A. J. Christensen, R. Martin, & J. Smyth (Eds.), *Encyclopedia of health psychology* (pp. 126–128). New York: Kluwer Academic.

Cruess, S. E., Antoni, M. H., Cruess, D. G, Fletcher, M. A., Ironson, G., Kumar, M., et al. (2000). Reductions in HSV-2 antibody titers during cognitive behavioral stress management and relationships with neuroendocrine function, relaxation skills, and social support in HIV+ men. *Psychosomatic Medicine, 7,* 160–182.

Cruess, D. G., Schneiderman, N., Antoni, M. H., & Penedo, F. (2004). Biobehavioral bases of disease processes. In R. C. Frank, A. Baum, & J. L. Wallander (Eds.), *Handbook of clinical health psychology* (pp. 31–79). Washington, DC: American Psychological Association.

Danzer, R. (2001). Cytokine-induced sickness behavior: Where do we stand? *Brain, Behavior, and Immunity, 15,* 7–24.

Dimeff, L. A., & Marlatt, G. A. (1998). Preventing relapse and maintaining change in addictive behaviors. *Clinical Psychology: Science and Practice, 5*(4), 513–525.

Ewart, C. K. (2004). How integrative behavioral theory can improve health promotion and disease prevention. In R. C. Frank, A. Baum, & J. L. Wallander (Eds.), *Handbook of clinical health psychology* (pp. 249–289). Washington, DC: American Psychological Association.

Fishbein, M. (1967). *Readings in attitudes theory measurement.* New York: Wiley.

Fishbein, M., & Ajzen, I. (1975). *Belief, attitude, intention, and behavior: An introduction to theory and research.* Reading, PA: Addison-Wesley.

Glueckauf, R. L, Nickelson, D. W., Whitton, J. D., & Loomis, J. S. (2004). Telehealth and health care psychology: Current developments in practice and research. In R. C. Frank, A. Baum, & J. L. Wallander (Eds.), *Handbook of clinical health psychology* (pp. 377–411). Washington, DC: American Psychological Association.

Hamilton, G., Cross, D., & Resnicow, K. (2000). Occasional cigarette smokers: Cue for harm reduction smoking education. *Addiction Research, 8,* 419–437.

Higgins, D. L, O'Reilly, K., Tashima, N., Crain, C., Beeker, C., Goldbaum, G., et al. (1996). Using formative research to lay the foundation for community level HIV prevention efforts: An example from the AIDS Community Demonstration Projects. *Public Health Reports, 111* (Suppl.), 28–35.

Hochbaum, G. M. (1956). Why people seek diagnostic x-rays. *Public Health Reports, 71,* 377–380.

Janz, N. K., & Becker, M. H. (1984). The health belief model: A decade later. *Health Education Quarterly, 11,* 1–47.

Leserman, J., Petitto, J. M., Goldon, R. N., Gaynes, B. N., Gu, H., Perkins, D. O., et al. (2000). Impact of stressful life events, depression, social support, coping and cortisol on progression to AIDS. *American Journal of Psychiatry, 157,* 1221–1228.

Leviton, L. C., & Raczynski, J. M. (2004). Interventions in community settings. In R. C. Frank, A. Baum, & J. L. Wallander (Eds.), *Handbook of*

*clinical health psychology* (pp. 501–548). Washington, DC: American Psychological Association.

Luepker, R. V., Raczynski, J. M., Osganian, S., Goldberg, R. J., Finnegan, J. R., Jr., Hedges, J. R., et al. (2000). Effect of a community intervention on patient delay and emergency medical service use in acute coronary heart disease: The Rapid Early Action for Coronary Treatment (REACT) Trial. *Journal of the American Medical Association, 284* (1), 60–67.

Marlatt, G. A., & Gordon, J. R. (1985). *Relapse prevention.* New York: The Guilford Press.

Marlatt, G. A., & Witkiewitz, K. (2004). Relapse prevention. In A. J. Christensen, R. Martin, J. Smyth (Eds.), *Encyclopedia of health psychology* (p. 245). New York: Kluwer Academic.

McKenzie, J. F., Neiger, B. L., & Smeltzer, J. L. (2005). *Planning, implementing, and evaluating health promotion programs? A primer* (4th ed.). San Francisco: Benjamin Cummings.

McGuire, M.T., Wing, R. R., Klem, M. L., Lang, W., & Hill, J. O. (1999). What predicts weight regain in a group of successful weight losers? *Journal of Consulting and Clinical Psychology, 67,* 177–185.

Melnikow, J., & Kiefe, C. (1994). Patient compliance and medical research: Issues in methodology. *Journal of General Internal Medicine, 9,* 96–105.

National Center for Health Statistics. (2005). Fewer Americans smoke, but fewer physically active in leisure time. Retrieved November 1, 2007 from http://www.cdc.gov/nchs/pressroom/05facts/earlyrelease200506.htm

National Center for Health Statistics. (2005). Death and death rates of leading causes of death: Death registration states, 1900–1940. 1900–1940 tables ranked in National Office of Vital Statistics, December 1947. Retrieved November 1, 2007 from http://www.cdc.gov/nchs/fastats/deaths.htm

National Office of Vital Statistics. (2008). Deaths/Mortality. Retrieved April 29, 2008 from http://www./cdc.gov/nchs/fastats/deaths.htm

Nathan, P. E. (1986). Outcomes of treatment for alcoholism: Current data. *Annals of Behavioral Medicine, 8*(2-3), 40-46.

Ockene, J. K., Emmons, K. N., Mermelstein, R. J., Perkins, K. A., Bonollo, D. S., Voorhees, C. C. et al. (2000). Relapse and maintenance issues for smoking cessation. *Health Psychology, 19,* 17-31.

Prochaska, J. O., & DiClemente, C. C. (1984). *The transtheoretical approach.* Chicago: Dow Jones-Irwin.

Prochaska, J. O., DiClemente, C. C., & Norcross, J. C. (1992). In search of how people change: Applications to addictive behaviors. *American Psychologist, 47,* 1102-1114.

Raczynski, J. M., Finnegan, J. R., Zapka, J. G., Meischke, H., Meshack, A., Stone, E. J., et al. (1999). REACT theory-based intervention to reduce treatment-seeking delay for acute MI. *American Journal of Preventive Medicine, 16,* 325-324.

Raczynski, J. M., Cornell, C. E., Stalker, V., Dignan, M., Pulley, L., Phillips, M., et al. (2001). Developing community capacity and improving health in African-American communities. *American Journal of Medical Science, 322,* 269-275.

Rand, C. S., & Weeks, K. (1998). Measuring adherence with medication regimens in clinical care and research. In S. A. Shumaker, E. B. Schron, J. K. Ockene, & W. L. McBee (Eds.), *The handbook of health behavior change* (2nd ed.) (pp. 114-135). New York: Springer.

Rosenstock, I. M. (1974). The health belief model and preventative health behavior. *Health Education Monographs, 2,* 354-386.

Sarafino, E. P. (2001). *Behavior modification: Principles of behavior change* (2nd ed). Mountain View, CA: Mayfield.

Schaub, A. F., Steiner, A., & Vetter, W. (1993). Compliance to treatment. *Clinical and Experimental Hypertension, 15,* 1121-1130.

Smith, T. W., & Ruiz, J. M. (2004). Personality theory and research in the study of health and behavior. In R. C. Frank, A. Baum, & J. L. Wallander (Eds.), *Handbook of clinical health psychology* (pp. 143-199). Washington, DC: American Psychological Association.

Steptoe, A., Doherty, S., Kerry, S., Rink, E., & Hilton, S. (2000). Sociodemographic and psychological predictors of changes in dietary fat consumption in adults with high blood cholesterol following counseling in primary care. *Health Psychology, 19,* 411-419.

Strecher, V. J., Seijts, G. H., Kok, G., Latham, G. P., Glasgow, R., DeVellis, B., et al. (1995). Goal setting as a strategy for health behavior change. *Health Education Quarterly, 22*(2), 190-200.

Taylor, S. E., Kemeny, M. E., Reed, G. M., Bower, J. E., Gruenewald, T. L. (2000). Psychological resources, positive illusion, and health. *American Psychologist,* pp. 99-109.

U.S. Department of Health and Human Services. (2007). *Healthy people 2010: Midcourse review.* Retrieved October 17, 2007 from http://www.healthypeople.gov

Watson, D. L., & Tharp, R. G. (1997). *Self-directed behavior: Self-modification for personal adjustment* (7th ed.) Pacific Grove, CA: Brooks/Cole.

Weinstein, N. D. (1982). Unrealistic optimism about susceptibility to health problems. *Journal of Behavioral Medicine, 5*(40), 441-460.

Weinstein, N. D., Rothman, A. J., & Sutton, S. R. (1998). Stage theories of health behavior: Conceptual and methodological issues, *Health Psychology, 11,* 170-180.

Westmaas, J. L., Gil-Rivas, V., & Silver, R. C. (2007). Designing and implementing interventions to promote health and prevent illness. In H. S. Friedman & R. C. Silver (Eds.), *Foundations of health psychology* (pp. 52-70). NY: Oxford University Press.

Williams, J. E., Paaton, C. C., Siegler, L. C., Eigenbrodt, M. L., Nietao, F. J., & Tyroler, H. A. (2000). Anger proneness predicts coronary heart disease risk: Prospective analysis form the Atherosclerosis Risk Communities (ARIC) Study. *Circulation, 101,* 2034-2039.

Zophy, J. W. (2000). Athletics/Sports. In A. M. Howard & F. M. Kavenik (Eds.), *Handbook of American Women's History* (pp. 46-47). Thousand Oaks, CA: Sage.

# Chapter 4

# Applications of Health Psychology to Exercise Behavior: Improving Health Through Exercise

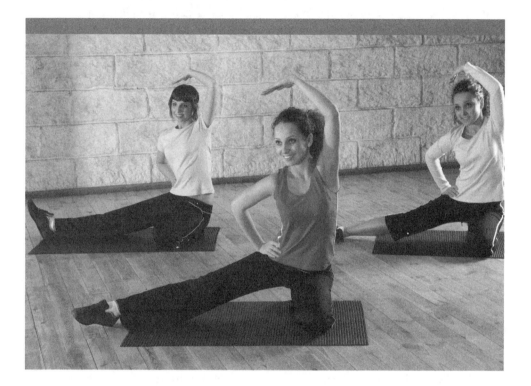

## Learning Objectives

After studying this chapter students will have the knowledge and skills to be able to:

1. Define, describe, and give examples of the three most useful types of exercise for improving biopsychosocial health.

2. Explain biological, psychological, and sociocultural factors that prevent people from maintaining health and fitness through exercise.

3. Discuss the biological, psychological, and sociocultural benefits of exercise.

4. Summarize recommendations on three types of exercise, including frequency, intensity, duration, training effects, injury avoidance, options, convenience, and safety issues.

5. Suggest ways to encourage exercise using theories common to the field of health psychology.

## Introduction

An abundance of scientific evidence demonstrates that regular **physical activity** improves biological and psychosocial health. When people increase their **exercise** levels, the likelihood of premature death decreases, energy levels rise, and emotional outlook improves. Studies of the positive effects of exercising come from many disciplines, including health psychology, epidemiology, behavioral medicine, and exercise physiology. Most people living in industrialized nations throughout the world are getting less exercise than ever before, and many eventually succumb to illnesses directly connected to their sedentary lifestyles. In fact, surveys indicate an epidemic of sedentary or non-exercising lifestyles (World Health Organization [WHO], 2007). Inactivity is partially due to technological advances that make it possible for people to earn a living without much physical movement or activity.

Inactivity puts us at risk of the major causes of death including heart disease, strokes, and some cancers. Many people attribute their deteriorating fitness and health to growing older, but physical activity can reverse declines due to aging. There are a variety of types of exercise, and each type has specific benefits. **Aerobic exercise** improves our cardiovascular and respiratory systems and the use of muscles and joints helps protect against loss of muscle and bone, which in turn helps prevent injuries, including falls. All types of physical activity reduce or prevent obesity, which is a risk factor for diabetes and many kinds of cancer. Exercise also improves psychological and social well-being (Cruess, Schneiderman, Antoni, & Penedo, 2004, p. 36). In national surveys, people say they believe exercise is good for their health, but the vast majority do not exercise regularly. In fact, only a small percentage of adults in the United States say they exercise regularly and only 15% do it for 5 or more days each week for 30 more minutes or more (Centers for Disease Control [CDC], 2000). Physical activity and fitness are the number one category among the national health promotion and disease prevention objectives of Healthy People 2010 (U.S. Department of Health and Human Services [DHHS], 2000).

In health psychology, exercise is viewed as a behavior, so theories of behavior change discussed earlier can be applied. Regular exercise is one of the most positive behaviors people can adopt to improve biological, psychological, and social health. This is true regardless of a person's age, gender, or level of ability. Students may think of exercise as something they did when they were younger or apply the term only to elite athletes, but from a health standpoint, this is too narrow a perspective. In this chapter, exercise is approached as a normal, everyday behavior aimed toward maintaining all three components of human health. The focus

**physical activity** Any movement or use of the musculoskeletal system.

**exercise** Physical activity done purposely to maintain or improve physical fitness and health.

**aerobic exercise** Any form of movement that elevates the rate of heartbeats and breathing.

is no longer on overly vigorous exercise, but on a wide range of physical activities (CDC, 2000). As **Figure 4.1** illustrates, even moving more during the workday and at leisure contributes to health-related fitness (Bouchard, Shepherd, Stephens, Sutton, & McPherson, 1990).

In order to apply healthy psychology theories to changing the behavior of exercise, students must first have a thorough grounding and clear understanding of definitions and types of exercise, exercise parameters including safety issues, as well as ways theories may be applied effectively and safely to this type of behavior modification. The role of health psychologists in exercise intervention activities includes their special expertise in behavioral theory and models. Theoretical models that appear most promising are social-cognitive theory, the stages of change model, and the relapse prevention model (Dubbert, King, Marcus, and Sallis, 2004). Exercise is a familiar term, but health psychologists also use the term *physical activity*. The behavioral risk factor is referred to as a sedentary lifestyle.

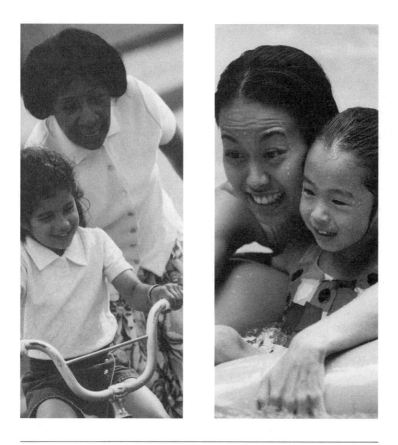

**Figure 4.1** Developing lifelong habits of fun and exercise with friends and family members promotes emotional, social, and physical health.

## Defining Movement and Exercise

Physical activity refers to any movement or use of the musculoskeletal system. You are physically active when you walk into a classroom, pick up a pencil or turn on a computer, and take notes during class. You use your musculoskeletal system when you turn pages of this textbook. You were physically active before birth, when you stirred in your birth mother's uterus. A few months after you were born, you learned to crawl. Later you stood upright and then walked a few toddling steps. You soon became capable of moving faster and further. In elementary school, you probably had physical education (PE) classes for exercise and skill development. That type of movement is identified as exercise because it is physical activity done purposely to maintain or improve physical fitness and health (Jamner, 2004). Perhaps you also participated in organized sports, rode your bike, or climbed trees as a child. All physical activity increases your metabolism or metabolic rate, which uses calories from the food you eat to a much greater extent than when you are sedentary or asleep.

When you drop your pencil on the floor and lean over to pick it up, you are doing a type of movement called **stretching**. When you lift a heavy backpack onto your shoulder, you are doing **strength training**. If you are slightly out of breath hurrying to class or work, your movement has become aerobic. This chapter focuses on applying health psychology behavior change theories to improving health through exercise.

Exercise involves several different body systems. When you move parts of your body you use muscles and other soft tissue, along with bones, lungs, and the cardiovascular system, which includes the heart, arteries, and blood. You use your nervous system, because your brain coordinates and monitors motor activity. When you exercise, your cells use the energy and nutrients from food. If you use all of the calories or energy circulating in your bloodstream, your body switches to another energy source through modification of stored fat. This is why exercise helps remove unwanted fat from the body.

Exercise is good for health for many reasons. It keeps the heart, lungs, and muscles physically fit. If we fail to move our joints, we eventually lose the ability to use them. If we fail to exercise, we lose muscle, bone, and cardiovascular health. If we continue to eat the same as when we were physically active, we begin to accumulate body fat or stored energy. Obesity is often the next step. This is why many people gain fat when they leave school and stop exercising in PE classes and playing sports. By becoming active again we can reduce the amount of stored fat on our bodies.

**stretching** Gentle movements to extend and relax muscles and joints; more safely accomplished when muscles are warmed by non-vigorous exercise, but may also follow a vigorous exercise session.

**strength training** Exercise to increase the strength of various muscles.

## Purposes of Movement and Exercise

Obviously we must move to get where we want to go, carrying what we will need when we arrive. We move to work and play. The ability to move quickly is important for avoiding injury and death. For example, when threatened, we can run from danger or prepare to defend ourselves. If we do not make a conscious effort to exercise we will gradually lose the ability to do so. Most college students move less than they did as children and as teenagers. We all know the saying, "Use it or lose it." This refers to the fitness and health of all body parts. Moreover, the less we move, the more fat (stored energy) we accumulate unless we also restrict our food intake. Obesity is a major health problem in many countries and reflects sedentary lifestyles. The next chapter addresses nutrition and ways to prevent obesity by changing eating behaviors through behavior modification. Both eating and exercise affect life expectancy and biological, psychological, and social aspects of health.

## Health Benefits of Exercise from a Biopsychosocial Perspective

### Biological Benefits of Exercise

This section reviews the biological benefits of exercise. For all people, exercise is the surest means to a longer and healthier life. Regular exercise reduces the risk of premature death and disability. If we want to avoid dying before our time or being bedridden toward the end of life, then our best bet is regular physical activity. Exercise reduces the risk of many specific debilitating diseases, including heart disease, strokes, diabetes, and some cancers (CDC, 2000). For example, an important sign of heart disease and a risk factor for premature death is high cholesterol levels. Regular exercise lowers cholesterol levels. Exercise also increases good cholesterol, or high-density lipoproteins (HDLs), in the blood. Find your healthy weight on the chart in **Table 4.1**.

Exercise helps maintain strong bones, making one less likely to develop osteoporosis and experience debilitating fractures in old age (CDC, 2000). Exercise maintains range of motion in joints and strengthens muscles so we can continue to do what we want to do throughout our lives. Exercise also helps our sense of balance, preventing falls. If we are fit, we are less likely to be seriously injured when we fall. There is considerable evidence that physical activity enhances the immune system by reducing stress and making people less likely to succumb to colds and other illnesses. Regular exercise improves our reaction time in emergencies. Obesity among children and teens is increasing in this country, but regular aerobic exercise can make obesity less likely. Regular exercise also reduces stress, which is distracting and often leads to injury (Weiss, 1989).

### Psychosocial Benefits of Exercise

Most people are happier if they can maintain their mental and physical capabilities as they age. This is more likely if they stay physically active all their lives. A considerable amount of research indicates that exercise also has immediate psychological benefits. After a meta-analysis, J. Anthony (1991) concluded that regular aerobic exercise reduces anxiety, distress,

# TABLE 4.1   Adult BMI Chart

| BMI | 19 | 20 | 21 | 22 | 23 | 24 | 25 | 26 | 27 | 28 | 29 | 30 | 31 | 32 | 33 | 34 | 35 |
|---|---|---|---|---|---|---|---|---|---|---|---|---|---|---|---|---|---|
| **Height** | | | | | | | **Weight in Pounds** | | | | | | | | | | |
| 4'10" | 91 | 96 | 100 | 105 | 110 | 115 | 119 | 124 | 129 | 134 | 138 | 143 | 148 | 153 | 158 | 162 | 167 |
| 4'11" | 94 | 99 | 104 | 109 | 114 | 119 | 124 | 128 | 133 | 138 | 143 | 148 | 153 | 158 | 163 | 168 | 173 |
| 5' | 97 | 102 | 107 | 112 | 118 | 123 | 128 | 133 | 138 | 143 | 148 | 153 | 158 | 163 | 158 | 174 | 179 |
| 5'1" | 100 | 106 | 111 | 116 | 122 | 127 | 132 | 137 | 143 | 148 | 153 | 158 | 164 | 169 | 174 | 180 | 185 |
| 5'2" | 104 | 109 | 115 | 120 | 126 | 131 | 136 | 142 | 147 | 153 | 158 | 164 | 169 | 175 | 180 | 186 | 191 |
| 5'3" | 107 | 113 | 118 | 124 | 130 | 135 | 141 | 146 | 152 | 158 | 163 | 169 | 175 | 180 | 186 | 191 | 197 |
| 5'4" | 110 | 116 | 122 | 128 | 134 | 140 | 145 | 151 | 157 | 163 | 169 | 174 | 180 | 186 | 192 | 197 | 204 |
| 5'5" | 114 | 120 | 126 | 132 | 138 | 144 | 150 | 156 | 162 | 168 | 174 | 180 | 186 | 192 | 198 | 204 | 210 |
| 5'6" | 118 | 124 | 130 | 136 | 142 | 148 | 155 | 161 | 167 | 173 | 179 | 186 | 192 | 198 | 204 | 210 | 216 |
| 5'7" | 121 | 127 | 134 | 140 | 146 | 153 | 159 | 166 | 172 | 178 | 185 | 19 | 198 | 204 | 211 | 217 | 223 |
| 5'8" | 125 | 131 | 138 | 144 | 151 | 158 | 164 | 171 | 177 | 184 | 190 | 197 | 203 | 210 | 216 | 223 | 230 |
| 5'9" | 128 | 135 | 142 | 149 | 155 | 162 | 169 | 176 | 182 | 189 | 196 | 203 | 209 | 216 | 223 | 230 | 236 |
| 5'10" | 132 | 139 | 146 | 153 | 160 | 167 | 174 | 181 | 188 | 195 | 202 | 209 | 216 | 222 | 229 | 236 | 243 |
| 5'11" | 136 | 143 | 150 | 157 | 165 | 172 | 179 | 186 | 193 | 200 | 208 | 215 | 222 | 229 | 236 | 243 | 250 |
| 6' | 140 | 147 | 154 | 162 | 169 | 177 | 184 | 191 | 199 | 206 | 213 | 221 | 228 | 235 | 242 | 250 | 258 |
| 6'1" | 144 | 151 | 159 | 166 | 174 | 182 | 189 | 197 | 204 | 212 | 219 | 227 | 235 | 242 | 250 | 257 | 265 |
| 6'2" | 148 | 155 | 163 | 171 | 179 | 186 | 194 | 202 | 210 | 218 | 225 | 233 | 241 | 249 | 256 | 264 | 272 |
| 6'3" | 152 | 160 | 168 | 176 | 184 | 192 | 200 | 208 | 216 | 224 | 232 | 240 | 248 | 256 | 264 | 272 | 279 |
| | **Healthy Weight** | | | | | | **Overweight** | | | | | **Obese** | | | | | |

Locate the height of interest in the leftmost column and read across the row for that height to the weight of interest. Follow the column of the weight up to the top row that lists the BMI. BMI of 19 to 24 is the healthy weight range. BMI of 25 to 29 is the overweight range, and BMI of 30 and above is in the obese range. Due to rounding, these ranges vary slightly from the NHLBI values.

*Source:* US Departments of Agriculture and Health and Human Services. *Dietary Guidelines for Americans.* 6th ed. Washington, DC: US Government Printing Office: 2005.

and depression. Additionally, exercise elevates mood, improves self-concept, and even increases intellectual functioning (Leith & Taylor, 1990). Exercise promotes emotional health by making us more resistant to stress. People who exercise regularly are less depressed and less anxious than they would be if they did not exercise (Phillips, Kiernan, & King, 2001). When we exercise, we trigger brain chemicals, including endorphins, that contribute to our feeling better about ourselves and decrease our sensitivity to pain. People who exercise tend to have better posture and muscle tone. They look and feel more confident. Exercise also increases our sense of well-being. When people choose favorite types of exercise, then exercise is also a source of fun and relaxation. The psychosocial benefits of exercising on a regular basis can be summed up as improvement in the quality of life.

The psychological benefits of exercise lead directly to social benefits. When we feel better about ourselves and our bodies, we have more energy and self-confidence. This is beneficial whether applying for jobs or making friends. By exercising on a regular basis, we have more stamina for both work and play. When we have strong and healthy muscles, bones, and cardiovascular systems, we have the ability to do just about anything we want to do. We can run to an airport carrying or rolling suitcases, and we can trot through subway systems wearing 40-pound backpacks. If the electricity is off, or there are no elevators in a building, we have the capacity to climb stairs to get to class, a job interview, or a medical appointment. If other people do not have to take care of us in our old age, we will be independent, happier, and less likely to be isolated. Social isolation has a negative effect on overall health. By reducing stress, regular exercise also makes us more tolerant of the faults of other people. Good social relationships are more likely when people are physically, intellectually, and emotionally fit. Older adults who exercise regularly are more likely to maintain their independence, which increases the likelihood of their continuing to mix socially (CDC, 2000).

## A Biopsychosocial Analysis: Why Are People Moving and Exercising Less and Less?

You are probably exercising less now than ever before in your life. People in this culture are moving less than at any other time in history. The reasons are biological, psychological, and sociocultural. The same thing is happening in most industrialized countries of the world. In many cases less movement is due to technological changes in cultures, but biology and psychology also play a part.

### Biological Factors Influencing Inactivity

An important biological factor affecting how frequently people exercise relates to the fact that people are living longer than ever before in history. Average life expectancy has increased markedly over the past centuries due to increases in knowledge, control of contagious disease, and improvements in medical care, and the availability of food. The older people become, the less likely they are to exercise, and there are now more elderly people than ever before in industrialized parts of the world (WHO, 2007). This means larger portions of the population are not exercising. Reflecting over your own lifetime, you realize you move less than you did when you were younger. You have lost aerobic capacity, strength, and flexibility, simply because you are spending your time differently. You probably use your mind more than you do your body. There are also psychological and social factors contributing to your being more sedentary.

## Psychological Factors Contributing to Inactivity

When asked why they do not exercise, most people indicate it is because they do not have time to exercise. College students often say they are too busy to exercise, because they have school, job, and family responsibilities. People believe they have too many obligations and priorities to take time off to exercise. Exercise does not seem as important as their other commitments. What many students do not understand is that exercise can actually save them time. When we exercise and become more fit, we become more efficient and have greater stamina or endurance. We also need less sleep. People who exercise generally sleep more deeply and for shorter periods of time than people who do not exercise (Sallis & Owen, 1999, p. 47). The reality is that many people are becoming weaker in their never-ending struggle to save time. Further, many people are becoming obese, and more tired because they are hauling around greater amounts of weight on less-fit bodies.

## Sociocultural Factors Affecting Inactivity

You could blame your lack of exercise on the Industrial Revolution with its abundance of labor-saving devices. Think about the simple act of sharpening a pencil, dialing a phone, or doing laundry. In school, your grandparents used a knife to sharpen pencils. Your parents put pencils into sharpeners and turned a crank. Today many children simply insert a pencil into an electric sharpener and let the machine do all the work or they use mechanical pencils. Others do not even use pencils, but write papers and take exams on computers. Pressing a computer key takes less effort, strength, and stamina than writing answers on a test paper.

The same can be said for dialing a phone. In old movies you see people using rotary dial telephones. That required more movement than punching in numbers. With cellphones, people do not even have to walk to get to a stationary phone and can just move their thumbs to dial or send text messages. Cellphones are getting smaller and lighter, which means as we downsize our communication gear, we lose physical strength and endurance. All over the world people are moving less than in previous civilizations due to labor-saving devices.

Machines now do your laundry. Think back to earlier cultures when people carried dirty clothes down to a river or stream, swished them in the water to remove the dirt, and spread the clothes to dry on rocks or grass before carrying them back up the river bank to their homes. In the 20th century, people had machines to do the washing, but clothes were still hung on clotheslines, requiring bending and stretching. Now, for many, the only physical effort required is moving wet clothes from a washing machine to a dryer or picking the clothes up at a commercial laundry or dry cleaners. These are just three examples of how our lack of movement and exercise is due to the widespread availability of labor-saving devices for most tasks of daily life.

This is also true at worksites. In the past, most occupations required movement and strength. With the inventions of power saws and hammers, carpenters no longer move as much as before. Fewer jobs require physical activity or movement for even 30 minutes a day. Examples of occupations still requiring a great deal of exercise are the jobs of lumberjack, ballet dancer, and rickshaw puller. You can get some exercise if you wait tables in a restaurant, teach aerobic dance, or dump refuse into garbage trucks. Most jobs in the United States are sedentary and require very little movement. Even during leisure time we are less active than ever before, because we mainly sit, watching television, DVDs, or movies, or playing video games.

Another sociocultural factor that may discourage exercise is gender. Many girls and women are reluctant to do strength training, because they fear they will become too muscled, which they regard as unfeminine. Women and girls often tell fitness trainers they want their muscles toned but not bulky. This is an unfortunate and false fear, because bulk is mainly due to hormonal differences between women and men. Strength training actually improves peoples' appearance by decreasing fat stored under the skin. Strength training increases bone density, which helps prevent osteoporosis—a major problem for older women (CDC, 2000). Osteoporosis weakens bones and puts people at greater risk of fracture. Thanks in part to legal changes, including the increased opportunities for girls and women that have resulted from the funding parity mandated by Title IX, more girls and women participate in sports at all levels (Snooks, 2000). Athletic scholarships and teams for women are more widely available, so more girls and women grow up benefiting from sports and exercise. Both women and men falsely believe they must buy memberships for gyms or fitness centers to exercise. Exercise can be done in the home or outdoors. Many communities need more safe and pleasant places for people to exercise particularly in urban areas (CDC, 2000).

## Types of Exercise

Exercise specialists write about three general types of exercise: aerobic, strength training, and stretching. From a health viewpoint, most is known about aerobic exercise and its biological, psychological, and social benefits. Aerobic exercise is any form of movement that elevates the rate of heartbeats and breathing. It improves many components of the body, but is especially valuable for cardiovascular health and endurance. Aerobic exercise is most beneficial when continued for 20 to 30 minutes at a time several days of the week (CDC, 2000). Strength training, or strengthening movements, is a second general form of exercise with many benefits. Regardless of what you may have heard from other sources, strengthening exercises are appropriate for both women and men at any age. **Flexibility** refers to using the

---

flexibility  The freedom to move joints through their full range of motion.

full range of motion of joints, and specific exercises increase and maintain flexibility. Arthritis, a common disability for many older people in the United States, can be improved by stretching for flexibility and strengthening exercises (CDC, 2000).

## Aerobic Exercise

Aerobic exercise specifically benefits hearts and blood vessels by increasing the rates of heartbeats and lung expansions. From a health viewpoint, it is the most important type of exercise we can do. Experts recommend that everyone, regardless of age or gender, exercise aerobically on a regular basis (CDC, 2000). If we can spend only 30 minutes on exercise each day, the exercise should be one that makes our heart and lungs work harder. Sweating is *not* required for aerobic exercise to be beneficial. It is true that aerobic exercise warms the muscles used in exercise, but sweating also results from ambient air temperature and humidity. Our bodies can produce sweat when we are just sitting at the beach or lying down in a backyard hammock. When breathing and heart rates increase we know we are getting aerobic exercise. This type of exercise is also referred to in research as endurance-type physical activity and involves repetitive movement of large muscle groups. Aerobic exercise has biopsychosocial benefits and improves physical, psychological, and social health.

### Biological Benefits of Aerobic Exercise

Physically active people live longer than people who are sedentary. This is demonstrated by epidemiological research carried out since the early 1950s. Aerobic exercise is the type of exercise most likely to reduce risks of premature death due to a variety of common health problems. The majority of people in the United States die of two cardiovascular events: heart attacks and strokes. The health of our vascular system depends largely on aerobic exercise. Regular aerobic exercise results in lower resting blood pressure, which helps prevent strokes (CDC, 2000). Aerobic exercise increases high-density lipoproteins (HDLs) or "good" cholesterol and lowers low-density lipoproteins (LDLs) or "bad" cholesterol. Exercise prevents obesity, making diabetes less likely (CDC, 2000). A further biological benefit is that exercise helps normalize insulin resistance (Cruess, Schneiderman, Antoni, et al., 2004, p. 36).

The biological benefits of exercise are well documented. As early as 1953, a British study reported that London bus conductors had fewer heart attacks than bus drivers. The scientists concluded it was because conductors walked the aisles and stairs of London's double-decker buses collecting fares all day long, while the bus drivers simply sat and drove (Sallis & Owen, 1999). In an early study of 17,000 male Harvard alumni, scientists reported that moderate but regular physical activity reduced the risk of death by about a third (Paffenbarger, Wing, & Hyde, 1978). They measured stair-climbing, walking city blocks, and sports play and found that physical activity representing about 2,000 or more calories of exercise per week was protective. Middle-aged men with high levels of physical activity were at lower risk of heart attack than sedentary former varsity athletes.

More recently scientists have studied the effects of exercise on the health of both women and men. They find that all physically fit people have lower death rates than those who are unfit (Blair et al., 1989). Moderate amounts and intensities of exercise are even beneficial to health; it does not matter what type of physical activity is performed as long as it is aerobic (Blair, Kohl, Gordon, & Paffenbarger, 1992). The greatest reduction in risk of heart disease occurs when sedentary people begin to exercise regularly (DHHS, 2000).

You can check the health of your cardiovascular system by taking your pulse. One way is by placing your index and middle fingers on your wrist near the thumb side of your hand. Using the second hand of a clock count the number of times your heart beats for 15 seconds and multiply by 4. That is an estimate of your resting heart rate, or the number of times your heart beats each minute. In general, the lower your heart rate, the healthier your cardiovascular system. The average adult's heart beats about 80 times per minute. If your heart beats less frequently, then you are healthier than the average adult. To get a more precise idea of your resting heart rate, count your pulse in the morning before you get out of bed. You can also have your heart rate taken at the student health center and compare the three numbers. Just before rising on your next birthday, check your resting heart rate again. If your heart is beating more frequently than it is today, then your cardiovascular system may be less fit. When you do regular aerobic exercise most days of the week, your cardiovascular system will become stronger and healthier. Your heart will beat less frequently at rest because it is stronger.

By helping to limit the accumulation of body fat and reducing blood glucose levels, exercise helps prevent and control diabetes (CDC, 2000). There is also evidence that aerobic exercise reduces the risks of some cancers (CDC, 2000). Further, muscles and bones used during aerobic exercises are strengthened in the process, which helps maintain balance and prevent osteoporosis, so bones are less likely to break in old age. Breaking a bone in old age often leads to premature death from pneumonia. Aerobic exercise also lowers stress and enhances immune function, making us more resistant to contagious diseases.

Psychosocial Benefits of Aerobic Exercise

Exercising aerobically on a regular basis has psychosocial benefits. Most people report they feel better immediately after exercising. Clearly there is mood improvement when we accomplish something we know is good for us. It helps if exercise is enjoyable rather than boring and burdensome. For psychosocial benefits, it also helps if exercise becomes a routine part of each day. Depression is a major health problem for about 20% of people living in the United States. Methodological and ethical issues limit research parameters, but psychological benefits in studies relate most directly to aerobic exercise.

The book *Physical Activity and Mental Health* (Morgan, 1997) includes about 900 references to research on the psychosocial benefits of exercise. Scientists concluded that for clinically depressed patients, aerobic exercise seems better than no treatment, and benefits are not significantly different from other interventions, including psychotherapy (Martinsen & Morgan, 1997). Other studies indicate that aerobic exercise relieves anxiety. Psychological benefits usually have positive effects on social relationships

Research about why improvements in emotional health occur provide several possible explanations. There are hypotheses that exercise affects neurotransmitters such as endorphins, norepinephrine, and serotonin, which may explain feelings of well-being reported following physical activity. Some authors show concern about overtraining and staleness associated with excessive exercise, but this appears likely only for professional athletes and others working toward maximizing their performance (O'Connor, 1997). In studies of athletic overtraining, it was beneficial for coaches to ensure that participants were having fun and avoiding monotony in training programs (Henschen, 1998).

Steptoe and Wardle (2004) report that physically active people report more positive mood profiles than those who are sedentary. They feel less tense, anxious, and depressed and have a greater capacity to cope with stress (p. 35).

### Examples of Aerobic Exercise

Any movement or exercise becomes aerobic when it elevates breathing and heart rates. This is accomplished by moving large muscle groups such as leg muscles, but it is possible to become aerobic moving only one's arms. The simplest form of aerobic exercise is walking briskly while swinging one's arms. The current recommendation is for 30 minutes of brisk walking at least 5 days a week for both children and adults (CDC, 2000). There are many other types of activities that can be aerobic, including wheelchair racing, jumping rope, rowing, swimming, cross country skiing, peddling a bicycle, tae bo, dancing (including but not limited to aerobic dance), jogging, and walking on treadmills or elliptical machines. Any physical activity that elevates our breathing and heart rate is aerobic and will result in all the biopsychosocial benefits discussed above.

### Important Characteristics of Aerobic Exercise

**The Training Effect** One important aspect of aerobic exercise is that, over time, exercise gradually becomes easier because our bodies adjust to the rigor of the activity. This is called the **training effect**. The effect occurs after a few weeks of regular exercise. Eventually most people find they must increase their effort to achieve the same heart rate benefits, because their bodies now find it too easy to exercise at the same rate.

**Duration** **Duration** refers to how long we exercise or the length of our aerobic workout. Several studies demonstrate that aerobic movement is more beneficial if it continues for at

**training effect** Aerobic exercise done on a regular basis gradually becomes easier, because the body adjusts to the rigor of the activity and is no longer stimulated at that level. One can gradually increase the vigor of exercise by moving faster or exercising for longer periods of time, resulting in a higher level of fitness.

**duration** The length of time one exercises; gradual increases in duration are recommended to safely increase fitness levels.

least 30 minutes each time. Some research suggests that the lower the intensity, the longer should be the duration of exercise (Blair, Kohl, & Gordon, 1992). There is research evidence that 3 separate sessions each day, each session lasting about 10 minutes, can improve health and a sense of well-being (DeBusk, Stenestrant, Sheehan, & Haskell, 1990). The hope is that sedentary people will be more likely to exercise aerobically for shorter periods of time without feeling overwhelmed by the idea of a 30-minute workout (Blair & Connelly, 1996). There is also research demonstrating that our bodies begin to use energy from stored fat after about 20 minutes of exercise. If fat loss is an important goal, it would be a clear advantage to exercise for more than 20 minutes per session. Duration, or time spent exercising, may be easier to measure than trying to figure out distances such as how far you walked.

**Injury Avoidance**  Avoiding injury is a major consideration, because overuse injuries are a common reason why people stop exercising. Overuse injuries occur because people fail to warm up muscles and joints before exercise or because they push themselves to do too much too soon. The best way to warm up is to do the chosen form of aerobic exercise at a slow pace or low level of intensity for the first 10 minutes of the session. This sends oxygen-filled blood to the muscles and other soft tissue used during exercise. A warm-up helps avoid muscle strain or tears. At the end of an exercise session, one should gradually reduce the intensity of movement to allow muscles to cool.

**Illness Avoidance**  It is important to avoid heat- and cold-related illness when exercising (American National Red Cross, 2005). You probably know your normal body temperature is about 98.6°F. That is the ideal temperature for your body to accomplish its metabolic functions. Exercising in extreme hot or cold can be dangerous to health. Exercise produces heat, so it can be perilous under conditions of high heat and high humidity. One of the mechanisms the body uses to cool itself is sweating. When sweat evaporates, it removes some heat from the body. If the air is very humid, such as over 80%, sweat will not evaporate and body heat increases. Heat-related illness may begin with painful muscle spasms, but if you continue to exercise you risk heat exhaustion and a life-threatening heat stroke. High humidity combined with high air temperature is the most common reason exercisers experience heat-related illnesses, but exercising in hot, dry conditions can also bring on heat-related illnesses. In very hot and humid weather, exercise indoors or during the coolest part of the day and carry water to drink while exercising.

Cold-related illness includes frostbite of exposed body parts and hypothermia, which occurs when the entire body becomes too cold (American National Red Cross, 2005). Air temperatures of 65°F and below can result in hypothermia. Wind chill exacerbates the cold, resulting in greater danger. When exercising in cold weather, wear layers of clothing that can be removed as muscles warm, such as sweatshirts that can be tied around the shoulders or waist. Frostbite occurs on exposed body parts such ears, nose, and hands. A great deal of body heat is lost through the head, so a hat or head scarf is recommended in cold weather. Regardless of air temperature, it is paramount to drink water before, during, and after exercising to maintain the necessary level of fluids in the body. Heat- and cold-related illnesses especially threaten older people, but people of any age are susceptible and might consider brisk walking indoors in malls or college buildings.

**Frequency and Intensity   Frequency** refers to how often we exercise. Again, the standard recommendation is all 7 days of the week, or at least 5 days each week. **Intensity** refers to the extent to which the heart and breathing rates are elevated. Exercise specialists suggest some mathematical formulas based on age and fitness level, but most require slowing down to time pulse rates. Formulas can be found in any fitness textbook. More recent studies indicate that intensity is less important for health than the total amount of calories expended during exercise, which is often related to duration more than intensity (Blair, Kohl, Gordon, & Paffenbarger, 1992; CDC, 2000). The American College of Sports Medicine (ACSM) and the Centers for Disease Control (CDC) recently revised their recommendations for intensity of exercise beneficial to health. What is currently recommended is 30 minutes of *light to moderate intensity* exercise on most days of the week. Unfortunately, few adults in the United States engage in regular moderate physical activity (USDHHS, 2000; USDHHS, 1996).

For purposes of simplicity, one may use **perceived exertion rate** to measure intensity. If one has sufficient breath to talk, but not to sing, the exercise is at an appropriate intensity. As people become more fit, they must move more quickly to reach the same level of intensity. This is due to the training effect.

Options for Aerobic Exercise
Exercise should be safe, fun, and interesting. Choosing types of exercise depends on personal preferences. The goal is to exercise aerobically on a regular basis for the rest of our lives, and this is more likely if we choose activities we enjoy. Research demonstrates it is helpful to exercise with other people rather than alone. Exercise partners encourage each other on days when one person is not very enthusiastic about exercising. It also helps to add variety to exercise routines to keep them interesting. For example, walkers can reverse directions or change routes for walking. Another way to add variety is to crosstrain or exercise aerobically in different ways during the week. Brisk walking is the simplest aerobic exercise, because it requires only supportive, comfortable shoes, and a safe, convenient route. Many people

**frequency** The regularity or incidence of exercise, usually measured in terms of the number of days each week one exercises.

**intensity** The extent to which the heart and breathing rates are elevated during exercise. Intensity can be measured by counting the number of heartbeats per minute after about 15 minutes of exercise. Mathematical formulas exist to measure intensity and to set goals for intensity according to age and desired levels of fitness.

**perceived exertion rate** A simple way to assess intensity; if people can talk, they are moving at the correct rate; if people can sing, then the intensity is too low to improve fitness.

walk at covered shopping malls for personal safety and protection from the weather. While in their 80s, an aunt and uncle of the author walked the hallways of their high-rise apartment building for 30 minutes each day. People who live or work in high-rise buildings can also climb stairs. They should warm up slowly and gradually increase the number of flights of stairs to climb each week. Television programs and videos are useful entertainment while exercising indoors on stationary devices such as treadmills or elliptical machines. Repetitive motion such as washing windows and cars, dusting furniture, and raking leaves can be aerobic if done rapidly enough. There are several other factors to think about when selecting types of aerobic exercise.

**Evaluate Safety Versus Risk** Safety issues relate to the type and intensity of exercise. "No pain, no gain" is an old, false, and dangerous adage. No current experts say exercise should be painful to achieve physical and psychosocial benefits. A basic rule is to gradually increase over many weeks the intensity, distance, or duration of the exercise session. To avoid injury, exercisers should increase their efforts by no more than 10% a week. For example, if your grandmother can walk 20 steps to and from her mailbox today, then increase her stamina the following week by having her walk 10% more, or 22 steps. If your grandfather can walk one block this week, then next week he can try a block and a tenth before he turns around to go back to his home. In the beginning it is easier to calculate the number of steps or blocks and eventually progress to miles. The 10%-increase rule is also applied to time. For example, if this week you can walk for 30 minutes, then next week you can try 33 minutes if you want to increase your stamina. When you are comfortable with that, you can increase to 36 minutes.

Injury is the most common reason people stop exercising. The American National Red Cross (2005) estimates about 1 in 12 people in the United States requires medical treatment for injuries each year. Injuries occur due to many factors, including the type of exercise activity, the physical condition and age of participants, and local geography. For example, skateboarding and rollerblading are very dangerous activities. Helmets, protective padding, and goggles should be worn for many kinds of exercise. Safety issues are also connected to where and when people exercise; riding a bicycle on paths may be more dangerous than walking those paths. Bicycling at night along streets and roads is more dangerous than during the day, because of reduced visibility. Uneven terrains and balance problems associated with bicycles make them more dangerous than stationary bikes. Other perils for walkers and bikers are unleashed dogs and lightning. Studies show that stress, personality characteristics, competitiveness, fatigue, and even substance use are related to sport and exercise injuries (Henschen, 1998). **Burnout** is related to mental fatigue and can occur even in children's sports activities (Anthony, 1991). It is usually related to feeling constantly

---

**burnout** A negative outcome of over-exercising or over-participation in sports. It may be related to feeling constantly pressured by oneself or others to improve physical performance. Participants may lose all sense of the purpose or fun of an exercise or sport.

pressured by yourself or others to improve performance. Burnout may result in participants' losing all sense of the purpose or fun of an exercise or sport.

**Convenience** Safety issues should be the first concern, but convenience runs a close second. Convenience is one of the most important factors influencing whether or not people maintain their exercise routines. Not having time to exercise is the major reason people give for not exercising, and convenience is part of this factor. If an exercise site is not convenient, people tend to skip the exercise. Many people pay monthly fees to exercise facilities but seldom use them. This usually means the facility is in an inconvenient location. Swimming is similar: People may have access to swimming pools, but rarely go because they think it is too much trouble to put on a swimsuit and go to a pool. Jumping rope is almost always convenient, because it requires minimal equipment and space.

**Enjoying Exercise** If people hate doing aerobic exercise, it is unlikely they will do it every day. Exercise should be so fun, interesting, and convenient that people look forward to it all day long. It is possible to read while utilizing some machines—elliptical trainers; stationary bikes— or to listen to music or books on a portable player. Many gyms have televisions, as well. All of these can stave off boredom and make the exercise fun.

**Cost** The cost of exercising is an important issue for most people. Belonging to a private fitness center may be costly, and even YMCAs and public facilities charge monthly fees. This is why people often choose mall walking. It is free, safe, requires little equipment, and provides a level surface, which may be important for people with balance issues. Some cities install and maintain paths through parks for walking and biking. Many neighborhoods are safe, have leash laws to control dogs, and provide sidewalks.

**Equipment** Exercise equipment can be costly or inexpensive. Jump ropes are relatively inexpensive compared to bicycles. Elliptical machines and treadmills are more expensive than bikes. Cross-country skiing is an aerobic exercise, but requires skis, poles, and snow. Ballroom and square dancing can be aerobic, if people do not rest very long between dances. For dancing there is usually a small fee attached, but the only equipment required is supportive, smooth-bottomed shoes.

**Limitations or Restrictions** Restrictions require adaptations. An injury may require a different form of exercise as well as rehabilitation. Chronic conditions such as arthritis may require adaptations, as well: For people with arthritis, exercise will help prevent further deterioration in joints, but some types of aerobic exercise may be too painful at first and should be avoided (CDC, 2000). Swimming is an excellent aerobic exercise for people with painful joints or injuries. Many towns have indoor pools for public use. Wheelchair racers quickly become aerobic using their hands and arms to propel the chair. Once you are definitely in the habit of 30 minutes of aerobic exercise 5 days each week, the next step is to begin strength training.

## Strengthening Exercises

When we stop using our muscles they begin to weaken. You may have lost strength since you were an adolescent, so you can imagine how weak you will be 30 or 40 years from now. It is frustrating not to have the strength to do what we want to do. Aerobic exercise strengthens the muscles and bones used in the exercise, but important muscles may not be involved. Strength training will help maintain and improve muscle capability. Running from a threat or through airports takes strength, as well as aerobic capacity. Are you able to lift two suitcases weighing 40 pounds each? Do you have sufficient hand strength to open a tightly sealed jar? Strength training will help people maintain the ability to do everything they want to do throughout their lives. It is easier to maintain muscle strength than it is to regain it once it is lost. The U.S. surgeon general suggests aerobic activity should be supplemented with strengthening exercises about twice a week for adults (USDHHS, 2000).

Strength-training exercises focus specifically on the muscles of the body rather than on the cardiovascular system. This type of exercise maintains and increases strength needed for work and play. Strength includes the amount of weight we can move and the amount of time we can use muscles without exhaustion. Core strength refers to the ability to hold ourselves upright with heads, spines, and abdomens positioned for good health. As they age, many people become bent, with slumping shoulders and protruding abdomens, indicating a lack of core strength. Perhaps you observe this in yourself when you are tired. Strength-training exercises are good for health regardless of age, gender, or ability.

### The Benefits of Strength-Training Exercises

**Biological and Psychosocial Explanations for Insufficient Strength**  From a biological viewpoint, many people lose strength as they grow older, simply because they stop using their muscles. As people age, they tend to do fewer activities requiring strength, both at work and during leisure time. After a period of disuse, muscles begin to **atrophy**. Eventually people do not even attempt to use their muscles, but ask for help or pay someone to do what they were once able to accomplish for themselves. This is particularly true of older women; age and gender are the two main biological factors resulting in loss of muscle strength. Gender-based sociocultural expectations continue to mean that most women and girls are neither expected nor encouraged to develop physical strength. Girls are less likely than boys to brag about their muscles or attempt to outperform peers with pullups or pushups. Increasingly, parents and teachers encourage girls to play sports that maintain and develop muscle strength.

**atrophy**  Wasting away and weakening of the musculoskeletal system due to lack of movement or exercise. This most noticeably occurs in muscles as people age if they do not make it a point to exercise.

From a sociocultural viewpoint, everyone has lost strength due to technological advances and the widespread use of labor-saving devices. The majority of jobs now available require very little muscle strength. People spend most of the day seated at a desk typing on a computer or talking on the phone. Many people start using the arms of their chairs to push themselves into a standing position. The result is a weakening of leg and back muscles. It is frustrating to be disabled by loss of strength. Eventually we feel helpless. Psychologically and socially we are more self-confident when we are strong enough to require little help from others. Strength is necessary to perform the tasks required by daily life.

**Biological and Psychosocial Benefits of Strength Training** Strength training is important to avoid deterioration due to aging, gender, and sociocultural factors such as sedentary jobs and leisure-time activities. Exercises are specific to muscles and other soft tissue such as ligaments and tendons. Bones are also strengthened by the stress of strength training. Life expectancy is greater than ever before and people are more likely to experience bone loss unless they make it a point to use their bones and muscles. Weakening of bones and muscles is the result of lifestyle choices. Some types of aerobic exercise, called **weight-bearing exercises**, stress bones of the legs and spine. Strength training helps bones and muscles too. Strength training also uses more calories than inactivity. Muscle cells use more calories than fat cells, even when we are inactive or asleep. **Body composition** is the muscle-to-fat ratio of our bodies. Being strong means we can work and play effectively and are less likely to be injured.

Types, Methods, and Aspects of Strength Training
Sports and other kinds of play can serve as strength-training exercises, including tennis, golf, soccer, volleyball, skating, football, baseball, bowling, skiing, cricket, etc. Many sports require both strength and aerobic fitness, but sports like bowling and shuffleboard are rarely aerobic, although they do use muscle groups. Many experts recommend concentrating on basic muscle groups in legs, arms, shoulders, back, and abdomen.

Everyone should maintain core strength, which includes abdominal muscles and those in the back, pelvis, and hips. Exercise specifically aimed at core strength does not require much movement. It involves holding one's body in one position for several minutes. The weight supported or resistance is the weight of the body against the pull of gravity. This strength-training exercise—the plank—involves holding one's body parallel to the ground in a straight

**weight-bearing exercises** Exercise that puts weight or stress on the muscles and bones of the feet, ankles, legs, and spine, helping to prevent osteoporosis. One weight-bearing exercise is walking. Swimming is not a weight-bearing exercise because the water supports most of the body's weight.

**body composition** Ratio of fat to muscle, bone, and water in the body. Regular exercise improves body composition by reducing fat weight.

**Figure 4.2**
The Plank: Strength training for arms, abdomen, back, shoulders, pelvis, and hips.

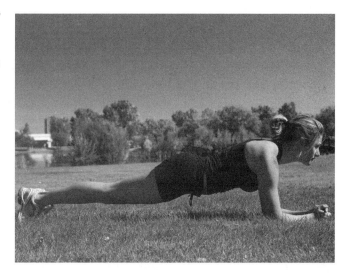

line (see **Figure 4.2**). Support for the body comes from the forearms, elbows, and feet. The arms are bent at the elbows with the hands and forearms on the floor. The lower half of the body is supported by the toes, with the feet bent at right angles about 2 inches apart. Pull stomach muscles toward the spine, and do not allow the back to bend or arch. Most people can only do this for a few seconds in the beginning and have to slowly work up to 5 minutes or more.

There are several types of strength-training exercises, but many elementary schools use **calisthenics**. Calisthenics require no equipment and can be done any time and in most places, from children's daycare centers to nursing homes. Calisthenics use muscles to move one's body weight. One example is the pushup: Lying face down on the floor, keeping the body rigid, you use arm and shoulder muscles to push your body off the floor. Return to the starting position to repeat the exercise.

Most calisthenics can be modified for beginning exercisers. Children frequently begin pushup exercises from bent knees rather than from feet. This reduces the amount of weight they must initially push off the ground. Weak-muscled people, such as people who have been inactive for a long time, can begin by leaning and pushing away from a wall. As their muscles grow stronger, they can move their hands closer and closer to the floor until they are doing pushups from their knees and then from their feet. An important advantage of calisthenics is they can be modified for everyone.

calisthenics  A simple form of exercise using the strength and weight of one's own body to increase fitness levels. One example is the pushup, an exercise in which people lie on the ground and use their arms to push their upper body off the ground.

**Free weights** can provide strength exercises; they are "free" because they are not attached to machines. One free weight is a barbell that is gripped by the hands and slowly raised. Resistance machines also provide strength training. Weights are stacked inside a frame and may be removed or added by the lifter. You may have heard the terms **reps** and **sets**. Reps refer to repetitions or the number of times a weight is moved. Sets are groups of reps. For example, if you lift a 1-pound barbell 10 times, or 10 reps, rest a minute, do 10 more reps, rest, and do 10 more reps you completed 3 sets of 10 reps by moving the weight 30 times. By counting moves and keeping records, people know they are making progress and becoming stronger. Mathematical formulas based on percentages of maximum strength may be calculated, but it is simpler to begin by moving a low amount of weight 5 times. Weights do not have to be commercial products. In elementary schools and nursing homes, weights are often cloth bags filled with beans or sand. Some people use canned goods as free weights but should avoid dropping them on their toes.

Safety Recommendations for Strength Training
As is true of aerobic exercise, there are safety issues connected with strength training. One important goal is to avoid injury, because injury stops exercise. To avoid injury, warm up muscles first by doing aerobic exercises or by repeating strength-training motions several times without actually moving any weight. A second safety issue involves high blood pressure. Older people should check with physicians before beginning strength training, because lifting or moving weight elevates blood pressure. Breathing is also important. Exhale as you lift or do the work such as the pushup, and inhale as your muscles relax. Experts recommend a gap of 48 hours between strength training sessions so muscles can recover. Some experts advise a training sequence of using large muscle groups first, such as the legs, and then chest, shoulders, back, and arms. If using weights, beginners should start with very light weights and gradually increase repetitions until they can do a set of 10. If people cannot do 10 reps, then the weight is probably too great for their current level of strength. One general safety rule is to limit increases in weights or repetitions by no more than 10% each week. For example, if you can do 10 pushups without strain this week, then next week you can try for 11 pushups. If you can lift a 1-pound weight 20 times this week, then you can try lifting it 22 times next week.

---

**free weight**  A quantity or mass, usually made of metal and not attached to a strength-training machine. A free weight is used to improve muscle strength by lifting or moving the weight through space for a certain number of times. One example of a free weight is the barbell.

**reps**  The number of repetitions or times a weight is moved through space.

**set**  A group of repetitions used in strength-training programs to improve fitness levels.

## Flexibility Exercises for Muscles and Joints

Flexibility exercises are the third type of exercise recommended for health. Flexibility refers to the freedom to move joints through their full range of motion. Loss of flexibility begins early in life. As we age we become less flexible due to our inactivity and due to patterns of movement. If we do not use our joints regularly, we eventually become stiff and lose the ability to move. We should do stretching exercises if work and leisure time activities do not require use of all joints. The biological benefit of doing flexibility exercises is the ability to move freely without stiffness or pain. There is also research evidence that stretching helps prevent lower back injuries, which are common in the United States (USDHHS, 2000). People lose flexibility when they are injured and must rest or wear a splint or cast for several weeks. Flexibility exercises are necessary to regain the use of joints after injury or surgery. Some people develop arthritis or bursitis and find it painful to move as they age. Unless they exercise, they may end life with a permanent limp or lose the ability to use the injured joint. Being flexible makes work and play easier, improves the quality of life, and helps prevent injuries.

Stretching refers to exercise to maintain and improve flexibility. Stretching affects ligaments, which are soft tissue surrounding joints and tendons that attach muscles to bones. Stretching is usually enjoyable. Stretching should be gentle and done only when the muscles and joints are warmed up by aerobic exercise. We can stretch every day.

How far, how fast, and the manner of stretching are safety issues. One should not strain soft tissue by stretching it beyond its capacity. We should hold a stretch for at least 10 breaths. Generally stretching does not involve bouncing motions. Many yoga and Pilates exercises are examples of stretching. People with pain in their lower backs often find stretching relieves pain. Stretching should never cause pain.

### Think About It!

#### Make a Commitment

A basic personal physical fitness program should include activities that enhance cardiorespiratory fitness, muscular strength and endurance, and flexibility. To develop an effective program, determine your needs, interests, and limitations. Answering the following questions can help you accomplish this step:

- How can I schedule my day's activities so I have time to exercise?
- Which physical activities am I most likely to enjoy and practice regularly for the rest of my life?
- Do I want to develop or enhance specific sports-related skills?
- Would I rather work out alone or with others?

*(continues)*

- Where will I exercise?
- Do I have physical limitations that require special equipment or rule out certain activities?

You need to choose enjoyable physical activities that will help you meet your fitness goals. As mentioned earlier, aerobic exercise is necessary for achieving cardiorespiratory fitness. Resistance training is important for increasing lean body mass and maintaining muscular strength and endurance. Warm-up and cool-down stretching exercises can improve range of motion.

Stop when you experience signs of exercise intolerance, such as pain or breathlessness, and note this in your log. A common problem encountered by enthusiastic but out-of-shape people is trying to do much to soon. By gradually increasing the intensity and duration of your physical activity, you can progressively overload your muscles and achieve your fitness goals.

Adding new activities prevents boredom with the workout program and develops different muscle groups or skills. Cross-training, incorporating a variety of aerobic activities into a fitness program, is an excellent way to maintain enthusiasm and interest. Working out in different environments can also add interest. Walking in parks or hiking on trails, for example, can be more interesting than walking around indoor tracks. By working out with friends or family members, you can enhance your physical as well as social health.

*Adapted from:* Alters, S., & Schiff, W. (2006). *Essential concepts for healthy living* (4th ed.) (pp. 302–303). Subbury, MA: Jones and Bartlett Publishers.

## Applications of Health Psychology to Exercise Behavior: What Factors Encourage People to Exercise?

Many theories of behavior change discussed in the previous chapter apply to exercise, including aerobic exercise, strength training, and flexibility. Physical activity is a behavior that most people must choose to do. People are more likely to maintain an exercise program if they enjoy it and expect it to be beneficial. Both factors are motivators for behavior change. Social support from family and friends is important and provides incentives for all behavior changes, including exercise. It is an even greater help if an exerciser is joined by friends or family members including spouses and children (see **Figure 4.3**).

### Behavior Change in Exercise and the Concept of Self-Efficacy

One important psychosocial determinant of regular exercise is **self-efficacy**, which is a central concept in health psychology. Self-efficacy refers to a belief in one's capability to exe-

**self-efficacy** A belief in one's capability to execute a course of action to achieve a goal, such as stopping the habit of smoking cigarettes or starting the daily habit of 30 minutes of brisk walking.

**Figure 4.3**
Brisk walking with a friend
or family member for 30
minutes each day improves
emotional, physical, and
relational health.
Convenient and enjoyable
exercise routines are more
likey to become permanent
behaviors.

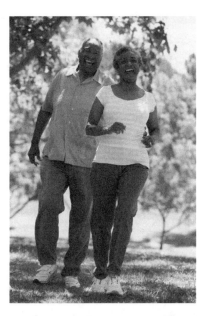

cute a course of action to achieve a goal (Bandura, 1997). Bandura's theory of perceived self-efficacy in relation to other theories has the strongest correlation with physical activity in every study that included it (Sallis & Owen, 1999). According to Bandura, helpful courses of action to encourage behavior change include changing one's environment, thinking, motivations, and emotional state. With regard to exercise behaviors, we would say we have self-efficacy if we strongly believe we are capable of regular exercise for aerobic fitness, strength, and flexibility.

## Interventions to Encourage Exercise Behavior

In health psychology, an **intervention** is an organized effort to help people change or modify their behavior. When there is an accumulation of research on specific topics, scientists often do a meta-analysis to summarize common threads among many studies. A meta-analysis of physical activity interventions revealed five characteristics that were effective in encouraging people to be physically active (Sallis & Owen, 1999).

1.  It helped most people to choose a low-to–moderate-intensity activity, such as brisk walking.

**intervention** An organized program designed to help people change or modify their behavior.

2. Using behavior modification techniques to motivate oneself to exercise was more effective than having a health risk appraisal or a medical checkup.

3. Mediated interventions were the third most helpful type of intervention. Mediated interventions are those in which helpful information and encouragement are delivered by mail, e-mail, or telephone. This also relates to friends or family members communicating about exercise dates.

4. Choosing to be more physically active during one's leisure time was helpful.

5. Being unsupervised in doing the activity was also helpful.

Researchers suggest other strategies to promote lifelong exercise behaviors. Setting achievable short-term goals is beneficial, such as, "One day this week I am going to walk briskly for 30 minutes." It also helps for people to monitor and record exercise behavior. For example, marking a calendar with a star for every day they exercise and looking back over each month to acknowledge consistency is a motivator. A sense of accomplishment may increase both interest and enjoyment. (See the Active Lifestyle Chart in **Figure 4.4**.)

## Theoretical Approaches to Change Exercise Behaviors

Most people who exercise report they like being fit, strong, and flexible. Many non-exercisers say they do not know how to go about starting an exercise program, which is why it is so important for those interested in encouraging behavior modification to become highly informed about all of the exercise parameters discussed above, including safety factors. Some non-exercisers report they know how to exercise, but do not have time for it. They can be reminded that studies show people get back the time they spend exercising aerobically, because they sleep more deeply and spend less time sleeping. Those who are fit, strong, and flexible are physically more comfortable and generally have more stamina for work and play. Listing and rereading the advantages of exercise often help to change behavior.

Behavior modification theories can be applied to exercise, because exercise or physical activity is a behavior. Health psychologists' theories explain what motivates people to change health-related behaviors such as exercising. Other theories provide plans for maintenance of exercise behavior. Most studies rely on self-reports.

### The Theories of Reasoned Action and Planned Behavior

Studies to change non-exercisers to regular exercisers used the theories of reasoned action and planned behavior (Cournehya, Keats, & Turner, 2000; Smith & Biddle, 1999; Courneya, Bobick, & Schinke, 1999). Operationalization of variables and research methods vary among these studies, but most conclude that attitudes and perceived behavioral control predict intentions, while intentions and control predict behavior change (Bogart & Delahanty, 2004, p. 215–216).

# Develop an Active Lifestyle

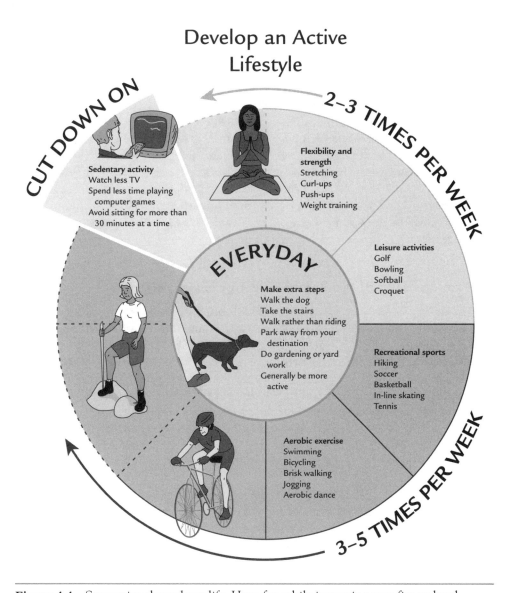

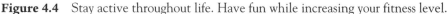

**Figure 4.4**  Stay active throughout life. Have fun while increasing your fitness level.

*Source:* Insel, P., Turner, R. E., & Ross, D. (2006). *Discovering nutrition* (2nd. ed.) (p. 447). Sudbury, MA: Jones and Bartlett Publishers.

## Ajzen's Theory of Planned Behavior Applied to Exercise

On his web site, Icek Ajzen applies the theory of planned behavior to exercising on a tread-mill (2008). Ajzen notes humans will consider 1) behavioral beliefs about the likely outcome, and the value of those outcomes, if their behavior changes, 2) normative beliefs about expectations of others and their own motivations to conform to those expectations, and 3) control beliefs about various things that may ease or obstruct the behavior change.

Attitudes about the behavior, expectations of others or the subjective norm, and perceptions about their control of their own behavior result in intentions to change a behavior and become antecedents to a behavior change. The behavior (exercise) is defined by its target, action, context, and time (TACT), including "walking (action) on a treadmill (target) in a physical fitness center (context) for at least 30 minutes each day in the forthcoming month (time)." On his web site Ajzen also gives examples of ways to measure intention, attitude, subjective norm, and perceived behavioral control.

## Application of the Health Belief Model to Exercise Behavior

The health belief model originated in the public health field when scientists were trying to understand what motivates people to take action to reduce their health risks (Becker, 1975; Becker & Maiman, 1975). According to the theory, if people believe they are susceptible to a serious health risk, they will do something to reduce the risk. Furthermore, when they believe their efforts will be worth the difficulties involved in taking action, they are more likely to make the effort. The main idea is that when people believe they are at risk of a serious illness, they will change their behavior if they believe the benefits of change outweigh the problems or barriers associated with change. Becker and Maiman added sociobehavioral determinants to this model when they recognized the influence of demographic variables such as age and gender, sociopsychological variables such a personality, and reference group pressure.

Think about how to relate the health belief model to changing exercise behaviors based on what you learned from this chapter and the previous chapter. Imagine yourself to be a person who does not exercise. Your life does not include aerobic, strength-training, or flexibility exercises. In fact, you describe yourself as a couch potato. You drive or ride to work, where you sit at a desk most of the day. When you get home, you plop down on a couch and spend the evening eating and watching television, movies, or DVDs. You follow a sedentary lifestyle, meaning minimal movement or exercise. Over the years you lose aerobic capacity. You know this because one day you tried to run one block from the bus stop to work in the rain and you ran out of breath (susceptibility to risk of being unable to run). You know you have lost strength, because a coworker asked for help moving his desk and you did not have the strength to help (susceptibility to risk of being weak). You know you lost flexibility, because when you drop a bag of chips off the couch it is difficult for you to lean over and pick it up, so you just kick it over to the couch and pick it up after you sit down to watch television (susceptibility to risk of joint stiffness and back pain).

Given this scenario, ask yourself about your beliefs. Do you have less stamina than ever before in your life? Do you believe your muscles are weaker and your joints are less flexible than when you were in high school? Do you believe you are likely or susceptible to becoming less and less physically fit the older you get? Do you believe this deterioration of your physical condition is seriously detrimental to your health and quality of life? If you answered "yes" to these questions, then you can move on to the next two questions based on the health belief model.

Now check for barriers or costs of beginning to exercise and benefits of exercise and list each separately. Under barriers or costs, write down all the reasons you can think of that keep you from exercising, for example, not enough time. Now list all the benefits of making changes to counteract your loss of stamina, strength, and flexibility. Third, compare the two lists and decide if the benefits of beginning to exercise exceed the barriers.

The health belief model suggests that changing from sedentary to active lifestyles will result in biological and psychosocial benefits. According to this theory, people make behavior changes if they believe benefits outweigh costs. Then they may begin thinking about scheduling time on most days of the week to exercise. They will choose activities to achieve the goal of becoming more aerobically fit, stronger, and more flexible. In addition to choosing a time and types of activity, they will make choices about safety issues, monetary costs, places to exercise, whether or not to include other people in the activity, appropriate clothing for the weather or exercising indoors, and buying or borrowing any necessary equipment.

Decisions about aerobic exercise are easier if the choice is brisk walking. Walking can be done outdoors in good weather, indoors in bad weather, and at any time, day or night. Very little equipment is needed. It would be important to have supportive flexible shoes. Most people exercise in old clothes, so no wardrobe purchases are necessary. Warm up and cool down are achieved by walking slowly at first, briskly during the longer aerobic middle period, and then slowly again to cool down. Upon arrival at home, people may add stretching for flexibility and calisthenics for strength.

For safety, if people find they are still tired one hour after exercising, it probably means they did too much and should shorten duration or lower intensity until endurance increases. Drink water before, during, and after exercise, and dress appropriately for the weather (barrier). This includes using sunblocks and wearing hats. If an unleashed dog (barrier) attacks, roll into a ball, protecting the back of the neck with the hands, and call animal control to report the location of the dog. If the dog bites (barrier), seek medical care.

## Application of the Transtheoretical Approach to Exercise Behavior

This model demonstrates that people can be identified by their exercise stage, and those in later stages have a lower body mass index and better cardiovascular fitness than those in earlier stages (Burke, Richards, Milligan, et al., 2000). Other research indicates that those in later stages perceive fewer barriers than those in earlier stages (Bogart & Delahanty, 2004, p. 217). This model for behavior change is credited to Prochaska and DiClemente (1984) and Prochaska, Norcross, and DiClemente (1994). The theory suggests that people changing a behavior go through six stages. After completing all stages, the behavior is persistent or habitual, or a relapse is possible.

While in the first stage, pre-contemplation, people do not consider exercising. This is the couch potato stage. After they become aware of shortness of breath when running for a bus, the inability to help a coworker move a desk, and helplessness in leaning over to pick up a bag of chips off the floor, they decide to start thinking about getting more exercise. They move on to stage 2, or contemplation. At this point they could compare barriers and benefits of exercising. Perhaps they decide to start a walking program, because exercise might relieve some of their problems. The third stage of the transtheoretical model is preparation. They decide to begin walking every afternoon after work. They plan to put on appropriate shoes and clothing and head out the door to walk. When they get back, they plan to mark the exercise outing on their calendars. Stage 4, the action stage, begins when they actually take their first brisk walk. They make it to the end of the block and back. The next day they repeat the block walk. During the following weeks, they increase the exercise time so they can now walk for 15 minutes straight. The walking becomes so habitual they look forward to it every afternoon when they get home from work. Psychologically, they are relieved and proud because they are finally doing something about their health and physical condition. They begin to notice other benefits, including the fact that their clothes are looser, which means they are losing fat; they sleep better at night; they have more energy; and when they run to catch a bus, they are not winded and wheezing when they sit down. After about 3 months, they discover they can walk briskly for 30 minutes at a time.

The fifth stage is maintenance. One day they experience what some experts call a lapse or relapse (Marlatt & Gordon, 1985). They go out to eat after work with friends, and by the time they get home it is dark outside. They decide they are too tired to walk that night. For about a week they return to the former couch potato habits, but then notice their daytime fatigue is returning and they are no longer sleeping well. They decide to get back into the exercise routine and devise ways to deal with causes of their lapse. It has been 5 years now and they have never lapsed again. They do not even think about neglecting to exercise. They are in termination. Congratulations are in order!

## Summary

Research from health psychology and related fields indicates that exercise is one of the most beneficial of all behaviors for maintaining and improving health. Today fewer people are physically active than ever before, due to technological changes over the last 100 years and increases in sedentary leisure-time activities. Students and faculty members in health psychology interested in applied interventions must be aware of a variety of factors specific to changing exercise behaviors, including motivation, frequency, intensity, training effect, duration, and injury and illness avoidance.

Among all types of exercise, regular aerobic exercise has the greatest potential for preventing heart disease, stroke, diabetes, and some cancers. The current minimum recommendation for everyone is 30 minutes of brisk walking at least 5 days a week. Strengthening exercises help preserve muscle, diminish the accumulation of stored fat, and can be as simple as calisthenics done at home. Stretching helps maintain flexibility and balance.

The health psychology construct of self-efficacy is applicable to a variety of behavioral changes, including exercise behaviors. Scientists in health psychology, epidemiology, and exercise science continue to develop interventions to promote exercise behavior. The health belief model predicts people are rational in decision making and will weigh the benefits against the costs before changing their exercise behavior. The theory of planned behavior posits that intentions to change are an outcome of beliefs and attitudes toward the behavior, normative beliefs or the subjective norm, and perceived behavioral control. The transtheoretical or stages-of-change model describes change as a series of steps or stages. Different kinds of interventions are beneficial at different stages.

## Review Questions

1. Name and briefly describe the three general kinds of exercise that are most useful for improving and maintaining health and fitness.

2. Discuss the purposes and health benefits of exercising.

3. Using the biopsychosocial approach, explain why people living today are not likely to get much exercise.

4. Using the health psychology approach, briefly explain the biological, psychological, and sociocultural benefits of exercise.

5. Answer the question, "Why are people living today less active than people who lived 100 years ago?"

6. Briefly explain the connection among calories eaten, the accumulation of fat on the body, and exercise.

7. What is the most important type of exercise? Justify or defend your answer.

8. What makes an exercise aerobic?

9. Explain what exercises for strength and flexibility accomplish and why they are important.

10. Define the following terms and make at least one important point about each with regard to exercise.

    a. Training effect

    b. Duration

    c. Intensity

    d. Safety

11. Explain how a person can avoid sports and exercise staleness and burnout.

12. How does strength training improve the body's use of calories stored as fat?

13. Describe core strength and explain how it can be improved.

14. Briefly describe how you could use the health belief model to decide on a strength-training exercise program.

15. Using the transtheoretical model, explain the stages you would probably go through if you started an exercise program to become more flexible.

## Student Activity

Using the transtheretical model of behavioral change, locate yourself with regard to exercise on one of the stages.

1. If you are not even thinking about daily exercise, use the health belief model to list the barriers and benefits of daily aerobic exercise based on the discussion in the text book.

   a. Write a paragraph explaining how the barriers may exceed the benefits and vice versa.

   b. If the benefits exceeded the costs and you are now thinking about starting a regular aerobic exercise program, list the type of exercise you intend to do,

the appropriate clothing, the time during the day you will exercise, and the location for the activity.

2. If you are already exercising on a regular basis, list the techniques you use and the benefits you have noticed from exercising. Share these with a classmate who is in the stage of pre-contemplation. Explain what gave you the self-efficacy to begin an exercise program.

3. If you have relapsed from regular aerobic exercise, write several paragraphs about when and how the relapse occurred. Explain what it would take to get you started in an exercise program again and how to avoid relapse in the future.

## References

American National Red Cross. (2005). *First aid: Responding to emergencies.* Yardley, PA: Stay-Well.

Anthony, J. (1991). Psychologic aspects of exercise. *Clinics in Sports Medicine, 10*(1), 171–180.

Ajzen, I. (2008). Retrieved January 4, 2008 from http://www.people.umass.edu/aizen/research.htm

Bandura, A. (1997). *Self-efficacy: The exercise of control.* NY: W. H. Freeman.

Becker, M. H. (1975). The health belief model and personal health behavior. *Health Education Monographs, 2*(4), 324–473.

Becker, M. H., & Maiman, L. A. (1975). Sociobehavioral determinants of compliance with health and medical care recommendations. *Medical Care, 13,* 10–24.

Blair, S. N., & Connelly, J. C. (1996). How much physical activity should we do? The case for moderate amounts and intensities of physical activity. *Research Quarterly for Exercise and Sport, 67* (2), 193–205.

Blair, S. N., Kohl, H. W., Gordon, N. F., & Paffenbarger, R. S. (1992). Physical activity and

health: A lifestyle approach. *Medicine, Exercise, Nutrition and Health, I,* 54–57.

Blair, S. N., Kohl, H. W., Paffenbarger, R. S., Clark, D. G., Cooper, K. H., & Gibbons, L. W. (1989). Physical fitness and all-cause mortality: A prospective study of healthy men and women. *Journal of the American Medical Association, 262,* 2395–2401.

Bogart, L. M., & Delahanty, D. L., (2004). Psychosocial models. In R. G. Frank, A. Baum, & J. L. Wallander (Eds.), *Handbook of clinical health psychology, Vol. 3,* (pp. 201–248). Washington, DC: American Psychological Association.

Bouchard, C., Shephard, R. J., Stephens, T., Sutton, Jr. R., & McPherson, B. D. (Eds.). (1990). *Exercise, fitness and health.* Champaign, IL: Human Kinetics Books.

Burke, B., Richards, J., Milligan, R. A. K., Beilin, L. J., Dunbar, D., & Gracey, M. P. (2000). Stages of change for health-related behaviors in 18-year-old Australians. *Psychology and Health, 14,* 1061–1075.

Centers for Disease Control and Prevention. (2000). Physical Activity and Fitness 2 (22).

*Healthy People 2010.* Retrieved May 5, 2007 from http://www.healthypeople.gov/Document/HTML/volume2/22Physical.html

Courneya, K. S., Bobick, T. M., & Schinke, R. J. (1999). Does the theory of planned behavior mediate the relation between personality and exercise behavior? *Basic and Applied Social Psychology, 21,* 317–324.

Courneya, K. S., Keats, M. R., & Turner, R. (2000). Social cognitive determinants of hospital-based exercise following high-dose chemotherapy and bone marrow transplant. *International Journal of Behavioral Medicine, 7,* 189–203.

Cruess, D. G., Schneiderman, N., Antoni, M. H., & Penedo, F. (2004). Biobehavioral bases of disease processes. In R. G. Frank, A. Baum, & J. L. Wallander (Eds.), *Handbook of clinical health psychology* (Vol. 3, pp. 31–79). Washington, DC: American Psychological Association.

DeBusk, R. F., Stenestrant, U., Sheehan, M., & Haskell, W. L. (1990). Training effects of long versus short bouts of exercise in healthy subjects. *American Journal of Cardiology, 65,* 1010–13.

Dubbert, P. M., King, A. C., Marcus, B. H., Bess, H., and Sallis, J. F. (2004). Promotion of physical activity through the life span, pp. 649–657. In Raczynski, J. M., & Leviton, L. C. *Handbook of Clinical Health Psychology, Volume 2, Disorders of Behavior and Health.* Washington, DC: American Psychological Association.

Henschen, K. P. (1998). Athletic staleness and burnout: Diagnosis, prevention, and treatment. In J. M. Williams (Ed.), *Applied sport psychology* (3rd ed., pp. 398–408). Mountain View, CA: Mayfield.

Jamner, M. S. (2004). Exercise, effects and benefits. In A. J. Christensen, R. Martin, & J. M. Smyth (Eds.), *Encyclopedia of health psychology* (pp. 104–106). New York: Kluwer Academic/Plenum.

Leith, L. M., & Taylor, A. H. (1990). Psychological aspects of exercise: A decade literature review. *Journal of Sport Behavior, 13,* 219–239.

Marlatt, G. A., & Gordon, J. R. (1985). *Relapse prevention: Maintenance strategies in the treatment of addictive behaviors.* New York: Guilford.

Martinsen, E. W., & Morgan, W. P. (1997). Antidepressant effects of physical activity. In W. P. Morgan (Ed.), *Physical activity and mental health* (pp. 93–106). Washington, DC: Taylor & Francis.

Morgan, W. P. (Ed.). (1997). *Physical activity and mental health.* Washington, DC: Taylor & Francis.

O'Connor, P. J. (1997). Overtraining and staleness. In W. P. Morgan (Ed.), *Physical activity and mental health* (pp. 145–160). Washington, DC: Taylor & Francis.

Paffenbarger, R. S., Wing, A. L. & Hyde, R. T. (1978). Physical activity as an index of heart attack risk in college alumni. *American Journal of Epidemiology, 108* (3), 161–175.

Phillips, W. T., Kiernan, M., & King, A. C. (2001). The effects of physical activity on physical and mental health. In A. Baum, T. Revenson, & J. Singer (Eds.), *Handbook of health psychology.* Mahwah, NJ: Erlbaum.

Prochaska, J. O., & DiClemente, C. C. (1984). *The transthoretical approach: Crossing traditional boundaries of therapy.* Chicago, IL: Dow Jones-Irwin.

Prochaska, J. O., Norcross, J. C., & DiClemente, C. C. (1994). *Changing for good: The revolutionary program that explains the six stages of change and teaches you how to free yourself from bad habits.* New York: William Morrow.

Sallis, J. F., & Owen, N. (1999). *Physical activity and behavioral medicine.* Thousand Oaks, CA: Sage Publications.

Smith, R. A., & Biddle, S. J. H. (1999). Attitudes and exercise adherence: Test of the theories of reasoned action and planned behavior. *Journal of Sports Sciences, 17,* 269–281.

Snooks, M. K. (2000). Title IX of the Education Codes. In A. H. Howard & F. M. Kavenik (Eds.), *Handbook of American women's history* (2nd ed., pp. 571–572). Thousand Oaks, CA: Sage Publications.

Steptoe, A., & Wardle, J. (2004). Health related behavior: Prevalence and links with disease. In A. Kaptein & J. Weinman, (Eds.), *Health Psychology,* pp. 25-51. Oxford, United Kingdom: Blackwell Publishing.

U.S. Department of Health and Human Services. (2000). *Healthy people 2010: National health promotion and disease prevention objectives.* Washington, DC: U.S. Government Printing Office.

U.S. Department of Health and Human Services. (1996). *Physical activity and health: A report of the surgeon general.* Atlanta, GA: Centers for Disease Control.

Weiss, J. M. (1989). Effects of exercise on the immune system: Relationship to stress. In R. S. Williams & A. G. Wallace (Eds.), *Biological effects of physical activity* (pp. 71-83). Champaign, IL: Human Kinetics.

William, J. M. (Ed.). (1998). *Applied Sport Psychology,* (pp. 447-448). Mountain View, CA: Mayfield Publishing Company.

World Health Organization. (2007). Physical inactivity: A global health problem. Retrieved August 4, 2008 from http://www.who.int/dietphysicalactivity/factsheet_inactivity/en/index.htm

# Applications of Health Psychology to Eating Behaviors: Improving Health Through Nutritional Changes

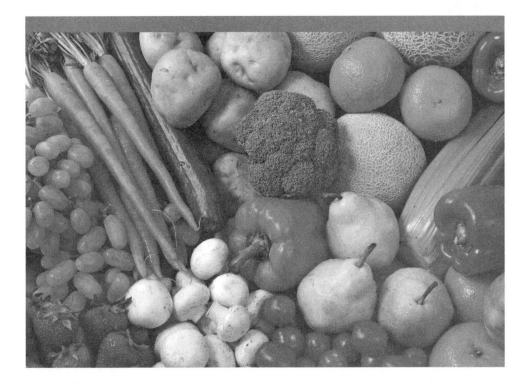

## Learning Objectives

After studying this chapter students will have the knowledge and skills to be able to:

1. Discuss outcomes of unhealthy eating behaviors.

2. Explain biological factors that influence eating.

3. Explain psychosocial factors that influence eating.

4. Identify basic components of healthy eating practices.

5. Compare their own eating patterns to current recommendations.

6. Explain why obesity is a health problem and the ideal ways to assess and eliminate obesity.

7. Identify the basic components of body composition and explain why sudden weight loss is not a healthy way to lose body fat.

8. Suggest interventions to encourage healthier eating practices using theories common to health psychology.

9. Discuss eating disorders and their outcomes for health.

## Introduction

As is true of exercise, eating is a behavior important for optimal health. Eating meets basic biological needs, yet many people suffer health problems due to poor eating choices. For example, some people eat too much food for their level of activity and gradually become obese. Others restrict their food intake severely, resulting in serious health problems and even death. Drastically limiting food intake is often motivated by psychosocial factors such as a misguided desire to improve physical appearance or to enhance athletic performance.

Good nutritional practices and weight control are two related but different issues in health psychology. Positive health behaviors include eating all necessary nutrients while preventing an accumulation of excess body fat. Body weight can be lost through starvation, but this is dangerous to health and results in undesirable losses of muscle and bone mass. Another important fact is that many adults who lose weight eventually regain it in the form of fat. This happens because they revert to previous eating and exercise patterns. Maintenance of a healthy body weight is central to good health.

## Eating Healthily Is a Lifelong Behavior

Students should think of eating as a chosen behavior, similar to the behavioral choices of exercising, smoking, and drinking alcohol. Eating is a learned behavior beginning in infancy. We make many choices about food consumption every day. We decide when we will eat, what we will eat, how we will eat, how much we will eat, where we will eat, and with whom we will eat. These choices affect our health. We eat to meet biological needs, but there are a multitude of additional choices and behaviors involved in eating. As is true of any behavior, food intake reflects biological, psychological, and sociocultural influences and parallels the biopsychosocial approach used in health psychology.

Some health psychologists and scientists in behavioral medicine and epidemiology specialize in the study of obesity, other eating problems, and interventions for people who habitually make poor nutritional choices. These scientists contribute hundreds of research reports each year examining both causes and solutions to poor nutritional behavior. To understand the science of healthy eating requires a thorough grounding in biopsychosocial influences on food intake, in the basic components of healthy eating behavior, and in ways to avoid unhealthy eating practices. Behavior change theories from health psychology can be applied to eating behavior to improve health.

## Obesity

Scientists and health professionals are most concerned with behaviors resulting in **obesity**. Epidemiologists refer to an epidemic of obesity in the United States and other industrialized nations (World Health Organization [WHO], 2008; Centers for Disease Control [CDC], 2003). Obesity is more prevalent among women, members of minority groups, and those with low incomes (U.S. Department of Health and Human Services [USDHHS], 2003). The physiology of obesity is fairly straightforward. It results from consuming more calories from food than the body can use. When people do not move or exercise sufficiently to use all the calories in the food they consumed, their bodies save the nutrients in the form of fat cells. Fat cells accumulate to the point of obesity. More than 44 million adults in the United States are obese, and about 15% of children and adolescents are overweight. The percentage has tripled over the past 20 years (Mokdad, Ford, Bowman, & Dietz, 2003; CDC, 2003). Obesity is a primary cause of deaths due to heart disease, strokes, and some cancers (American Heart Association [AHA], 2006; American Cancer Society [ACS], 2006). Type II diabetes is directly related to obesity and may result in blindness, amputations, kidney failure, and death (American Dietetic Association [ADA], 2008). Solutions to obesity rest in changing both eating and exercise behaviors.

## Other Outcomes of Unhealthy Eating Practices

Due to socioeconomic conditions, there are millions of impoverished people who suffer from **malnutrition** or the lack of sufficient nutrients. In the United States people may become malnourished as a result of factors that include low income, inadequate education, age, and debilitating health conditions. Solutions to these problems require economic, political, and social change, along with changes in individual behaviors.

Unhealthy eating behavior includes inadequate intake of calories, vitamins, minerals, water, and fiber. Hypertension, high cholesterol levels, kidney stones, osteoporosis, and gout result from faulty eating behavior. Nutrition during pregnancy is crucial to the health of

**obesity** A body composition that includes fat at too high a percentage for good health. Obesity is usually determined by comparing one's height and weight to body mass index tables designed for this purpose. Obesity is a risk factor for many serious diseases, including heart disease and diabetes.

**malnutrition** Inadequate nutrient intake or taking in too few nutrients from food or by intravenous feeding. Malnutrition may lead to sickness and death. Socioeconomic levels and geographic location often result in malnutrition due to famine, war, or natural disasters resulting in the widespread lack of food products for a population. People diagnosed with anorexia nervosa often suffer from malnutrition.

both mother and child. Many clinical health psychologists specialize in the study and treatment of disordered eating practices such as anorexia nervosa and bulimia nervosa. Both cause health problems and may result in death. Good nutritional practices are basic and important to health, but many people never consider changing their eating behavior.

This chapter focuses on the behavior of people who have access to a variety of foods, but still make unhealthy food choices. It considers eating behavior from five perspectives or viewpoints. The first part of the chapter examines biological and psychosocial factors that influence eating behavior. Many current trends result in faulty food choices and prevent optimal health. A second section focuses on the basic components and current recommendations for healthy eating behavior. The third part of the chapter explores the health problems of obesity, and a fourth section discusses disordered eating practices based in popular fad diets, bulimia nervosa, and anorexia nervosa. Anorexia and bulimia are problems for a limited segment of the population, especially young women and some athletes. The fifth and final section of the chapter summarizes applications of health psychology theories to improving eating behavior.

## Biological and Psychosocial Factors Influencing Eating Behaviors

### Biological Factors Influencing Eating Behavior

There are five biological purposes for eating. We eat to continue to live; to grow when we are young; for energy, so we can do what we want to do; to repair damaged body tissue; and to prevent disease. Studies indicate people may also eat in response to hormonal changes, medications, and to specific types of tumors.

#### Starvation and Hunger

A basic biological reason for eating is to continue to live. **Starvation** results when no nourishment, either solid or liquid, is taken into the body. Starvation eventually results in death. **Hunger** refers to a biological or physiological state. It is often described as an unpleasant, even painful, sense of an urge to eat. Similarly, thirst is believed to be based in the body's need for liquids such as water. Thirst arises when our bodies become dehydrated or we consume too much salt. Experts consider both hunger and thirst to be physiological drives resulting from biological needs of the body. Hunger is also affected by stomach distension, hormones, and insulin. We will not have the energy to accomplish what we want to do if we are hungry. Even though hunger is biological in origin, it is affected by sociocultural and psychological

---

**starvation** The process of suffering from lack of food or nourishment.

**hunger** Hunger refers to a biological or physiological state. It is often described as an unpleasant, even painful, sense of the need to eat.

factors. For example, do we lose the desire to eat when we see a roach crawl across our plate of food? That is a reaction based in the culture. We also know from historical accounts that when people are extremely hungry, they eat things they would not ordinarily eat including dirt and other people. Hunger can overcome psychosocial values when survival is at risk. **Pica** is a condition of craving and eating non-food items such as clay, chalk, and laundry starch. Some nutritionists believe humans crave certain substances because they contain nutrients needed by the body. The craving of specific foods or odd combinations of foods during pregnancy may be both biological and psychosocial in origin.

### Satiety

**Satiety** is a biologically based feeling that the stomach is full and is related to hunger. Studies show when people overeat frequently, their stomachs stretch or enlarge to accommodate greater and greater amounts of food. This is why some people have their stomachs stapled or banded to prevent overeating. They hope to achieve a sense of satiety before they eat more food than their body needs. Cultural events, such as Thanksgiving, are occasions when people eat beyond satiety. Have you ever had someone you love, like your mother or aunt, insist you eat more food even though you say you are full? Many people also consume specific foods for sociocultural and psychological reasons, including the fact that they enjoy the sensation of eating a food such as candy or ice cream.

### Energy

We get energy or calories from foods and liquids. All humans need energy to live and do what they want to do, including work and play. We also need reserve energy for emergencies. Energy is measured by the number of calories or kilocalories in food. In addition to calories, our bodies need water and specific nutrients, including carbohydrates, fats, proteins, vitamins, minerals, and fiber.

### Nutritional Needs Vary by Age

Age is a biological factor affecting nutritional need. Adequate nutrition involves taking in a sufficient number of calories and nutrients to survive and grow when we are young. Optimal growth includes the achievement of maximum brain size, skeletal growth, and bone density within the limits of genetic background. Nutritional needs are extremely important during infancy and childhood. As infants we first consumed milk, from breast or bottle. There is evidence that breast milk is the ideal food for infants, because allergic reactions are less likely to occur than with other sources of milk. Lactation is the ability of a woman to produce milk after pregnancy. It is a biological response to childbirth and hormonal

---

**pica** A condition of craving and eating non-food items such as clay, chalk, and laundry starch.

**satiety** A biologically based feeling that the stomach is full.

## Think About It!

### Better Nutrition Beginning in Infancy

Breast milk can be collected through the use of breast pumps, stored, and later put into bottles for feeding. This is a choice made by many women who must be absent from their infants during the day due to employment or school, but choose to collect, chill, and store milk to be given when their infants are not available to them for feeding. It is still unusual for companies in the United States to allow mothers to bring their infants to work for feeding during the day. Some companies do have "lactation rooms" where employees can collect and store milk during the day.

changes. There are many reasons why women do not breastfeed. Unfortunately, some women cannot breastfeed due to health problems such as AIDS/HIV or the necessity of being away from their infants for long periods of time. Alternatives to breast milk are commercial formulas made for infants. A mother's milk and most commercial formulas supply the calories and other nutrients needed for an infant to live and grow.

Eventually children need more nutrients than can be provided by milk, so other foods are introduced. Many infants are first given solid food in the form of very liquid cereal products. Cereals are least likely to cause an allergic reaction, although some infants are allergic to grains such as wheat. Following the successful introduction and acceptance of cereal, most parents enlarge infants' diets to include pureed fruits, vegetables, and meats. Nutrition continues to be important throughout childhood and adolescence. Unfortunately more and more children and teens are becoming obese due to taking in excessive numbers of calories. This puts them at risk of diabetes.

By their middle 20s, most people reach maximum height, but many continue to consume the same number of calories as when they were younger and growing. This is more food than their bodies need. Excess calories no longer needed for growth are stored in the body in the form of fat. Some stored fat is required for good health, because fat insulates and helps control body temperature. Fat is also available for energy when people cannot take in necessary nutrients due to injury, illness, or surgery. Unfortunately many adults take in more calories than they need and become overweight and obese.

## Psychosocial Factors Influencing Eating Behavior

We learn what to eat and how to eat from family members and friends at home, school, and work. Fairly early in life toddlers show preferences for certain foods. We may have heard hilarious stories about our rejection of new foods when we were toddlers. Food preferences are not well understood, but may be due to varying senses of taste among children. Psychosocial factors play an important part. Most food preferences are learned behaviors. Sometimes toddlers see their older siblings reject food and copy the behavior. Food preferences change during childhood, when we are teenagers, and again during adulthood. In old age, our eating behavior may change again for economic reasons such as low income or biological reasons such as poor chewing ability. Some elderly people return to eating soft foods similar to those eaten by infants.

It is difficult to separate psychological from sociocultural influences. For example, research reveals that people eat more food than normal or eat specific foods when they are under the influence of strong emotions such as anger. Many people report they eat in unhealthy ways when they are bored, sad, tired, anxious, or depressed. Many of these emotional states or moods are individually or psychologically based, but some can be traced back to earlier life experiences. For example, if our caregiver distracted us from a hurt knee with a cookie, we may now find comfort in the taste of something sweet when we are in pain, unhappy, or anxious. Some people report they consume unhealthy foods when they are lonely or need comfort. Others say they overeat when they are under a great deal of stress.

Eating patterns have sociocultural origins associated with birthdays, earning good report cards in school, and achievements on the job. Vacations and holidays are often accompanied by changes in eating behavior. Some people reward themselves with food. Just seeing or smelling some food may trigger eating even when there is no hunger. **Appetite** is different from hunger. Appetite is the desire to eat or drink. It is mainly influenced by sociocultural and psychological factors, rather than by biological factors. Different foods and liquids have different textures and appearances. Foods may be desired for the pleasure of anticipated flavors such as sweet, sour, bitterness, or saltiness. Sometimes a food's density or mouthfeel, such as softness, hardness, crispness, or creaminess, is appealing to our appetites.

Appetites can be stimulated by the odor and appearance of food. Foods are often described as "mouth-watering" or "finger-licking good." Some people say they have a "sweet tooth" meaning they always have an appetite for sweet food. Others say they need lots of salt or everything tastes bland. Some substances found in food, such as caffeine, can make us more alert, although too much caffeine can make us nervous and restless. Alcoholic beverages may help us feel relaxed due to their sedative effect on the nervous system. Appetite is also influenced by environmental factors such as heat and cold, as well as by what is available to eat. We say we lack an appetite for certain foods due to past unpleasant experiences including food poisoning or allergic reactions to a food. Appetite stimulates eating behaviors and is based on psychosocial factors.

Childhood Experiences with Food

Food and liquids meet biological needs, but specific eating and drinking behaviors are learned. For most people this occurs first in a social setting such as the family. Family eating patterns reflect the general culture and influence children's eating behavior. Most of us

---

**appetite**  The desire to eat or drink.

have good and bad memories of foods consumed as children. Behavioral demands were made on us while we ate. We learned proper eating patterns. In this culture, it is likely we were urged to eat vegetables, avoid sweets before meals, use a napkin, chew quietly with our mouths closed, say please and thank you, keep our elbows off the table, and so forth. Sometimes the rules about eating took precedence over the food and made meals an unpleasant experience. Some children are praised if they eat every morsel on their plate, which can develop into a habit of continuing to eat even after we feel full in order to earn dessert and caregiver approval. Something sweet becomes a reward for doing as parents or caregivers wished us to do.

Our eating practices broaden when we start school, watch television, and visit outside the family and neighborhood. We are exposed to other ideas about food and eating behavior. Children often trade food in the school cafeteria. They learn some foods are socially acceptable and others are "yucky." At this stage children throw away food they dislike or give it to pets.

Other Psychosocial Influences

Scientific reports in newspapers, magazines, and on television influence eating behavior. From the 1940s to the 1960s, parents were told that their children's level of intelligence depended mainly on their intake of protein. The result was that many children developed the habit of eating too much protein, mainly from meat and eggs. High-protein foods are often high in fat, so children learned to consume more fat than they needed. Many continue to follow the pattern as adults.

As we grow older, sociocultural factors have a greater influence on what, where, when, how, and with whom we eat. Ethnicity, religion, historical traditions, advertising, and regional and global availability of food also shape eating behavior. Ethnicity is a sociocultural factor influencing eating and reflecting the availability of foods in different regions of the world. Due to immigration and international travel, many foods once unique to one population are now eaten and enjoyed on a worldwide basis. On the other hand, the smell and sight of certain foods may be offensive to some members of ethnic or religious groups. For example, people from India who honor cattle may find the odor of cooking beef and animal fat repugnant. People growing up in the United States may find the odors of spices used in Asian countries nauseating. Rural areas often have access to foods not available in the city, and vice versa. People now visit farmers' markets to buy farm-fresh organically grown food. **Figure 5.1** shows many factors that affect food choice.

Religion influences eating behavior in other ways. Followers of the Muslim and Jewish faiths have many dietary rules, including ingredients that cannot be eaten or time periods during which no food is allowed. For many years, Roman Catholics were to avoid eating meat on Fridays. Many continue to observe rules of controlled eating during Lent, and many people forego a specific food, such as chocolate or alcohol, during the 40 days before Easter. Many specific foods and recipes are associated with religious customs.

There are common national holiday eating patterns. In the United States, Thanksgiving Day is a national holiday and meals on that day often include turkey, dressing, cranberry

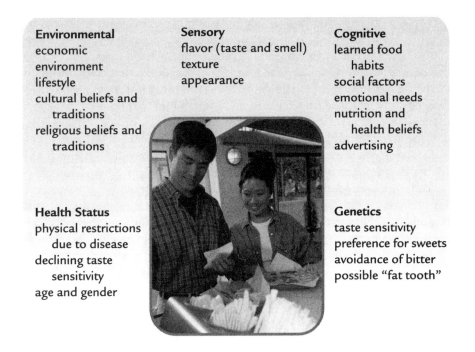

| Environmental | Sensory | Cognitive |
|---|---|---|
| economic | flavor (taste and smell) | learned food |
| environment | texture | habits |
| lifestyle | appearance | social factors |
| cultural beliefs and | | emotional needs |
|    traditions | | nutrition and |
| religious beliefs and | |    health beliefs |
|    traditions | | advertising |

**Health Status**
physical restrictions
   due to disease
declining taste
   sensitivity
age and gender

**Genetics**
taste sensitivity
preference for sweets
avoidance of bitter
possible "fat tooth"

**Figure 5.1** As we grow older many factors affect our choice of foods.

*Source:* Insel, P., Turner, R. E., & Ross, D. (2007) *Nutrition* (3rd ed.). Sudbury, MA: Jones and Bartlett Publishers.

sauce, and pumpkin pie. The spring celebration of Easter may include new clothes, dyeing hardboiled eggs, and eating baked ham or lamb. New Year's Eve and the next day are celebrated with champagne or other liquor and in some areas of the country, by eating black-eyed peas for luck. Special events such as birthdays are often accompanied by cakes with candles for the celebrant to blow out after making a wish. Halloween is associated with costumed children going through neighborhoods collecting candy. Valentine's Day cards may be accompanied by boxes of chocolate candy. These are all traditions based in the culture and passed on in families, schools, and through the media. All influence eating behavior.

Advertising encourages specific eating behaviors by making foods appealing. Many people in the United States grow up liking the smell and taste of cooked fat, and salivate when they smell French fries or hamburgers cooking. Others associate eating at fast food restaurants with happy occasions when the whole family was together. Some advertisements relate foods like ice cream with special family occasions, such as the return of a soldier from war. Other ads recommend we eat in certain restaurants as a way to relax after a hard work week, or in bars to drink beer and meet other people like ourselves. Additional advertising comes from the diet food industry and reflects currently popular fads about healthy eating. The Food and Drug Administration (FDA) has established criteria for food to be labeled "low fat" or "high fiber." Food labeled "low fat" is sometimes not very nutritional because it contains large amounts of sugar. For example, all of the calories in soft drinks come from sugar. Processed sugar lacks protein, fats, vitamins, minerals, and fiber.

Types of food, and the frequency and timing of eating, also reflect occupations. In early history, the United States was basically an agrarian economy. Most people worked on farms and were self-sufficient. They raised plants and animals for food. Their eating behavior reflected the types of food they produced and the timing of their work day. This is the likely origin of the hearty American breakfast consisting of eggs, bacon or sausage, and bread. Many of us still expect this kind of breakfast even though we will never touch a shovel, plow, or tractor. In fact, most jobs no longer require much physical labor, although we continue to consume hearty American breakfasts like farm-based cultures.

Culture affects eating in other ways. Most of us expect to eat three meals a day, with mid-morning and midafternoon breaks that often include doughnuts or sweet rolls. This may result in our consuming more sugar and fat calories than we need based on our activity level. Many people work long hours and come home tired and hungry. When this happens, there is a tendency to overeat or consume too many calories. Where we eat also reflects sociocultural lifestyles. Many people lead rushed lives, with long commutes to and from work in cars, buses, or trains. One outcome is people grab food that is easy to eat en route. People also eat while watching television or reading the paper. Nutritionists believe this behavior is detrimental, because people are more likely to overeat when they are distracted while eating.

Socioeconomic factors such as income affect eating patterns, including eating at home, which is generally less expensive than eating in restaurants or drive-through eateries. Education, including knowledge of nutrition, affects eating behavior, although many people say they know better than to eat certain foods they love. Some people believe hard work deserves indulgence in food and drink. Types of jobs also affect eating behavior. Some people pack a lunch, eat a hearty workingman's lunch, or take 2 hours for a business lunch that includes alcohol. Construction workers often buy food from portable canteens near worksites. Children hear music from ice cream trucks and run to buy sugary treats. A multitude of other psychosocial factors affect eating behavior and health. It is important to learn the basic components of healthy eating in order to understand the health issues involved and the influence of psychosocial factors.

## Basic Components of Healthy Eating

Most adults are involved in many activities, including work, school, spending time with family and friends, and participating in various forms of recreation. In order to do all these things, people need a healthy diet and adequate sleep. Most activities require energy and health achieved through food and exercise. A well-chosen diet with necessary calories, vitamins, minerals, and fiber helps us avoid sick days and spending time and money at medical facilities. The biological benefits of healthy eating are to live, grow, have energy to do what we want to do, and maintain good health through old age. As adults, we must consume enough calories and other nutrients to sustain life, to have adequate energy, and to have reserve energy in case of an emergency. We need stored fat for energy in situations when we cannot eat due to illness or injury.

Health psychologists interested in research and clinical practices have a thorough grounding in the science of nutrition and healthy eating behavior in addition to understanding theories about ways to change eating behavior. In the science of nutrition, there are standard terms and recommendations. Food refers to both solids and liquids including beverages. **Diet** describes typical eating patterns. For example, the study of an animal's diet would examine its typical feeding behavior. There is confusion about the word "diet" because it is often used to describe various plans for losing weight and implies restrictions in normal eating patterns. Our diet is simply the food we eat on a daily basis. There are special diets when people are ill or have surgery. For example, there are liquid diets and salt-free diets. General recommendations for healthy eating for all adults include adequacy, balance, and variety.

## Adequacy

Taking in sufficient amounts of food and liquids is the first imperative for dietary intake. Nutritional recommendations reflect age, activity level, and general health requirements. **Adequacy** refers to eating sufficient amounts and types of foods to consume the correct number of calories and all necessary nutrients. Adequacy is a minimum standard. Nutrition scientists have many recommendations about nutrition for both genders and different ages. From time to time the Food and Nutrition Board of the National Academy of Sciences recommends changes based on new scientific findings (Insel, Turner, & Ross, 2006). The **recommended dietary allowances (RDAs)** and **dietary reference intakes (DRIs)** specify recommendations about calories, protein, fats, fiber, and some vitamins and minerals. RDAs and DRIs can be found on the inside cover or in the appendices of most nutrition

**diet** A person's usual eating practice or pattern.

**adequacy** Eating sufficient amounts and types of foods to consume the correct number of calories and all necessary nutrients.

**recommended dietary allowances (RDAs)** These specify recommendations about calories, protein, fats, fiber, and some vitamins and minerals that meet the needs of most healthy individuals by life-stage and gender. RDAs and DRIs can usually be found on the inside cover or in the appendices of most nutrition textbooks.

**dietary reference intakes (DRIs)** Suggested by the Food and Nutrition Board of the National Academy of Sciences. There are targets for intake by healthy individuals and include vitamins, minerals, water, carbohydrates, fiber, fat, linoleic acid, and alpha-linolenic acid protein. The DRIs include the RDAs.

textbooks. Some requirements are explained on food labels of commercially prepared foods. An ideal diet is called **optimal**. Optimal means we are taking in all the nutrients we need for the best possible health regardless of age.

Our diet should contain enough calories to avoid fatigue and illness. Level of activity influences the ideal range of calories. Physically active people such as soccer players and gymnasts need more calories than office workers. People who stand all day need more calories than people who sit all day. When we are sick or injured we may need more calories than when we are well. For example, if we are badly injured in an automobile accident, experience a bad burn, or have surgery, then we need more of some nutrients until we recover although relative inactivity may necessitate lower caloric intake. Needs fluctuate throughout life, but always include a balance of carbohydrates, protein, fats, vitamins, minerals, and fiber.

Complex Carbohydrates

Calories come from foods containing carbohydrates, proteins, and fats or lipids. Foods containing **complex carbohydrates** should be our major energy source and include grains, vegetables, fruit, and milk. Food containing carbohydrates is especially important for the brain and other parts of the nervous system. If we skip breakfast and get a headache, it is probably from lack of adequate carbohydrate for fuel. Carbohydrates are very important to health, even though some fad diets suggest avoidance. Eating too many calories, regardless of the type of food it comes from, will result in obesity. Most of the calories we take in on a daily basis should come from carbohydrates.

Nutritionists say that if we do not take in enough calories from carbohydrates, our bodies will degrade or metabolize lean body mass (muscle) and stored fat to provide energy. Metabolizing stored fat may sound like a good idea, but the process can damage our kidneys.

Carbohydrates should be complex rather than simple to include vitamins, minerals, and fiber along with energy. Nutritionists emphasize the role of fiber in health, because it helps prevent health problems in the colon. In the battle with obesity, the bulkiness of fiber helps fill stomachs and takes longer to digest. We are less likely to overeat if we consume fiber with each meal. Imagine eating an orange and compare that experience to consuming a soft drink or a beer with the same number of calories. We get hungry sooner when calories come from simple sugars or alcohol than when we eat high-fiber foods such as oranges. In most cases, sugar is a simple carbohydrate and provides calories, but no vitamins, minerals, or fiber.

**optimal** An ideal diet.

**complex carbohydrate** A food containing carbohydrates for energy along with other important nutrients and fiber. Dietary guidelines for Americans encourage intake of complex carbohydrates by increasing consumption of fruit, vegetables, whole grains, and low-fat milk. Chemically, the term refers to chains of two or more monosaccharides to differentiate them from simple carbohydrates or sugar molecules.

For that reason sugar is known as an "empty" calorie. The typical cola drink contains 8 teaspoons of sugar. Sugar contributes to obesity and tooth decay. In the United States we consume more than 100 pounds of sugar per person each year.

### Protein

The **protein** found in food is important for building and repairing body tissue, as well as for many biochemical processes. Muscle is mostly protein. Protein is derived from food groups that include meat, eggs, nuts, and fish, but also from legumes or beans. Iron is an important mineral we get from meats, eggs, and some vegetables. Milk products also contain protein, along with a very important mineral, calcium. Most adults should choose low-fat or fat-free proteins.

### Oils and Fats

Dietary fat is an important nutrient, because it provides a sense of satiety or fullness. Stored fat insulates the body from temperature changes, and pads of fat protect body parts from injury. Important vitamins are found in fats and essential fatty acids must be included for good health. Most people in the United States take in too many calories from fat compared to their calories from carbohydrates and protein. Per gram, fats and oils have twice the calories of carbohydrate and protein.

## Balance and Variety

Our eating patterns should represent a balance among the major nutrients. Dietary recommendations include percentages of daily caloric intake from carbohydrate (45% to 65%), fats (20% to 35%), and protein (10% to 35%) plus small amounts of fatty acids (Institute of Medicine, Food and Nutrition Board, 2002). A major issue in the United States today is the lack of balance in food intake. Most people consume food with too few calories from complex carbohydrates, and too many calories from proteins, simple carbohydrates, and fats.

Eating a variety of foods helps ensure consumption of essential nutrients, including all known vitamins and minerals, and helps achieve balance. Variety also helps us to avoid excessive amounts of harmful additives, contaminants, or toxins found in food. This is why eating exactly the same foods every day is not recommended.

In addition to providing carbohydrate, protein, and fat, the foods we eat should contain vitamins, minerals, and fiber. Drinking water is also essential to good health, as is exposure

---

**protein**  A large complex compound consisting of amino acids that provide nutrients to the body for growth and repair of body tissue. Examples of foods containing sizeable amounts of protein are meat, poultry, milk, eggs, fish, and some vegetables and grains. Burns, surgery, fevers, and infections require greater amounts of protein than normal to maintain health.

to sunlight so the body can manufacture vitamin D. In addition to eating an adequate diet we should also eat a balanced diet.

## The Ideal Diet

We may wonder about the ideal diet for eating behavior. This is an important question, and the answer is that an optimal eating pattern depends on multiple factors, including individual characteristics. When we were children, teens, and younger adults, we needed extra nutrients to support growth. When we stop growing, we no longer need the same amount of calories. In addition, age affects metabolic rate, or the rate at which we use calories. Generally, metabolic rates slow as we age, meaning we need fewer calories. An exception is when we are sick or injured.

## Deficiencies

Vitamin, mineral, and fiber deficiencies occur even if we consume sufficient calories. Many nutrition-related health problems were not understood until vitamins and their food sources were identified. Up until the late 18th century, seamen experienced and died from scurvy caused by lack of vitamin C. Deficiency in vitamin C causes depression, hysteria, bleeding gums, loosened teeth, and failure of wounds to heal. Vitamin A deficiency still results in blindness in children all over the world. If we have difficulty seeing at night, it could be due to a vitamin A deficiency. This deficiency also results in dry, rough, scaly skin and contributes to leg cramps. The processing used to create the flour for commercially produced white bread removed most of the nutrients found in whole grains and in flours typically used in home-baked breads. When vitamin B deficiencies were understood, the U.S. government compelled commercial food producers to enrich bread and cereal products. Today food processors must ensure that nutrients are included in the foods they sell. They are required to provide detailed labels of nutrient values so consumers can make healthier choices.

Many people in the United States suffer from malnutrition. Nutritionists say low levels of calcium, vitamin D, protein, and fiber often occur in the general population. Low levels of calcium lead to bone loss, which contributes to osteoporosis. Osteoporosis contributes, in turn, to more easily broken bones, particularly in older women and men. Elderly people also experience bone loss due to the lack of adequate vitamin D from sunlight. The legs of children and adults lacking vitamin D often become bent or bowed.

Adequate fiber helps people avoid constipation, diverticulosis, and some types of colon cancer. Dental health depends on an adequate supply of several vitamins and minerals, including calcium. Protein is important for blood cell production and protecting muscle mass. The lack of niacin and folate or folic acid contributes to diarrhea, irritability, dizziness, confusion, and neural tube defects. Anemia and abnormal brain-wave patterns are associated with the lack of vitamin B6. Many people in the United States rely on fast food, which may be deficient in important vitamins and minerals.

The absence of needed nutrients and water affects biopsychosocial health. Dehydration, or the lack of adequate water, may result in headaches. When we lack sufficient nutrients and calories we do not have the energy to work, play, or even be pleasant to people at home or at work. When important relationships are disrupted, we are more likely to become depressed and anxious. There are other psychological problems specifically connected with the absence of certain nutrients. Weakness and confusion follow inadequate magnesium and potassium intake. Lack of salt can result in mental apathy. Iron deficiency anemia, the most common deficiency in the world, results in weakness, headaches, and the inability to concentrate. High sugar intake is associated with obesity and must be avoided by people who have diabetes or who are at risk of diabetes. In some people, high blood pressure or hypertension is associated with excessive salt intake. Alcohol also contributes to hypertension and strokes. High-fat diets contribute to cardiovascular disease, diabetes, and some cancers. Fortunately we have good sources of information about ways to improve nutritional choices.

## Guidelines for Healthy Eating Behavior

There are many ways to analyze eating behaviors. Current research suggests that the four food groups of a generation ago were too simple. Recommended dietary allowances (RDAs) may be too complex for daily use. A simpler approach to assessing eating habits is the food guide pyramid (U.S. Department of Agriculture [USDA], 2007). It is based on current knowledge about adequacy, balance, and variety. The first food guide pyramid, introduced in 1992, was an effort by the USDA to simplify nutrition recommendations for all adults.

That pyramid was divided into six zones and graphically showed which food groups should make up the bulk of food intake. For example, the bread, cereal, rice, and pasta group was the largest area at the base of the pyramid. At least six servings are recommended per day for adults. A minimum of three vegetable servings and two fruit servings are in the next zones. At least two servings each day should come from the milk, yogurt, and cheese group. Two servings of the meat, poultry, fish, dry beans, eggs, and nut group are recommended daily. The pyramid recommends using fats, oils, and sweets sparingly, as seasonings and in cooking (**Figure 5.2**). The pyramid also defines what counts as a serving.

The pyramid looks simple but may not be sufficient for our purposes. For example, many foods, such as casseroles, are combinations of food groups. Also it is difficult for some people to calculate the size of servings without actually measuring them. Measuring is tedious and hot food becomes cold before it can be eaten. Nevertheless, the pyramid is a great advance over previous efforts to make understandable dietary recommendations. The U.S. population includes many ethnic and nationality groups, so nutritionists devised a Mediterranean diet pyramid, a Latin American diet pyramid, and an Asian diet pyramid. Key recommendations pertain to adequate nutrients within caloric limits, weight management, and physical activity, and include information about food safety and alcohol consumption.

The USDA introduced MyPyramid (USDA, 2007), a more personalized approach for those with access to the Internet. It emphasizes physical activity, moderation in food choices,

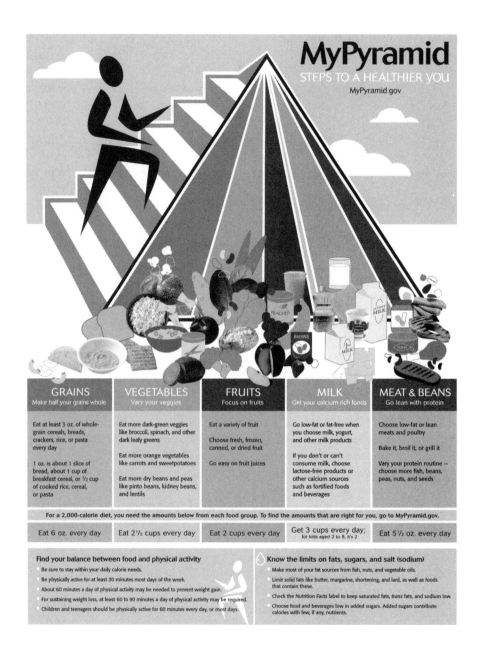

**Figure 5.2** Compare your eating patterns over the past 24 hours with the recommendations on the pyramid. Did you eat recommended amounts from the five categories before eating any extra food?

*Source:* U.S. Department of Agriculture, www.mypyramid.gov

and recommends changes in typical diets. For example, cereals should be whole grains, and serving size is specific for the grain group. "Amounts of food" for each group are more specific than "serving size," because they include ounces for grains and the meat/bean groups. Cups are used for vegetables, fruits, and milk. Users can go to the web site, enter their age, gender, and level of physical activity. Based upon this input, the program will calculate the number of appropriate calories for the individual. A recommended eating plan based on seven food groups can then be printed out and used. If level of activity changes, caloric needs will change, and users can recalculate recommendations.

## Health Problems Associated with Obesity

In addition to eating a healthy diet, everyone should also have a healthy body weight. Overeating, or consuming more calories than can be used in a day, leads to the common and serious health risk of obesity. People in the United States tend to gradually add fat weight to their bodies as they grow older. In 2003 and 2004, 32.2% of adults (over 66 million) were obese and almost 5% of those were extremely obese. At the same time 17% of children and adolescents 2–19 years of age (more than 12 million) were overweight (Centers for Disease Control, 2006). Obesity is a risk factor for cardiovascular disease, diabetes, and some cancers. An additional point to remember is that people can be obese and still be deficient in nutrients. For example, if people eat only beef, bread, and ice cream, then they are taking in too many calories from protein, fat, and simple carbohydrates, but lack important nutrients found in vegetables and fruits. Fats and sugar contribute to satiety, but crowd out or displace other important nutrients from a diet. Fibrous foods, such as fruits, vegetables, and some plant-based sources of protein take more time to digest, so they stay in the stomach longer, producing a sense of satiety and prevent hunger pangs.

The major causes of death in the United States are cardiovascular disease (CVD) and cancer, so researchers interested in these illnesses focus on identification of their causes. The previous chapter examined the evidence that daily, moderate, aerobic exercise reduces risks of CVD, diabetes, and some cancers. This chapter examines additional solutions related to eating behaviors found in people living in industrialized countries.

Excessive intake of fat and low intake of fiber are believed to be major contributors to obesity, CVD, diabetes, and cancer. Epidemiologists studying countries with low rates of cardiovascular disease discovered that in those countries most diets were based on whole grains. They concluded that excessive amounts of meat and animal-based fats contribute to high rates of cardiovascular disease. They noted lower levels of colon cancer in those countries, as well, and concluded that fiber helps prevent colon cancer. In Japan, less animal fat is consumed than in the United States, and Japanese women have lower rates of breast cancer than U.S. women. Japanese men have lower rates of heart disease until they move to the United States. Many scientists suggest that eating more plant-based food, such as grains, vegetables, and fruits, might lower the high rates of obesity, CVD, and cancer in the United States.

## What Is a Healthy Body Size?

Many people ask but cannot find a definitive answer to this question. If our health is good, we are not weak from hunger, and we are neither gaining nor losing weight, then our eating behavior and weight are probably appropriate for our age and current activity level. Caloric intake and activity levels are balanced. If we stop our physical activity but continue to eat in our usual way, we will begin to gain fat weight. For example, when people retire they are usually less active, and gain fat weight because they are eating the same amount and types of food as when they were employed. If they add daily exercise, then caloric intake and energy use will again be in balance. (See **Figure 5.3** about balancing caloric intake with energy output.)

Our body stores any calories we eat but do not use or burn. Fat is energy held in reserve, and too much body fat is defined as obesity. Several components contribute to body weight. This is known as body composition.

### Body Composition

Body weight includes the combined weight of water, bone, muscle, and fat. Among these four elements, only excess fat is considered unhealthy. Most nutrition books contain charts recommending appropriate weights based on age, gender, and height. Unfortunately, these charts do not distinguish among the four components. From a health viewpoint, it is very important to maintain adequate amounts of water, muscle, and bone in the body. Fat is the only component we should ever try to lose through exercise and dietary behavior change. It is possible to be very thin and still have too much fat, because very-low-calorie intake reduces bone and muscle mass, changing our body composition. See **Figure 5.4** to understand the effect of body composition on appearance.

### Body Mass Index

Some scientists use the calculation of **body mass index (BMI)** to indicate healthy weight ranges. BMI is based on height and weight, but does not tell us about body composition. BMI is used because weight and height are simple to measure and understood by most adults, but the index does not give a complete picture for purposes of health. BMI is based on total weight, but fails to distinguish among weight from fat, muscle, bone, and water. There are several complex ways to compare weight from fat to weight from lean body mass (bone and muscle), but they require complicated and expensive measurement techniques done by trained personnel. Two examples are underwater weighing and biological impedance measurements.

> **body mass index (BMI)** Body weight in kilograms divided by the square of height in meters. BMI tables suggest appropriate, healthy weight for height for men and women.

**Figure 5.3**
When energy intake equals energy used then body weight stays the same.

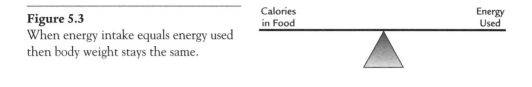

## Waist-to-Hip Ratio, a Simple Measure

Some scientists believe that fat around the waistline, or central obesity, is more dangerous for health than fat carried elsewhere on the body. One easy way to measure this distribution of fat is to compare the distance around the waist to the distance around the hips. A string will do, but a measuring tape makes it easier. In general, we are healthier if the distance around our hips (measured 7 to 9 inches below the waist) is longer than the distance around the waist. If the waist measurement is greater than the hip measurement, the person may be obese and is eating more calories than he or she needs based on his or her level of activity. Divide waist measurement by hip measurement. Women whose ratio is greater than 0.90 and men whose ratio is greater than 0.80 are probably at increased risk for health problems.

The best solution is two-pronged: increase activity level through exercise, and analyze eating behaviors to make sure all necessary food groups are represented properly. Lower-calorie foods such as vegetables or fruit can be substituted for higher-calorie foods such as ice cream or hamburgers and fries. A related but even simpler way to assess whether or not we are gaining fat weight is to compare waist measurements over the past few years. If we are letting our belt out a notch, or cannot snap or zip up jeans, then we have probably added fat to our waistline and body weight.

**Figure 5.4**
The man on the left has a healthier body composition than the man on the right even though they are the same weight.

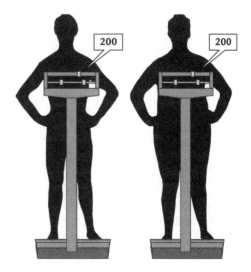

## Suggestions to Encourage Healthier Eating Behavior

Health psychologists apply the process of behavior modification to change habitual acts such as exercise and eating. In the previous chapter, behavior modification techniques and theories from health psychology were applied to improving exercise behavior. The logic used in the health belief model, the theories of planned behavior and reasoned action, and the transtheoretical model can also be applied to modification of eating behavior. There are hundreds of books on eating behavior, and most are called diet books. Outside of closed residential treatment programs, such as at weight-loss spas, it is difficult for most people to change food consumption habits on their own. Fortunately, there are useful recommendations based on scientific studies from the field of health psychology. Most people cannot suddenly change lifelong eating patterns, so clinical health psychologists and nutrition counselors suggest making gradual changes when altering eating behavior. They discovered a number of useful recommendations in addition to gradual change. Most recommend recording all eating behaviors.

### Record and Evaluate Eating Behavior

The first step in changing a behavior is to record and understand the behavior. Often what we actually do is different from what we think we are doing. There are a variety of record-keeping formats available. **Retrospective records** rely on memory of past food consumption. Retrospective food records usually focus on the last 3 days or the last 24 hours of eating. This provides a quick look at eating patterns (Snooks & Hall, 2002). Many nutritionists, clinical psychologists, and weight-loss groups begin sessions by using retrospective records, weighing and measuring their clients, and then making recommendations for changes before the next session. The initial meeting is followed by weekly sessions, with measurement and discussions of the past week's behavior and recommended changes for the coming week. This approach is also used by most commercial weight-loss groups.

**Prospective records** are kept at the time one actually consumes a food. Some studies indicate that recording everything we eat actually reduces food intake, because it is tiresome to write everything down and also because it is embarrassing to report eating an entire package of cookies. Prospective eating diaries are more likely to be accurate, because food is mea-

**retrospective records** Records of past eating, exercise, or other behaviors relying on the memory of intervention participants. For example, retrospective food records usually focus on the last 3 days or the last 24 hours of eating. This provides a quick assessment of eating patterns.

**prospective records** Records of eating, exercise, smoking, or other behaviors written at the time the behavior occurs. Analysis makes it possible to set up a plan for changes in eating, exercise, or smoking behavior.

sured before it is eaten. Keeping a record of everything eaten for a year or even for a month is burdensome. Eventually people get tired of keeping records, stop analyzing their behavior, and cancel appointments with clinicians or stop attending group sessions.

One solution to this attrition is to use a shorter time frame for recordkeeping. Many people are able to keep accurate records for 7 consecutive days, but most settle for 3-day records based on 2 week days and 1 day of a weekend. For simplicity, the recommendation is to record food and drink consumed at the time it takes place. The 3 days should be when routines are followed and not times of special events like birthdays. It is important to record both the food and the amount eaten. It is best to measure the amount of food or drink before it is consumed rather than estimate the amount.

Some restaurants, including fast food places, provide brochures with the food they serve, number of calories in each type, and the division of calories among fat, carbohydrate, and protein (McDonalds, 2008; Wendy's, 2008). The label on most food packages provides serving size, nutritional composition, and calories. Students can also learn more about serving size by studying the food guide pyramid on the Internet.

## Compare Food Records to the Ideal Diet

People can find the structure of an ideal diet for their age and activity level on the web site and then compare what they eat to what is recommended. For most people, the food guide pyramid's servings, or the more recent MyPyramid, with ounces and cups, make this step easy. In the United States, most people eat too many servings from the meat and fat group and not enough from the vegetable group. Comparing actual consumption to an ideal diet that takes individual factors into account enables one to determine what food groups should be added and which should be reduced.

## Record and Evaluate Moods and Thoughts Associated with Eating Behavior

Many clinical health psychologists and counselors recommend recording not only what we eat, but where, when, and why we chose that food and the amount. Some therapists also ask clients to record the extent of their hunger and their feelings or emotional states before and after eating to give individuals a better understanding of eating behavior.

## Choose One Serving of One Food Group to Add to the Daily Routine

Most experts recommend making one simple change at a time until the behavior becomes habitual. From a behavior modification viewpoint, it may be simpler to add food rather than take away something we like and avoid feeling deprived. When one food change becomes routine, then a second can be made. Adding servings from the vegetable group is a good place to start because adding one vegetable to the daily diet adds variety, vitamins, minerals, carbohydrates, and fiber. All improve health. Once the behavior change is established, a second vegetable serving could be added until the recommended three servings per day are habitual. Next people might choose another food group to change. Fruit is a good idea, because it is sweet.

## Other Possible Changes

After adding food groups to the daily diet, people can use behavior modification to eat less of the meat group, because most people in the United States consume too much meat. This can be accomplished by smaller or fewer servings. For example, if someone habitually eats a Big Mac every day, the person could opt one day a week for a different sandwich or have one meat patty rather than two. A McDonalds hamburger contains 260 calories with about 4 grams of fat, while a Big Mac contains 560 calories with about 11.5 grams of fat (McDonalds, 2008). Wendy's Junior hamburger has 280 calories, including 80 calories from fat, while a Classic Single with Everything has 420 calories, including 180 calories from fat (Wendy's, 2008). People can avoid feeling hungry by adding servings from the cereal, vegetable, fruit, or milk groups.

## Writing Prospective Eating Plans

Some health promotion specialists recommend following a specific plan and not worrying about past behavior. If we educate ourselves about nutrition and are highly motivated, we can use a standard, such as the new food guide pyramid, to devise daily menus. This approach provides an idea of what nutrients are missing from our diets. We can add servings of healthy food groups and eliminate servings of food groups being overeaten.

## Prepared Foods and Commercial Programs

Many commercial weight-loss programs sell meals precisely planned and prepared to control caloric and nutritional intake. Most require adding fresh fruit, vegetables, and milk to meals. These meals are more expensive than the do-it-yourself modifications suggested above, but are less expensive than eating out. One risk of this approach may be losing weight so quickly that muscle and bone are lost along with fat. Exercising aerobically and strength training help maintain lean body tissue.

## Prevention of Relapse

A basic problem with any behavior change is reverting or returning to old habits (Marlatt & Gordon, 1985). This occurs with modification of both eating and exercise behaviors. One particular complication is that food has social and psychological value in addition to its biological benefits. Many people use food as a way to deal with problems or unpleasant emotions. Records and analysis of eating patterns may reveal a tendency to eat unhealthily when experiencing fatigue or negative emotional states such as anxiety or depression. Many peo-

**Figure 5.5**

Planning and implementing self-management of exercise and eating behaviors will result in healthy fat weight loss.

*Source:* Insel, P., Turner, R. E., & Ross, D. (2007) *Nutrition* (3rd ed.). Sudbury, MA: Jones and Bartlett Publishers.

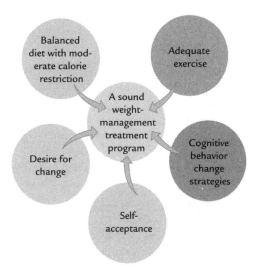

ple eat because they think they need more energy when they are simply tired and need sleep, rest, or relaxation. Others grab something sweet, such as a candy bar, when they see a bad test grade or after meeting with supervisors about poor work productivity. Another common tendency is to control caloric intake with friends or family, but overeat in private. In those cases solutions may be to eat more at meals and to have healthy snacks available for between-meal hunger when alone. (See **Figure 5.5** for components of a healthy weight management program.)

## Theoretical Approaches to Changing Eating Behavior

Eating behavior is a more complicated behavior to change than exercise, for several reasons. First, there are a variety of ways to improve health through nutritional choices. For example, some studies focus on increasing consumption of fruits and vegetables, others on lowering fat intake. Secondly, obesity reflects dieting and exercise behaviors rather than just one or the other. A third difficulty is that motivation to lose weight should include improvement in physical appearance. Changing only for health reasons may not succeed. A fourth research complication is people may not value health or appearance more than the pleasure of eating. Eating-behavior-modification theory includes analyses of records, attitudes, decision making, cognitions or thoughts, social actions, self-change processes, motivations, social interaction, social environments, health beliefs, modeling, and other causal pathways to predict behavior change for both weight loss and dietary modification (Ewart, 2004).

Based in systems theory, social action theory (SAT) examines behaviors as highly routine actions followed daily. Health-protective behaviors are more likely to become habitual if they are compatible with existing lifestyle routines. In designing interventions for behavioral change, SAT researchers focus on interpersonal interaction sequences, including the impact of cultural factors. The processes of taking action to protect health include motivations and expectations, self-efficacy, goals, problem solving, considering alternative behaviors, and other factors (Ewart, 2004, p. 265).

Students will recall the health belief model included the concepts of health beliefs (eating more healthily), perceptions of threats to health (heart disease, stroke, and cancer), susceptibility to those threats, and comparisons of the costs versus the benefits of making a change especially in terms of the time and effort required to change. The transtheoretical or stages of change model can be applied to eating behavior, whether it is to increase intake of fibrous foods or decrease fat intake (Rosen, 2000).

Some health psychologists combine theories to help people change nutritional practices. For example, Steptoe, Doherty, Kerry, Rink, and Hilton (2000) used the health belief model, self-efficacy, and stages of change theories to test an intervention to increase consumption of lower-fat foods among people with high cholesterol levels. In the study, self-efficacy and perceived benefits of low-fat eating predicted behavior change. Study participants who made larger reductions in fat intake reported greater self-efficacy and perceived benefits. Povey, Conner, Sparks, James, and Shepherd (2000) examined stages of change for three nutritional goals ranked from general to specific: eating a healthy diet, eating a low-fat diet, and eating five servings of fruits and vegetables each day. The more general the behavior, the more likely participants were to be in action or maintenance stages. In another study, the theory of planned behavior served as a predictor of dietary change and revealed the effects of attitudes and perceived behavioral control were larger than the effects of subjective norms (Bogart & Delahanty, 2004, pp. 218–219).

## An Experiment That Reduced Risks of Cardiovascular Disease

It is often difficult to make comprehensive changes in eating and exercise behaviors unless people are living in controlled situations. Ornish (2001), a physician, sequestered volunteer cardiac patients in a hotel and controlled their food intake and exercise behavior in a closely supervised experiment. His plant-based diet was designed to reduce risks of cardiovascular disease without resorting to surgery. Changes in eating habits, along with exercise and stress management, reversed existing heart disease, as demonstrated by improvements on arteriograms. Patients who switched from meat and eggs to legumes and grains lost more weight and felt better than those who made only moderate changes to their diets. For this reason, Ornish believes comprehensive dietary changes are easier to make than gradual minor modifications. His Advantage Ten program benefits most people, because it is low in cholesterol and fat, which are known risk factors for artery disease. His eating plan is also high in antioxidants believed to be protective against cancer. A somewhat unusual aspect of his diet is the avoidance of fats and oils of all kinds, including oils from avocados, olives, nuts, and seeds. Ornish also suggests avoiding alcohol and simple sugars. He contends that people who follow his diet will lose weight safely, improve their health, and still eat abundantly. The majority of calories in his plan come from complex carbohydrates including beans, legumes, grains, fruits, vegetables, and non-fat dairy products. (Legumes are plants

## Think About It!

### Another Challenge: Will You Do It?

| Behavior | Actions to Modify Behavior |
|---|---|
| Identify faulty eating behaviors and eliminate or ignore improper eating cues. | • Keep daily food records to identify problem foods.<br>• Use a shopping list and do not buy problem foods.<br>• Eat fruit or a meal before shopping for food.<br>• Discard problem foods.<br>• While at home, restrict eating to the kitchen or dining room.<br>• Do not eat while watching TV, reading, or talking on the phone.<br>• Avoid places with vending machines.<br>• Avoid fast-food restaurants that do not sell low-fat foods. |
| Reduce caloric intake. | • Serve meals on smaller plates.<br>• Prepare smaller amounts of foods to reduce the likelihood of "seconds."<br>• Avoid buffet-style or all-you-can-eat restaurants.<br>• Eat a low-fat high-fiber snack such as a piece of fruit or vegetable before a meal.<br>• Keep fruit and vegetables on hand to snack on when hungry.<br>• Ask for salad dressing "on the side" at restaurants.<br>• Prepare low-calorie lunches and snacks to take to work or school.<br>• Substitute fresh fruit or yogurt for rich desserts.<br>• Read nutrition labels to identify high-calorie foods.<br>• Learn to leave some food on your plate. |
| Stay focused on weight-loss goal. | • Set reasonable incremental goals, such as losing 5 pounds in 5 weeks.<br>• Place a picture of yourself on the refrigerator, pantry door, or bedroom mirror. |

*(continues)*

|                                      | • Measure your waistline once a week.<br>• Place exercise equipment and walking shoes where you can see them.<br>• Buy new pants that are one size smaller and hang them where you can see them.<br>• Ask your friends and family to support your efforts. Give them examples of how they can help. |
| Practice appropriate behaviors.      | • Find ways to move around while at work, school, or home. For example, take the stairs instead of the elevator.<br>• If you relapse, tell yourself that this is normal. Do not label yourself a failure. Ask yourself what you can learn from the experience so it is less likely to affect your eating again. Minor occasional indulgences will not affect your weight. Continue to focus on your weight loss goal.<br>• Set aside at least 30 minutes each day to engage in an enjoyable physical activity. Gradually increase the duration of the activity to 45 to 60 minutes daily. |
| Use nonfood rewards for behaviors    | • Praise yourself frequently for exercising or taking smaller servings of high-calorie appropriate foods.<br>• Buy a desired item such as a new CD, DVD, or an item of clothing.<br>• Take a walk or ride a bike through a park. |

Source: Alters, S., & Schiff, W. (2009). *Essential concepts for healthy living* (5th ed.). Sudbury, MA: Jones and Bartlett Publishers, LLC.

with edible seeds, and include peas, soybeans, and lentils.) Legumes provide protein with little fat, calories for energy, and fiber. In addition to legumes, Ornish emphasizes grains (eg, wheat, corn, and rice). Plant-based foods do not stay in the stomach as long as fat or protein, so hunger results sooner than it does following meals containing fat. People on plant-based diets may have to eat more frequently to avoid feeling hungry.

## Dieting and Eating Disorders

### Yo-Yo Dieting, Crash Diets, and Fad Diets

There are health risks to severe dietary restrictions even if obesity is reduced. Drastically limiting food intake is not a healthy behavior. It may lead to poorer health, because such diets often lack important nutrients. Generally, people make poor nutritional choices and eat too much when they are very hungry. There is evidence that weight cycling or **yo-yo dieting** (a pattern of losing weight, gaining weight, and losing again) may be more harmful than just being slightly overweight (Brownell & Rodin, 1996). When people regain weight they generally have a higher percentage of body fat than when they started unless they have consistently exercised.

Unfortunately, the word "diet" has come to mean restricted eating occurring for short periods of time to achieve loss of body weight. A typical psychosocial situation occurs when people plan to attend class reunions. They want to appear attractive to former classmates and believe the way to do this is by losing many pounds of body weight very quickly on drastic crash diets. Unfortunately health is damaged by this practice. First, when someone takes in too few calories for his or her level of activity, the person becomes hungry and irritable with family and friends. Second, when people lose weight by drastic means, they lose muscle and bone along with fat. It is very difficult for adults to replace lost muscle and bone. Third, when calories are restricted, the body assumes the person is starving and slows metabolism to compensate. This means the body uses fewer calories even at rest. Fourth, drastic behavior change is usually not permanent. As soon as the high school reunion is over, most people return to their former eating patterns. What they gain back is fat, not muscle or bone, so they end up with a higher percentage of body fat than when they started restricting food intake.

The majority of adults in the United States report they are dieting to lose weight. Following restrictive eating plans may lead to deficiencies in specific nutrients as well as hunger and fatigue. The truth is, the most healthful way to lose fat weight from the body is to exercise aerobically, as discussed in the previous chapter. The increased activity has the added benefit of maintaining or even increasing lean muscle mass and bone strength. When we use more calories through exercise, our body composition improves. If people decide they consume too many calories each day for good health, then they can reduce the number of calories while increasing exercise. The important point is to decrease caloric intake in such a way that health is protected.

Dieting to lose weight is an enormously popular topic. There are over 600 diet books currently on the market. The most widely sold usually present innovative approaches to eating that become fads. These books become wildly popular and then fall out of favor when another new diet book appears on the market. Most plans result in a loss of weight because people are eating fewer calories. There is nothing magic about any particular kind of food, and general nutrition recommendations should be followed to maintain health. Over the

---

**yo-yo dieting** An eating pattern of alternating limiting food intake (dieting), followed by regaining weight, followed by a repetition of dieting and weight loss. This pattern is believed to be detrimental to health, because one's total percentage of body fat tends to increase each time because muscle and bone are lost due to dieting.

past several years, popular fad diets included high-fat, no-carbohydrate; no sugar or white flour; eggs and grapefruit only; and fruit-only plans. Fruit-only diets are so high in fiber they often result in diarrhea and dehydration.

Early diets based on liquid proteins and on drugs ended in death. Many people trying to lose weight with prescription drugs experience heart damage as a side effect. Psychological side effects of fad diets include feeling irritable and deprived. These two negative emotional states jeopardize relationships with family, friends, and coworkers.

## Eating Disorders Are Serious Health Risks

In the United States and other industrialized countries, the majority of health problems with food involve consuming too many calories for a person's level of activity. Obesity, with its attendant problems, is the result. Other eating problems involve taking in too few calories for good health. This behavior pattern is not well understood, but probably happens for a variety of reasons. Motivation for extreme thinness includes an obsession with body size. A culture may put pressure on young women and men who literally starve themselves. The American Psychiatric Association considers **anorexia nervosa** and **bulimia nervosa** to be psychological disorders associated with excessive concern about body size (American Psychiatric Association, 2000). Anorexia nervosa is diagnosed based on a body weight of 15% below normal due to weight loss and refusal to gain weight. People with this disorder have a distorted body image. They believe themselves to be fat when in reality there is very little fat on their bodies. Their low body weight is due to low-calorie diets and/or excessive exercise or both.

The distinguishing characteristic for a diagnosis of bulimia nervosa is a pattern of eating followed by extreme dieting, purging by vomiting, or using laxatives. The American Dietetic Association (2003) notes that both patterns result in serious health problems, including weakened heart muscles, kidney failure, iron-deficiency anemia, and abnormal electrical activity in the brain. Victims of the disorder may experience amenorrhea, or cessation of menstruation, resulting from a very low percentage of body fat. Due to low levels of estrogen, premature osteoporosis may begin with its corresponding loss of bone mineral density. This may also happen to female athletes (Insel, Turner, & Ross, 2006, p. 274). Weakened bones make stress fractures more likely and bone loss is often irreversible. Vomiting may result in erosion of tooth enamel and rupture of the esophagus. In many cases, hospitalization is required to prevent death. Athletes, both male and female, sometimes diet extensively

---

**anorexia nervosa** A disordered eating pattern consisting of repeated dieting and/or overexercising, with the result that body weight falls below healthy levels.

**bulimia nervosa** A disordered or unhealthy pattern consisting of eating followed by vomiting or purging with laxatives.

or purge to improve performance. For example, some jockeys and boxers vomit to meet weight requirements for competition. Ballet dancers may be threatened with expulsion from the ballet company if their weight exceeds certain levels, even if most of their weight is bone and muscle rather than fat.

## Summary

Good nutritional practices are essential to health. Eating the correct kinds and amounts of food provides sufficient energy and enhances immune systems to aid in resistance to disease. Food makes it possible for us to grow and thrive when we are young. Once we reach maximum height, many of us continue to eat as though we are still growing. This practice may result in obesity, or excess body fat, putting us at risk for cardiovascular disease, diabetes, and some cancers. A fewer number of people, including teens and adults, risk ill health and death by starving their bodies.

This chapter examines biological, psychological, and sociocultural factors influencing eating behavior. Nutritional needs are greatest for infants, children, and teens. Important psychological factors influencing eating behavior are moods such as boredom, loneliness, or depression. Appetite is a desire to eat or drink. It can be affected by biology, but is mainly psychological and sociocultural in origin. Other sociocultural influences on eating behavior include childhood experiences, ethnicity, religion, advertising, and historical traditions.

A diet is a habitual eating pattern. Diets must be adequate and include carbohydrates, protein, fat, vitamins, minerals, and fiber. Diets should be balanced and include variety to maintain good health. The food guide pyramid and web site, www.MyPyramid.gov, are excellent sources of current information on good nutrition. Obesity, or too much fat on the body, is a serious health risk and often results from too little exercise and from eating too many calories. Our bodies are composed of bone, water, muscle, and fat. Fat is the only part of the body that puts our health at risk.

Using theories and models of behavior modification may help people develop healthier eating behaviors. Recording and analyzing eating behavior, followed by adding recommended food groups, is one path to healthier eating and body composition. Fad diets and crash diets are popular in the United States, but often result in loss of muscle and bone along with fat. The eating disorders of anorexia and bulimia nervosa can damage health and end in death. These disorders are best treated by trained clinicians.

## Review Questions

1. Identify the basic biological reasons for healthy eating practices.

2. Summarize psychological and sociocultural influences on eating behavior.

3. List five factors that most influence your own eating behaviors, giving an example of each.

4. Explain the three major sources of calories in our diet and give an idea of the percentage of each that should be included on a daily basis.

5. Describe one source of reliable information on nutritional practices, including food groups and serving sizes.

6. Discuss the major causes of obesity in this country.

7. Describe healthful solutions to this problem.

8. Explain how it is possible to be obese but malnourished.

9. Discuss ways to measure obesity. What is the problem with calculations such as BMI? What is the simplest method to determine if we are obese?

10. Of the steps for behavior modification discussed in this chapter, which do you think would be the most difficult and why?

11. After reading this chapter, decide if gradual single changes or drastic multiple changes are the better way to change eating patterns.

12. Explain the health problems involved with fad diets and crash diets.

13. Describe two eating disorders, how they are diagnosed, and the best approach to their treatment.

14. Challenge one idea from this chapter that goes against something else you have learned or experienced.

## Student Activity

Use what you know about health psychology and behavior modification to accomplish the following:

1. Keep a 3-day record of all the food and drink you consume.

2. Estimate the amount by serving size, or measure the food/drink prior to consumption.

3. Using the food guide pyramid, sort your foods and liquids into the five major food groups.

4. Compare your pyramid to the food guide pyramid in terms of number of servings from each group.

5. Make a list of what food groups you are missing and how many servings you should add from each group.

6. Choose one food group to change and add one serving of that food every day for a week.

7. At the end of the week analyze your success. Give yourself 100 points for each day you ate one serving from the chosen food group.

8. Look at your score. It can range from 0 to 700 points. Give yourself a grade based on your score.

9. Write an analysis of how successful you were at modifying your behavior. Include a list of what helped and hindered your efforts.

10. Identify the origins of what helped and hindered, stating whether the causes were biological, psychological, or sociocultural in origin.

11. Write a report containing all the information listed above.

# References

American Cancer Society. (2006). *Cancer prevention and early detection facts and figures 2006.* Retrieved January 10, 2008 from http://www.cancer.org

American Dietetic Association. (2003). Position of the American Dietetic Association: Nutrition intervention in the treatment of anorexia nervosa, bulimia nervosa, and eating disorders not otherwise specified (EDNOS). *Journal of the American Dietetic Association, 103,* 748–765.

American Heart Association. (2006). *Our 2006 diet and lifestyle recommendations.* Retrieved January 10, 2008 from http://www.americanheart.org

American Psychiatric Association. (2000). *Diagnostic and statistical manual of mental disorders,* (4th ed.), DSM-IV-TR. Washington, DC: American Psychiatric Association.

Bogart, L. M., & Delahanty, D. L. (2004). Psychosocial models. In R. G. Frank, A. Baum, & J. L. Wallander (Eds.), *Handbook of clinical health psychology* (Vol. 3, pp. 201–248). Washington, DC: American Psychological Association.

Brownell, K. D., & Rodin, J. (1996). The dieting maelstrom: Is it possible and advisable to lose weight? *American Psychologist, 41,* 781–791.

Centers for Disease Control and Prevention. (2003). *Physical activity and good nutrition: Essential elements to prevent chronic diseases and obesity.* Atlanta, GA: U.S. Department of Health and Human Services.

Centers for Disease Control and Prevention. (2006). *Obesity still a major problem.* Retrieved November 1, 2007 from http://www.cdc.gov/nchs/pressroom/06facts/obesity03_04.htm

Ewart, C. K. (2004). How integrative behavioral theory can improve health promotion and disease prevention. In R. G. Frank, A. Baum, & J. L. Wallander (Eds.), *Handbook of clinical health psychology* (Vol. 3, pp. 249–289). Washington, DC: American Psychological Association.

Insel, P., Turner, R. E., & Ross, D. (2006). *Discovering nutrition* (2nd Edition). Sudbury, MA: Jones and Bartlett.

Institute of Medicine, Food and Nutrition Board (2002). *Dietary reference intakes for energy, carbohydrate, fiber, fat, fatty acids, cholesterol, protein, and amino acids.* Washington, DC: National Academy Press.

Marlatt, G. A., & Gordon, J. R. (1985). *Relapse prevention: Maintenance strategies in the treatment of addictive behaviors.* New York: The Guilford Press.

McDonalds. (2008). Nutrition information chart: Find out about your favorites.

Mokdad, A. H., Ford, E. S., Bowman, B. A., & Dietz, W. H. (2003). Prevalence of obesity, diabetes, and obesity-related health risk factors. *Journal of the American Medical Association, 289,* 76–79.

Ornish, D. (2001). *Eat more, weigh less.* New York: HarperCollins.

Povey, R., Conner, M., Sparks, P., James, R., & Shepherd, R. (2000). Application of the theory of planned behavior to dietary behaviours: Roles of perceived control and self-efficacy. *British Journal of Health Psychology, 5,* 121–139.

Rosen, C. S. (2000). Is the sequencing of change processes by stage consistent across health problems? A meta-analysis. *Health Psychology, 19,* 593–604.

Snooks, M. K., & Hall, S. K. (2002). Body image and self-esteem in three ethnic groups. *Health Care for Women International, 23*(5), 460–466.

Steptoe, A., Doherty, S., Kerry, S., Rink, E., & Hilton, S. (2000). Sociodemographic and psychological predictors of changes in dietary fat consumption in adults with high blood cholesterol following counseling in primary care. *Health Psychology, 19,* 411–419.

U.S. Department of Agriculture. (2007). *Steps to a healthier we.* Retrieved January 11, 2008 from http://www.MyPyramid.gov

U.S. Department of Health and Human Services. (2003). *Healthy People 2010*. Retrieved January 9, 2008 from http://www.health.gov/healthypeople

U.S. Department of Health & Human Services, Office of Disease Prevention & Health Promotion. (2005). *A healthier we: Based on the dietary guidelines for Americans*. Washington, DC: Author.

Wendy's. (2008). Your guide to nutrition at Wendy's.

World Health Organization. (2006). *What is obesity, and why does it matter?* Retrieved January 11, 2008 from http://www.euro.who.int/obesity

# Chapter 6

# Applications of Health Psychology to Harmful Addictive Behaviors

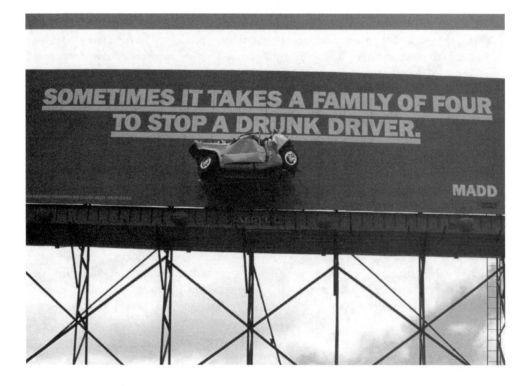

## Learning Objectives

After studying this chapter students will have the knowledge and skills to be able to:

1. Analyze and discuss the biological effects of psychoactive substances.

2. Describe current patterns of tobacco use in the United States.

3. Analyze and discuss the biological effects of using tobacco.

4. Analyze and discuss the psychosocial impact of tobacco use.

5. Discuss methods for ending tobacco use.

6. Describe current patterns of alcohol use in the United States.

7. Discuss the biological effects of alcohol use and abuse.

8. Explain the psychosocial effects of alcohol use and abuse.

9. Explain treatments for ending alcohol abuse.

## Introduction

Addictions to harmful substances have biological, psychological, and sociocultural origins. Addictive substances also cause biological, psychological, and sociocultural harm. We previously discussed how theories and models of behavior change can be used to improve exercise and eating behaviors. Similarly, behavior change models developed in health psychology can also be applied to reducing substance abuse.

**Psychoactive substances** are chemical compounds affecting the nervous system and especially the brain. One group of substances, **stimulants**, makes people feel more alert. These include caffeine, nicotine, cocaine, and amphetamines. Other substances have **depressant** effects and sedate the central nervous system (CNS). Many were first used by physicians to relieve pain and encourage sleep. Sedatives include alcohol, barbiturates, and opiates, such as morphine and heroin. A third class of substances, hallucinogens, produces illusions and hallucinations, sometimes including feelings of well-being. Psilocybin, peyote, and LSD are examples. Combinations of substances, or so-called **designer drugs**, are also available. Illegally making, distributing, selling, buying, and using psychogenic substances is a major social problem in the United States, associated with premature death, birth defects, criminal activity, and the spread of disease.

This chapter focuses on two psychoactive substances, **nicotine** and alcohol, because they are commonly used, leading causes of preventable death, and widely researched. Both are addictive, legal only after a certain age, widely available, heavily advertised, and harmful to health. As is true of exercise and eating, the use of tobacco and alcohol is a lifestyle choice or behavior. Nicotine and alcohol use have biological, psychological, and sociocultural origins and harmful outcomes. Using both tobacco and alcohol is amenable to behavior modification, and has long been of interest to health psychology researchers and clinicians.

**psychoactive substances** Chemical compounds affecting the nervous system, especially the brain. Such substances affect mood and perception. Examples are alcohol and nicotine.

**stimulant** A psychoactive substance that speeds up or quickens central nervous system processing, increasing physical and mental activity. Stimulants may provide temporary feelings of alertness and suppress appetite. Caffeine and amphetamines are examples.

**depressant** A psychoactive substance that slows down the central nervous system, decreasing physical and mental activity. Depressants may relieve anxiety and promote sleep, but also impair coordination, judgment, and respiration.

**designer drugs** Combinations of psychoactive substances that may result in unpredictable and dangerous effects such as euphoria, paranoia, and mood swings.

**nicotine** A chemical stimulant found in tobacco products

# A Biopsychosocial Analysis of Tobacco Use

Tobacco use is the leading preventable cause of premature death in the United States (Centers for Disease Control [CDC], 2002a). Smoking and other forms of tobacco use cause deaths from cancer, chronic obstructive lung disease, coronary heart disease, and stroke. More than 450,000 deaths per year, or 1,200 deaths each day, are attributed to tobacco-related disease (Henderson & Baum, 2002). More women die from lung cancer than breast cancer (American Cancer Society [ACS], 2006).

Tobacco sales are controversial. The health branches of government urge all Americans to stop using tobacco products, while tobacco growers continue to receive government subsidies. The tobacco industry lobby is very effective with Congress, and especially effective with representatives from tobacco-producing states. The industry spends millions each year marketing its products. It may surprise students to know that as early as the 1920s smoking was advertised to women as a way to stay thin (Lovell, 2002). The tobacco industry later linked cigarette smoking to women's liberation by offering cigarettes under trade names such as Virginia Slims, Eve, and Satin. Billboards with the theme "You've come a long way baby" were common. Marketing is currently limited by government regulations, but is now specifically aimed at poorly educated and low-income minority citizens in the United States and throughout the world. Tobacco production and distribution is a multi-billion-dollar business. The United States is the leading producer of tobacco in the world.

The use of tobacco is a learned behavior. Most smokers begin during adolescence and become addicted after a short period of time. About 23% of high school students report current cigarette smoking (CDC, 2006a). Some teens smoke to feel more adult, others use smoking to rebel against adult control, or to achieve an image of toughness. Once people start smoking they usually continue because they become addicted quickly; nicotine is extremely addictive. Many women worry about weight gain. They believe nicotine boosts their metabolism and suppresses their appetite, because tobacco may reduce the senses of smell and taste. Many people report using tobacco as a way to cope with stress at school, work, and home.

## Background of Tobacco Use in the United States

Tobacco was used in South America and the Caribbean at the time of Columbus. It was introduced in Europe by American colonists in the early 1600s. Originally tobacco leaves were used mainly in the form of snuff, for pipe smoking, and chewing. When the tuberculosis (TB) germ was discovered in the 1880s, health specialists believed it was spread through saliva in tobacco spit. Spittoons appeared in bars, offices, and court houses. It appeared healthier to smoke tobacco leaves. Today more tobacco is smoked in cigarettes than in any other form.

As early as the 1950s smoking was identified as a likely cause of lung cancer, and in 1964 the U. S. Surgeon General issued a 387-page report summarizing scientific evidence that tobacco use was harmful to health (U.S. Public Health Service, 1964; Fisher, Brownson, Heath, Luke, & Sumner, 2004). At that time over 4,000 cigarettes were smoked each year for every person 18 years or older living in the United States or about 524 billion cigarettes annually

(USPHS, 2000). About half of all men smoked. In spite of proven threats to health, tobacco is still highly popular and profitable. The percentage of smokers in the population has decreased to about 21%, but population size has increased, so 45 million people now smoke (CDC, 2006b).

## Biological Effects of Tobacco Use

There are both short- and long-term biological effects from using tobacco. Nicotine, the major substance found in tobacco, is a highly addictive stimulant. It elevates heart rate and blood pressure and restricts the flow of blood. All three effects increase the likelihood of clots, contributing to heart attacks and strokes. Smoking damages nearly every area of the body and is even a risk factor for bone loss or osteoporosis. Immediate biological effects include irritation of nasal passages, burning sensation in the eyes, and coughing due to irritation of the lungs. Carbon monoxide poisoning is a toxic side effect of tobacco use. Carbon monoxide takes up space on red blood cells ordinarily occupied by oxygen. This results in fatigue and shortness of breath.

Tobacco contains many cancer-causing substances, including more than 60 known carcinogens and thousands of other chemical agents, including tar, arsenic, and lead. Environmental tobacco smoke (ETS), or secondhand smoke, is a combination of smoke rising from burning ends of cigarettes and smoke exhaled by smokers. ETS increases risks of lung cancer and heart disease in nonsmokers and contributes to respiratory illnesses and ear infections in children (CDC, 2003). Smoking cigars is associated with cancers of the mouth, larynx, esophagus, lungs, and bladder and with chronic obstructive lung disease. At one time baseball players who routinely chewed tobacco reported being stimulated to better athletic performances by nicotine. Users of chewing tobacco and snuff are more likely to develop cancers of the tongue and gums.

## Types of Tobacco-Related Damage to Health

The **dose-response relationship** refers to the biology of tobacco in that the greater the number of cigarettes smoked, the greater the damage to the body. The extent of damage to health also reflects age at first exposure, puffing behaviors, and inhalation patterns. **Synergistic effects** refer to the fact that chemicals in tobacco interact with other substances, increasing damage to health; for example, air pollution is more damaging to smokers than

**dose-response relationship**  Refers to the body's reaction to the dosage or amount of substances put into it. For example, the greater the number of cigarettes smoked, the greater the damage to the body.

**synergistic effects**  Chemicals in tobacco interacting with other substances, increasing damage to the health of users.

to nonsmokers. When alcohol use and tobacco smoke are combined, there is greater damage to body cells, especially in the mouth and throat. Nicotine exacerbates cholesterol levels by reducing good cholesterol or high density lipoproteins (HDLs). Tobacco causes premature death in users (see **Figure 6.1**).

A recent study showed that among men, 41% of heavy smokers died in middle age compared to 14% who never smoked. Among middle-aged women, 26% of heavy smokers died, compared to 9% of those who never smoked (USDHHS, 2006). Cigarette smoking causes 87% of lung cancer deaths. Smoking is also responsible for most cancers of the larynx, oral cavity, esophagus, and bladder. Women smokers have three times the risk of breast cancer as nonsmokers. Smoking by women is also related to rates of cervical cancer, early menopause,

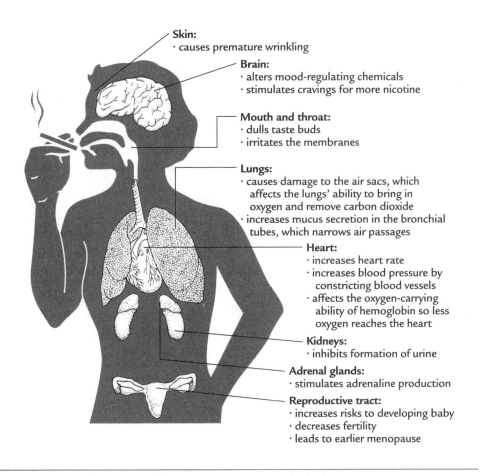

**Skin:**
· causes premature wrinkling

**Brain:**
· alters mood-regulating chemicals
· stimulates cravings for more nicotine

**Mouth and throat:**
· dulls taste buds
· irritates the membranes

**Lungs:**
· causes damage to the air sacs, which affects the lungs' ability to bring in oxygen and remove carbon dioxide
· increases mucus secretion in the bronchial tubes, which narrows air passages

**Heart:**
· increases heart rate
· increases blood pressure by constricting blood vessels
· affects the oxygen-carrying ability of hemoglobin so less oxygen reaches the heart

**Kidneys:**
· inhibits formation of urine

**Adrenal glands:**
· stimulates adrenaline production

**Reproductive tract:**
· increases risks to developing baby
· decreases fertility
· leads to earlier menopause

**Figure 6.1**   Smoking causes damage to many areas in the body.

*Source:* Alexander, L., LaRosa, J., Bader, H., & Garfield, S. (2008). *New Dimensions in Women's Health* (4th ed.). Sudbury, MA: Jones and Bartlett Publishers.

and urinary incontinence. Tobacco interacts with medications. It decreases the effects of acetaminophen, antidepressants, estrogen, insulin, and beta blockers. When combined with oral contraceptives, tobacco use increases risks of heart disease and blood clots.

## Psychosocial Effects of Tobacco Use

Psychologically and biologically, tobacco acts as a stimulant on the nervous system. This is why most users report feeling less tired and more alert after smoking. Nicotine reaches the brain within seconds of inhaling smoke. It is addictive, so the sense of relaxation reported after starting to smoke may be due to no longer feeling stress from the absence of nicotine in the blood stream.

Tobacco-related sickness and death affects families. About 8.6 million people in the United States have at least one serious illness caused by smoking. Chronic bronchitis is the most prevalent condition, followed by emphysema (CDC, 2003). In 2002, direct medical costs from smoking were estimated to be $75 billion a year, plus $82 billion in lost productivity (CDC, 2002b). Where smoking is allowed, spouses, children, and coworkers are exposed to damaging health effects from ETS. Secondhand smoke causes 3,000 deaths from lung cancer each year among nonsmokers (U. S. Environmental Protection Agency, 1992). Fire deaths and nicotine poisoning in children are additional causes of tobacco-related deaths. For example, toddlers fall victim to nicotine poisoning after eating leftover cigarette butts. Convulsions, vomiting, depressed breathing, and cardiac arrhythmias result from swallowing tobacco.

Tobacco use during pregnancy can retard fetal growth and increase the likelihood of miscarriages, stillborn births, and low birth weight in infants (CDC, 2004b). Smoking is a risk factor for ectopic pregnancies or the implantation of fertilized eggs outside the uterus. Smoking also interferes with the production of breast milk. Smoking reduces fertility and contributes to sudden infant death syndrome (SIDS). (See **Figure 6.2** for dangers associated with smoking during pregnancy.)

Tobacco use becomes an important part of users' lifestyles. When discussing smoking, users report feeling energized, which is a combination of biological and psychological effects. Smoking with coworkers and spouses adds social benefits, especially if the activity is forbidden inside workplaces or restaurants. Many smokers report that handling the cigarettes and other paraphernalia contributes to their pleasure. Smoking cessation or stopping tobacco use is difficult because nicotine is highly addictive and the behavioral habit has biological, psychological, and social reinforcements for smokers.

## Interventions for Smoking Cessation

Biopsychosocial factors influence the origins of tobacco use behaviors, the continuation of the behaviors, and returning to use after stopping (Ockene et al., 2000). Cigarette smoking receives considerable attention from researchers and clinicians. The Agency for Health Care Policy and Research (AHCPR) recommends smoking cessation interventions involving

**Figure 6.2**
Using tobacco, alcohol, or drugs before and during pregnancy puts the infant at risk. If you use these substances, stop before becoming pregnant.

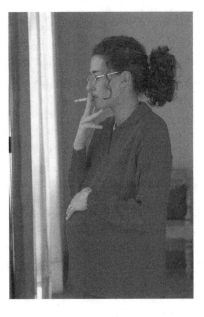

medical providers, social support from fellow smokers, training with print guides, the use of nicotine patches and gum, and counseling over the phone or Internet (USPHS, 2000). Unfortunately only 20% to 30% of smokers use formal treatment programs (Orleans & Alper, 2002).

The **American Stop Smoking Intervention Study (ASSIST)** was a government-funded demonstration project to help states develop strategies to reduce smoking, in particular, "to change social, cultural, economic, and environmental factors that promote smoking" (National Institutes of Health, National Cancer Institute [NCI], 2004, p. 1). Smoking prevalence declined among adults in ASSIST states compared to non-ASSIST states. Reduction in smoking prevalence was associated with policy changes, tobacco control infrastructure in state health departments, and strong interagency relationships.

Motivations to cease smoking vary from person to person. Some decide to quit smoking because their clothes and homes smell smoky, they have bad breath and stained teeth, or they begin to notice wrinkles around their mouths and eyes due to sucking and squinting. Others quit on doctor's orders, due to diagnoses of lung cancer, bladder cancer, or cardiovascular disease. Older women and heavy smokers (two or more packs a day) have greater difficulty

**American Stop Smoking Intervention Study (ASSIST)** A U.S. government–funded demonstration project to help states develop strategies to reduce smoking. One goal was to change social, cultural, economic, and environmental factors that promote smoking.

quitting than others. This may be due to greater physical and emotional dependence on nicotine. Many people lack social support for quitting, especially if spouses, coworkers, or friends smoke.

Tobacco users face choices when they want to quit. There are a variety of ways to stop smoking, but most people find it difficult to quit due to the addictive effects of nicotine. Quitting "cold turkey" refers to suddenly stopping tobacco use. Studies indicate that people are able to quit by themselves, but usually stop several times before successfully quitting. Cognitive-behavioral strategies from health psychology produce a 25% to 30% long-term quit rate, and nicotine replacement therapy nearly doubles the quit rate (Orleans, Ulmer, & Gruman, 2004).

Intervention research shows it helps to record each cigarette smoked, including the time of day, site or location, and one's emotional state before and after smoking. Some people use behavioral changes, such as smoking only half of each cigarette, or buying packs rather than cartons, making smoking more expensive. Nicotine reduces sensations of hunger, and many who want to quit report they become hungrier sooner than before quitting. The senses of smell and taste return, so food becomes more appetizing. For these reasons, some smokers gain weight. Exercise and careful eating patterns as suggested in the two previous chapters are solutions to weight gain. Blood gases change to healthier levels when people stop using tobacco, because there is more space for oxygen on the red blood cells. For some, this causes a period of discomfort that is relieved by aerobic exercise such as brisk walking. For some users, the effects of nicotine withdrawal include anxiety, headaches, fatigue, and irritability. Aerobic exercise helps reduce stress by producing endorphins in the blood stream.

Pharmacological aids include transdermal patches that gradually release nicotine into the bloodstream, chewing gum containing nicotine, or using smokeless inhalers that provide nicotine. Patches and gum are available over the counter (OTC) and may be helpful for gradual withdrawal. If one smokes when using these products, there is a risk of nicotine poisoning. Sprays, inhalers, and antidepressants are available by prescription.

Smoking cessation programs recommend a number of strategies that may be helpful. Behavior modification theories and models discussed in earlier chapters apply to cessation of tobacco use. Some people find it easier to taper cigarette use, by smoking fewer cigarettes each day to gradually reduce the need for nicotine. Others quit cold turkey. In both cases, setting a quit date is helpful. Commercial programs exist in a variety of forms including self-help packets and small group sessions. Smoking cessation programs are available as tapes, videos, workbooks, on the Internet, and through hotlines from the American Cancer Society and the American Lung Association (2008). Health professionals at hospitals and in private practice offer smoking cessation programs, including support groups. Some programs include connection to a buddy to call when participants are tempted to smoke or chew. Relaxation techniques, stress management training, and practical advice about keeping track of tobacco use and weight gain are part of many interventions. Health insurance may pay all or part of the costs of smoking cessation programs.

Most programs emphasize the benefits of changing the behavior, including immediate health benefits on the cardiovascular and respiratory systems. Quitting decreases the risk of cancer, cardiovascular disease, and chronic lung disease. The earlier a person quits, the better it is for health, due to the dose-response relationship discussed earlier. Quitting before age 50 cuts in half the risk of dying over the next 15 years (ACS, 2004). Orleans (2000) suggests more research is needed to further reduce tobacco use.

## Smoking Prevention for Teens and Young Adults

Smoking prevention is important to health in the United States because thousands of teenagers begin smoking during high school (CDC, 2006a). Current prevention efforts include educational programs connected to health classes and counseling centers in schools. Mass media campaigns can be funded at state levels when states successfully sue tobacco companies. Cutting funding for anti-tobacco youth campaigns increases susceptibility of young people to tobacco use (CDC, 2006c). Excise tax increases by governments make cigarettes more expensive and less available to teenagers. Beneficial school-based prevention interventions, including resistance skills training, parent involvement, and community organization, are showing promise (Dishion, Kavanaugh, & Kiesner, 2003).

A random-digit-dialed computer-assisted telephone interview of young smokers in New York State indicated that talking with a nurse, doctor, or dentist was used by at least 20% of the age group. Unassisted strategies are also successful. Data from the National Youth Smoking Cessation Survey indicated that smokers aged 16–24 were more likely to make unassisted quit attempts. Frequently used strategies include limiting the number of cigarettes smoked and not buying more, exercise, quitting with a friend, telling others they no longer smoke, and switching to cigarettes with less nicotine (Giovino, Barker, & Tworek, 2004).

# A Biopsychosocial Analysis of Alcohol Use and Abuse

Excessive alcohol use is the third leading preventable cause of death in the United States (CDC, 2004a). Excessive alcohol use includes **heavy drinking** and **binge drinking**. Heavy drinking is defined as more than two drinks per day for men and more than one drink per day for women. (See **Figure 6.3** for what is considered moderate drinking.)

**heavy drinking** Consuming more than two drinks per day for men and more than one drink per day for women.

**binge drinking** Consuming more than four drinks on one occasion for men and more than three drinks on one occasion for women.

**Figure 6.3**

Many people plan to drink moderately, but due to the effects of alcohol on their brain they lose count.

*Source:* USDA Center for Nutrition Policy and Promotion and Insel, P., Turner, R. E., & Ross, D. (2007). *Nutrition* (3rd ed.). Sudbury, MA: Jones and Bartlett Publishers.

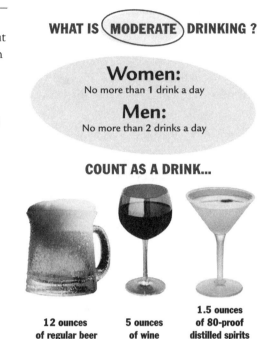

Binge drinking refers to more than four drinks on one occasion for men and more than three drinks on a single occasion for women. About 5% of the total population reports drinking heavily and 15% say they binge drink (CDC, 2006d). Fifty-two percent of binge drinkers are 18 to 20 years of age (Serdula, Brewer, Gillespie, Denny, & Mokdad, 2004). Both heavy drinking and binge drinking lead to many health risks and injuries. **Alcohol abuse** accounts for about 75,766 deaths each year (CDC, 2004a). The deaths include liver disease and unintentional injuries.

In health psychology, discussions of alcohol abuse are often linked to other psychoactive substances under the heading "substance abuse disorders." This discussion focuses only on alcohol because it is the most commonly abused of all substances, it is legal after a certain age in the United States so it can be monitored and studied, and because public interventions for alcohol abuse existed as early as the 1930s. It is difficult to know precisely the extent of alcohol use in this country, because it is measured by taxes collected on legal sales. National surveys indicate that over half of all adults drank alcohol in the past 30 days (CDC, 2006d).

Alcohol abuse generates many health and safety problems, resulting in extensive biological, psychological, and sociocultural harm in the lives of individuals and those interacting

**alcohol abuse** Excessive and habitual consumption of alcohol.

with them. Millions of Americans have problems with alcohol. This addiction costs billions of dollars each year, including cost of medical care for alcohol-associated illness and injury. On the average, about 30 years of life are lost per alcohol-attributable death (Mokdad, Marks, Stroup, & Gerberding, 2004). Motor vehicle-related injury is the leading cause of death in the United States for young people (1 to 34 years) and at least 40% of traffic deaths are alcohol related (Quinlan et al., 2005). (See **Figure 6.4** for some of the dangers of using alcohol and other drugs.)

## Biological Effects of Alcohol Use

Alcohol is a volatile organic compound named ethanol or ethyl alcohol. One drink is defined as the consumption of 10 to 16 grams of ethyl alcohol in beer, wine, or liquor. Each drink contains 0.5 ounces or 12 grams of alcohol. Alcohol abuse, the name given to excessive and habitual consumption of alcohol, poses both chronic and acute threats to health. Acute threats include deaths from falls, firearms, and alcohol poisoning. Chronic diseases include liver destruction, cancers, and strokes. Prolonged use of alcohol damages heart muscles, increases the likelihood of diabetes, and is carcinogenic, particularly in cells of the mouth, esophagus, rectum, and lungs. Alcohol contributes to osteoporosis due to liver damage causing excessive loss of calcium and vitamin D from the body. Health care costs are 100% to 300% higher for alcohol abusers than others, but treatment costs would offset medical costs (Orleans, Ulmer, & Gruman, 2004).

Alcohol acts first on the nervous system, affecting physical and mental activity, including speech, vision, and voluntary muscle movement. About 20% of alcohol is rapidly absorbed through the stomach wall, especially if the stomach is empty. The tiny alcohol molecule quickly moves into the bloodstream and reaches the brain in seconds. It produces feelings of well-being or euphoria by affecting judgment and reasoning centers. After only one drink, many people are convinced they are smarter, more charming, and more attractive than ever before. Some people say they drink before going to a party to feel more confident.

---

**Figure 6.4**
Violence and unintentional injuries and death are associated with the use of alcohol and other psychoactive substances.

*Source:* National Clearinghouse for Alcohol and Drug Information. (1995). Making the Link [Fact Sheets]. Rockville, MD: Author; and McKenzie, J., Pinger, R., & Kotecki, J. (2008). *An Introduction to Community Health* (6th ed.). Sudbury, MA: Jones and Bartlett Publishers.

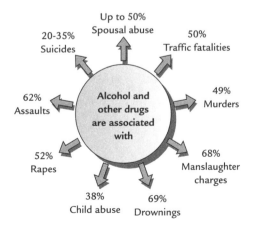

Alcohol and other drugs are associated with

- Up to 50% Spousal abuse
- 20-35% Suicides
- 50% Traffic fatalities
- 62% Assaults
- 49% Murders
- 52% Rapes
- 68% Manslaughter charges
- 38% Child abuse
- 69% Drownings

Several specific terms are applied in discussions and analyses of alcohol use. **Addiction** is the compulsive use of substances that can be harmful to health due to negative physical, social, or cultural effects. **Physical dependence** occurs when a decline in the usual level of a substance in the bloodstream results in unpleasant psychological and physical symptoms. Some experts draw a line between addiction and dependence by suggesting that addiction refers to an overwhelming desire to use a substance, while dependence is a condition of habitual craving.

**Tolerance** is a biologically based response to substance use and refers to the fact that consistent use of many substances requires larger and larger amounts to attain the same psychogenic effects. Similar to nicotine users, alcohol abusers become uncomfortable and anxious when concentration of the substance in their bloodstream diminishes. Tolerance is due to the ability of the body to achieve and maintain homeostasis, or a stable state, in heart rate, respiration, temperature, and electrolyte balance. Heavy drinkers may need to increase the amount they consume to feel the same effects. Their bodies have gradually adjusted to the level of alcohol in their bloodstream and more of the substance is needed to achieve the desired effect. Abusers can tolerate much higher percentages of alcohol in their bloodstream than occasional drinkers. Alcohol, barbiturates, and stimulants such as tobacco are known for the likelihood of developing tolerance, and users often experience withdrawal symptoms when use is discontinued.

**Withdrawal effects** are unpleasant physical and psychological symptoms that occur when the substance of abuse is absent. Depending on the extent of abuse, the withdrawal process from alcohol may be life threatening. The effects of withdrawal vary but usually include nausea and vomiting, restlessness, sleeplessness, and depression. **Delirium tremens (DTs)** are severe physical and mental symptoms that occur when heavy drinkers stop using alcohol. Symptoms include sweating, shaking, anxiety, and frightening hallucinations. Delirium tremens is life threatening, and withdrawal should occur only under medical supervision.

Deaths due to acute alcohol poisoning occur when people quickly drink large amounts of alcohol over a short period of time. This is most common in the United States during

**addiction** Physical and psychological dependence on a behavior. The term is generally applied to compulsive use of substances harmful to health, such as alcohol.

**physical dependence** When a decline in the usual level of a substance in the bloodstream results in unpleasant psychological and physical symptoms.

**tolerance** A biologically based response to a substance. Consistent use of many substances requires larger amounts to attain the same psychogenic effects.

**withdrawal effects** Unpleasant physical and psychological symptoms due to decreases in the usual level of substances in the body of addicted persons.

**delirium tremens (DTs)** Severe physical and mental disorders occurring when alcohol is withdrawn from heavy users.

high school and college initiations and drinking contests. The practice results in death because respiration is suppressed and breathing ceases. In most social drinking situations, people drink slowly and ordinarily go to sleep before they drink enough to cause respiratory collapse.

The **alcohol dehydrogenase enzyme (ADE)** metabolizes alcohol in the body. It is present to varying degrees depending on gender and ethnicity. For example, women have about a half to a fourth of the amount of the enzyme as men. This means women absorb alcohol into their bloodstream more quickly than men. Alcohol absorption by the body is also affected by genetic background, ethnicity, age, health, weight, family history, previous experience with alcohol, and the amount of food in the stomach. In general, a person weighing 140 pounds can metabolize one drink in about 2.2 hours. Coffee has no effect on the length of time it takes to become sober after drinking. Becoming sober requires time for the body to process the toxin.

**Blood alcohol concentration (BAC)** refers to the concentration of alcohol in the bloodstream. Legal parameters determine whether someone is driving under the influence (DUI) or driving while intoxicated (DWI). Having a BAC of 0.10 means there are 10 parts of alcohol to 10,000 blood components. Higher BAC levels significantly affect the ability to drive by influencing vision, perception, reaction time, judgment, and the ability to assess and control speed. This is why public safety experts warn against drinking and driving.

From a nutritional standpoint, alcohol has short- and long-term effects. It is rapidly absorbed and moves ahead of other nutrients in the gastrointestinal (GI) tract. The body treats alcohol as a poison and works quickly to clear the bloodstream of the toxin. Liver cells remove alcohol from the blood, but fatty acids begin to accumulate. Eventually liver cells die, forming scar tissue. **Fibrosis** is the early stage of liver damage due to alcohol; cirrhosis, the late stage, makes the regeneration of liver cells impossible. Alcohol inflames stomach tissue so the GI tract is unable to absorb vitamins, leading to vitamin deficiencies. Alcohol abuse contributes to gout and alters protein metabolism, damaging the immune system. From a caloric standpoint, alcohol is an empty calorie, because it contains 7 calories per gram, but has no other nutritional value. Those habituated to alcohol are less likely to maintain adequate nutritional intake because alcohol sedates the sense of hunger. It also acts as a diuretic, dehydrating the body of necessary water and causing mineral loss through rapid excretion of urine. Many abusers sense thirst but misread the body signal and order another

---

**alcohol dehydrogenase enzyme (ADE)**  An enzyme found in the stomach that assists in metabolizing alcohol molecules. In general, women appear to have less of the enzyme than men.

**blood alcohol concentration (BAC)**  The concentration of alcohol in the bloodstream.

**fibrosis**  The early stage of liver damage due to alcohol; cirrhosis, the later stage, makes the regeneration of liver cells impossible.

drink rather than water. Eating salty snacks exacerbates the problem of dehydration and thirst.

Research on biological benefits of **moderate drinking** is interesting and controversial. Clearly, excessive amounts of alcohol are detrimental to cardiac health, but some studies suggest benefits from moderate alcohol intake in reducing cardiovascular disease (Klatsky, Armstrong, & Friedman, 1990, 1992; Marmot & Brunner, 1991). Moderate drinking is two or fewer drinks per day for men and one or fewer drinks per day for women. One followup study confirmed a J-shaped relationship between mortality and alcohol, meaning there was reduced risk for moderate drinkers, but an increased risk for people having more than 3 drinks per day (Klatsky & Udalstova, 2007). Other studies found neither damaging nor protective effects of moderate consumption (Shaper & Wannamethee, 2000). The subject remains controversial, and few, if any, health professionals would recommend using alcohol to benefit cardiovascular health. A recent article in the *American Journal of Preventive Medicine* concluded, "These findings suggest that some or all of the apparent protective effect of moderate alcohol consumption on CVD may be due to residual or unmeasured confounding factors" (Naimi et al., 2005). The authors further suggest that given the limitations, all nonrandomized studies about the health effects of moderate drinking should be interpreted with caution. Regardless of possible cardiovascular benefits for moderate drinking, other health risks remain, including motor vehicle crashes, interactions with medications, birth defects, cancer, and some forms of stroke.

## Psychosocial Effects of Alcohol Use and Abuse

Alcoholism or alcohol-dependent behavior is more common than any other addiction in this culture, even though it is often detrimental to health and a threat to public safety. Residual problems occur in both health care settings and courts of law. Abuse puts at risk the health and safety of family members, coworkers, friends, and abusers' educational and occupational goals. For example, about 60% of job loss is due to alcoholism (CDC, 2006d).

Alcohol use is learned the same way smoking behavior is learned, from family and friends, usually during adolescence. Alcohol is widely available, relatively inexpensive in most forms, and highly advertised in all media. Alcohol is a common part of television shows and movies. Drinking and drunk characters are usually viewed as happy and amusing. The impact of these social and cultural influences is powerful, as evidenced by the fact that there is less of a problem with alcohol abuse in countries where alcohol is forbidden for religious reasons.

**moderate drinking** Men drinking two or fewer drinks each day, and women having one drink or less each day.

Deaths of loved ones and friends from any cause are psychologically and socially disruptive. Alcohol-attributable deaths and injuries include liver disease and vehicle accidents (Midanik et al., 2004). Both take a considerable toll on families and friends of the victims. Other alcohol-related deaths are due to psychosis, esophageal and pancreatic cancers, ischemic heart disease, prostate and breast cancers, and stroke. Unintentional causes of death are drowning, falls, fires, and freezing. Intentional causes of alcohol-related death are homicides, suicides, and poisoning. Alcohol reduces inhibitions and self-discipline, so criminal activity is often associated with its use. All deaths, accidents, and crimes create economic and legal problems for survivors, along with psychosocial difficulties.

Alcohol use is especially damaging during pregnancy. It may harm a developing fetus before a woman knows she is pregnant and result in **fetal alcohol spectrum disorders (FASDs)** (CDC, 2001). There is no known safe amount for alcohol consumption during pregnancy. In surveys of women who might become pregnant (ages 18 to 44), more than half reported alcohol use and 12% reported binge drinking (CDC, 2004c). In an earlier survey of pregnant women, about 21% reported drinking alcohol after they learned of their pregnancies (CDC, 1995).

FASDs are a leading preventable cause of mental retardation and birth defects in children. FASDs are permanent conditions characterized by abnormal facial features, growth deficiencies, and CNS problems affecting learning, memory, communication, vision, and hearing. Alcohol-use risks also include placental attachment disorder, miscarriage, and preterm delivery. Five or more drinks each week decreases fertility in women.

Alcohol use by teens contributes to unintended pregnancy, sexually transmitted disease, rape, interference with brain growth, fighting, and auto accidents. States prohibit the purchase of alcohol by youth under the age of 21. This change was recommended by health experts based on data showing the human brain continues to grow throughout the teen years and growth may be limited due to exposure to alcohol. About 52% of 18- to 20-year-olds binge drink (Serdula et al., 2004) and 26% of high school students report heavy drinking (CDC, 2006d). Many researchers contend that maturational processes and societal contexts including family and peers contribute to alcohol problems among adolescents (Boyd, Howard, & Zucker, 1995).

Family disruption, trauma, and homelessness are associated with alcohol abuse. People under the influence of alcohol are more likely to drown, kill their children, and commit suicide (Midanik et al., 2004). Domestic or family violence including the abuse of spouses

**fetal alcohol spectrum disorders (FASDs)** The leading preventable cause of mental retardation and birth defects in children whose mothers drank alcohol during their pregnancy.

## Think About It!

### Is This Your Own Experience?

Having three or more of the following symptoms over a year usually indicates alcohol dependence syndrome:

- A strong desire or compulsion to drink
- Difficulty in controlling the amount of alcohol consumed and when it is consumed
- Withdrawal symptoms when alcohol is not consumed, or consuming alcohol to avoid withdrawal symptoms
- Evidence of tolerance, that is, increased amounts of alcohol are needed to achieve the effects originally produced by lower amounts
- Progressive neglect of other interests because of drinking, while spending an increased amount of time obtaining and drinking alcohol, and recovering from its effects
- Continued use of alcohol despite clear evidence of its physical and/or psychological effects on the user

*Source:* Alters, S., & Schiff, W. (2009). *Essential concepts for healthy living* (5th ed.). Sudbury, MA: Jones and Bartlett Publishers.

and children are often connected to alcohol use (Greenfield, 1998). Professional athletes experience pressure to perform and may use substances to allay that pressure (**Figure 6.5**).

## Interventions for Alcohol Abuse

Causes of alcohol abuse are not well understood and most researchers take a multivariable approach, citing biological, psychological, and sociocultural contributing factors (Maisto, 2004). Many view substance abuse as a mental disorder, and some studies show genetic influences. Some researchers suggest that about 50% of the risks for addiction in humans are genetic (Wenzel & Glanz, 2004, p. 117). Another perception is that alcohol abuse is a disease to be treated medically. In the early part of the 20th century, the American Medical Association applied the word alcoholism to alcohol abuse, suggesting it is a disease. One effect of this perspective was that people with alcohol problems were viewed as sick, rather than as immoral or sinful. It was assumed alcoholics would be more likely to seek help if alcohol abuse was defined as a disease rather than as a character flaw, thus removing the stigma and encouraging abusers to seek treatment.

Due to continuing censure by society, women still hide alcohol addiction, although about one third of alcoholics in this country are women. Women tend to conceal alcohol abuse because they are still more widely condemned than men when drunk and are under-

**Figure 6.5**
All-Star third baseman Ken Caminiti fought drug and alcohol problems for much of his adult life. The substances he took are thought to have weakened his heart. He died of a heart attack at age 41.

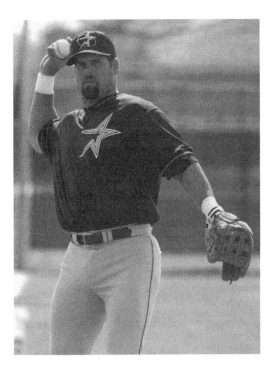

represented in clinical samples of substance abusers (Schober & Annis, 1996). Women are uniquely at risk of not seeking treatment for abuse because of issues associated with child-rearing obligations, lack of insurance and transportation, spousal abuse, and poverty (Milby, Schumacher, & Tucker, 2004).

Behavior modification interventions and individual-level approaches from health psychology include counseling, cognitive behavioral treatment, self-help programs, and pharmacologic treatments, or combinations of all of the above (Orleans, Ulmer, & Gruman, 2004). One general view in health psychology is that alcohol abuse can be improved by mental health counseling and is amenable to change through various interventions or behavior modification approaches (Moos, Finney, & Conkite, 1990). There are varieties of interventions for alcohol-related problems, but no single effective treatment has been identified for all patients (Milby, Schumacher, & Tucker, 2004, p. 55). Interventions range from public health approaches to clinical treatments for mental health disorders (Humphreys & Tucker, 2002).

One assumption is that clinical treatment can be complemented by lower-threshold interventions offered within and outside traditional health care systems. Counseling for improved self-control, social skills, marital and family relations, identification of motivations, stress management, aversion therapy, medications, and behavioral contracts may be effective for many (Milby, Schumacher, & Tucker, 2004, pp. 55–59). Guided self-change interventions designed by Sobell and Sobell (1998) and motivational interviewing techniques are used for some problem drinkers. More succinct interventions include the goal of reduction in drinking and improvements in health, rather than total abstinence from alcohol (Burke, Arkowitz, & Dunn, 2002).

**Alcoholics Anonymous (AA)** and its 12-step program began in the United States in 1935. It is a worldwide self-help group providing social support for avoiding alcohol and staying sober. AA utilizes the medical disease model of substance abuse. It is difficult to study the effectiveness of AA, because names are not used and data are confidential. Two of the early steps in this voluntary treatment program are acknowledging powerlessness over alcohol, and appealing to a higher power for help. Later steps include making amends for past misbehaviors that occurred while under the influence of alcohol. Participants speak openly at AA meetings about drinking and sobriety. Two other self-help organizations include Women for Sobriety and Self-Management and Recovery Training (SMART).

Medical treatment interventions include psychotherapy and chemical approaches. The first step is detoxification in a medical setting, because withdrawal can range from mild to severe and may be life threatening. Aversive therapy includes pairing drinking behaviors with unpleasant experiences. For example, substances such as naltrexone and disulfiram make patients ill if they consume any alcohol. The difficulty is that patients are not consistent about taking an aversive drug. Talking with a therapist, participating in support groups, learning stress management techniques, and avoiding cues that trigger alcohol use are all part of treatment systems that include both pharmacological and psychosocial interventions. Many can be implemented on an outpatient basis or in residential settings. Counseling usually includes family members.

Relapse refers to reversion to a previous behavior and is a common occurrence in substance abuse. Relapse prevention refers to strategies designed to prevent this from happening. Marlatt and Gordon (1985) described multiple approaches to relapse prevention. They view abuse as an overlearned habit pattern rather than as a disease, and believe patterns can be changed through self-management techniques, including identifying high-risk situations, coping, self-efficacy, developing new attitudes, finding nondestructive ways to obtain gratification, and relying on coping techniques other than alcohol use. Relapse prevention may include detoxification followed by social-learning interventions (McCrady, Dean, Dubreuil, & Swanson, 1985). Outside of a hospital or treatment clinic, patients will be exposed to ordinary social environments such as family, work, and leisure, including situations that may trigger relapses. Relapse prevention programs help patients acknowledge their problem, identify antecedents to drinking, and become skilled at maintaining abstinence in high-risk situations. Drink refusal and assertiveness training are included. Spouses and other family members, employers, and self-help groups, including AA, are encouraged for relapse preven-

**Alcoholics Anonymous (AA)**  A worldwide self-help group providing social support for avoiding alcohol and staying sober.

tion. In the United Kingdom, researchers believe that problem drinkers can successfully practice low-risk drinking and that problem drinking is a learned behavioral disorder that can be biological, psychological, or social in nature (Heather & Robertson, 1997). British clinicians apply social learning theory to treat problem drinking. In the United States there is some support for moderation management treatments, and some individuals have even stopped abusing alcohol on their own (Maisto, 2004). (See **Figure 6.6.**)

## Summary

Nicotine and alcohol are commonly used psychoactive substances. Their use may result in dependencies or addictions, including compulsive and habitual use. In research, substance abuse is explained by many factors, including genetic background, biological tendencies, family practices, advertising, general customs, and the influence of subcultures. For people who are addicted, when alcohol or nicotine levels drop in the bloodstream, unpleasant physical and psychological side effects often occur. The frequent use of psychoactive substances often results in tolerance, meaning a larger amount of the substance is required to achieve the desired effects. Millions try to stop abusing alcohol and using tobacco and many experience relapse in their efforts.

   The use of tobacco, especially the practice of smoking cigarettes, is the leading preventable cause of death in the United States. Lung cancer, heart disease, and strokes result from tobacco use. In 1964, the U.S. Surgeon General issued a scientific report demonstrating the dangers of tobacco. Nicotine in tobacco is a stimulant to the central nervous system. Smoke in the environment is a risk for cancer, heart disease, and respiratory illness among nonsmokers. The greater the number of cigarettes smoked, the greater the damage to the body. Tobacco use is especially dangerous during pregnancy, both for the fetus and the mother. After birth, smoking is a risk factor for sudden infant death syndrome and ear infections in

**Figure 6.6**
Parental behavior influences children's decisions to use alcohol, tobacco, and other substances.

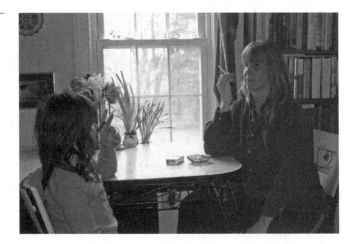

children. Many people successfully stop smoking, but quitting may require several attempts. Smoking cessation programs are available from national health agencies such as the American Cancer Society and from hospitals, private therapists, and commercial organizations.

Alcohol is the psychoactive substance most likely to be used in the United States and is a leading risk for illness, injury, and death. Alcohol has a depressant effect on the nervous system affecting judgment and response time. Drinking alcohol during pregnancy contributes to birth defects. Abrupt withdrawal from alcohol may cause severe symptoms and even death. Alcohol affects nutritional health and causes brain, liver, and pancreatic damage. Alcohol abuse is detrimental from the biological, psychological, and social viewpoints used in health psychology. Treatment for alcohol addiction is available in self-help organizations such as Alcoholics Anonymous, in medical clinics, and with therapists.

## Review Questions

1. Define substance abuse and list probable causes of the behavior.

2. Explain the concepts of tolerance, withdrawal, and relapse as they relate to substance use and abuse.

3. Describe current patterns of tobacco use in the United States.

4. Discuss the biological and psychosocial effects of using tobacco.

5. Explain interventions available for decreasing or ending tobacco use.

6. Describe current patterns of alcohol use in the United States.

7. Discuss the biological and psychosocial effects of alcohol use and abuse.

8. Explain interventions for reducing alcohol use and abuse.

## Student Activity

1. Interview someone who currently uses alcohol or tobacco products, but be certain to conceal the identity of your respondent in your verbal discussions and written reports. Discover the origins of their use, including childhood and school-related experiences. Ask about biological effects and why they use the substance. Discuss any impact the use has on family members, friends, and coworkers. Ask about the impact of the use on their health. Have them describe any attempts to quit using the substance. Why do they believe quitting is such a difficult process? Ask what they would recommend to a friend or family member who is considering using the substance.

   If you cannot find a respondent who currently uses a substance, try to find someone who was once a user of tobacco or alcohol and ask similar questions.

2. Students should sort their interviews into two groups, tobacco or alcohol use. Based on the information given in this textbook and by the professor during class, codify the answers given on the interviews and report to the class the most common findings.

# References

American Cancer Society. (2006). *Cancer facts and figures*. Retrieved January 18, 2008 from http://AmericanCancer.org

American Cancer Society. (2008). *Quit Smoking 101*. Retrieved January 18, 2008 from http://AmericanCancer.org

American Lung Association. (2008). *Quit Smoking*. Retrieved January 18, 2008 from http://www.lung.usa.org

Boyd, G. M., Howard, J., & Zucker, A. (Eds.). (1995). *Alcohol problems among adolescents: Current directions in prevention research*. Hillsdale, NJ: Lawrence Erlbaum Associates.

Burke, B. L., Arkowitz, H., & Dunn, C. (2002). The efficacy of motivational interviewing and its adaptations: What we know so far. In W. R. Miller and S. Rollnick (Eds.), *Motivational interviewing: Preparing people for change* (2nd ed., pp. 217–250). New York: Guilford.

Centers for Disease Control. (1995). Sociodemographic and behavioral characteristics associated with alcohol consumption during pregnancy—United States, 1988. *Morbidity & Mortality Weekly Reports, 44*(13), 261–264.

Centers for Disease Control. (2001). *Fetal alcohol spectrum disorders*. Retrieved April 15, 2007 from http://www.cdc.gov.ncbdd/fas

Centers for Disease Control. (2002a). Targeting tobacco use: The nation's leading cause of death 2004. *Morbidity & Mortality Weekly Reports, 51*, 409–412.

Centers for Disease Control. (2002b). Annual smoking-attributable mortality, years of potential life lost, and economic costs—United States, 1995–1999. *Morbidity & Mortality Weekly Reports, 51*, 300–303.

Centers for Disease Control. (2003). Cigarette smoking-attributable morbidity—United States, 2000. *Morbidity & Mortality Weekly Reports, 52*(35), 842–844.

Centers for Disease Control. (2004a). Alcohol-attributable deaths and years of potential life lost—United States, 2001. *Morbidity & Mortality Weekly Report, 53*(37), 866–870.

Centers for Disease Control. (2004b). Smoking during pregnancy—United States, 1990–2002. *Morbidity & Mortality Weekly Report, 53*(39), 911–915.

Centers for Disease Control. (2004c). Alcohol consumption among women who are pregnant or who might become pregnant—United States, 2002. *Morbidity & Mortality Weekly Report, 53*(50), 1178–1181.

Centers for Disease Control. (2005). Annual smoking-attributable mortality, years of potential life lost, and productivity losses—United States, 1997–2001. *Morbidity & Mortality Weekly Report*.

Centers for Disease Control. (2006a). Youth risk behavior surveillance—United States, 2005. *Morbidity & Mortality Weekly Report, 55*(SS-5), 1–108.

Centers for Disease Control. (2006b). Tobacco use among adults—United States, 2005. *Morbidity & Mortality Weekly Report, 55*(42), 1145–1148.

Centers for Disease Control. (2006c). Cigarette use among high school students—United States, 2006. *Morbidity & Mortality Weekly Report, 55*(26), 724–726.

Centers for Disease Control. (2006d). *Alcohol and public health*. Retrieved June 25, 2007 from http://www.cdc.gov/alcohol/index.htm

Dishion, T. J., Kavanaugh, K., & Kiesner, J. (2003). Prevention of early adolescent substance abuse among high risk youth: A multiple gating approach to parent intervention. *NIDA Monograph 177*, 208–228.

Fisher, E. B., Brownson, R. C., Heath, A. C., Luke, D. A., & Sumner, W. (2004). Cigarette smoking. In J. M Racznski & L. C. Leviton (Eds), *Handbook of clinical health psychology* (Vol. 2, pp. 75–120). Washington, DC: American Psychological Association.

Giovino, G., Barker, D. C., & Tworek, C. (2004). *The national youth smoking cessation survey*. Retrieved August 5, 2008 from http://www.rwjr.org/publichealth/products

Greenfield, L. A. (1998). *Alcohol and crime: An analysis of national data on the prevalence of alcohol involvement in crime.* Report prepared for the Assistant Attorney General's national symposium on alcohol abuse and crime. Washington, DC: U.S. Department of Justice.

Heather, N., & Robertson, I. (1997). *Problem drinking* (3rd Edition). Oxford, UK: Oxford University Press.

Henderson, B. N., & Baum, A. (2004). Neoplasms. In S. B. Johnson, N. W. Perry, & R. H. Rozensky (Eds.), *Handbook of Clinical Health Psychology* (Vol. I, pp. 37-64). Washington, DC: American Psychological Association.

Humphries, K., & Tucker, J. A. (2002). Toward more responsive and effective intervention systems for alcohol-related problems. *Addiction, 97,* 91-104.

Klatsky, A. L., Armstrong, M. A., & Friedman, G. D. (1990). Risk of cardiovascular mortality in alcohol drinkers, ex-drinkers, and nondrinkers. *American Journal of Cardiology, 66,* 1237-1242.

Klatsky, A. L., Armstrong, M. A., & Friedman, G. D. (1992). Alcohol and mortality. *Annals of Internal Medicine, 117*(8), 646-54.

Klatsky, A. L., & Udalstova, N. (2007). Alcohol drinking and total morality risk. *Annals of Epidemiology, 17*(Suppl.5), S63-7.

Lovell, G. (2002). *You are the target, big tobacco: Lies, scams—now the truth.* Vancouver, BC: Chryan Communications.

Maisto, S. A. (2004). Alcoholism. In A. J. Christensen, R. Martin & J. M. Smyth (Eds.), *Encyclopedia of health psychology* (pp. 9-13). New York: Kluwer Academic.

Marlatt, G. A., & Gordon, J. R. (Eds.). (1985). *Relapse prevention.* New York: Guilford Press.

Marmot, M., & Brunner, L. E. (1991). Alcohol and cardiovascular disease: The status of the U-shaped curve. *British Medical Journal, 303,* 565-568.

McCrady, B. S., Dean, L., Dubreuil, E., & Swanson, S. (1985). The problem drinkers' project: A programmatic application of social-learning-based treatment. In G. A. Marlatt &

J. R. Gordon (Eds.), *Relapse prevention* (pp. 417-471). New York: The Guilford Press.

Midanik, L. T., Chaloupka, F. J., Saitz, R., Toomey, T. L., Fellows, J. L., Dufour, et al. (2004). Alcohol-attributable deaths and years of potential life lost—United States, 2001. *Morbidity & Mortality Weekly Report, 53*(37), 866-870.

Milby, J. B., Schmacher, J.E., & Tucker, J. A. (2004). In J. M Racznski & L. C. Leviton (Eds.), *Handbook of clinical health psychology* (Vol. 2, pp. 43-74). Washington, DC: American Psychological Association.

Mokdad, A., Marks, J., Stroup, D., & Gerberding, J. (2004). Actual causes of death in the United States, 2000. *Journal of the American Medical Association, 291,* 1238-1245.

Moos, R. H., Finney, J. W., & Conkite, R. C. (1990). *Alcoholism treatment: Context, process, and outcome.* New York: Oxford University Press.

Naimi, T. S., Brown, D. W., Brewer, R. D., Giles, W. H., Mensah, G., Serdula, M. K., et al. (2005). Cardiovascular risk factors and confounders among nondrinking and moderate-drinking U. S. adults. *American Journal of Preventive Medicine, 28*(4), 369-73.

Ockene, J., Emmons, K., Mermelstein, R., Perkins, K., Bonollo, D., Voorhees, C., et al., (2000). Relapse and maintenance issues for smoking cessation. *Health Psychology, 19,* 17-31.

Orleans, C. T. (2000). Promoting the maintenance of health behavior change: Recommendations for the next generation of research and practice. *Health Psychology, 19,* 76-83.

Orleans, C.T., Ulmer, C. C., & Gruman, J. C. (2004). The role of behavioral factors in achieving national health outcomes. In R. G. Frank, A. Baum, & J. L. Wallander (Eds.), *Handbook of clinical health psychology* (Vol. 3, pp. 465-499). Washington, DC: American Psychological Association.

Orleans, C. T., & Alper, J. (2002). Helping addicted smokers quit. In S. Isaacs & J. Knickman (Eds.), *To improve health and health care: The Robert Wood Johnson Foundation Anthology*

(Vol. 7, pp. 125-149). San Francisco: Jossey-Bass.

Quinlan, K. P., Brewer, R. D., Siegel, P., Sleet, D. A., Mokdad, A. H., Shults, R. A., et al. (2005). Alcohol-impaired driving among U.S. adults, 1993-2002. *American Journal of Preventive Medicine.* May 28 (4), 346-350.

Rimm, E. (2000). Moderate alcohol intake and lower risk of coronary heart disease: Meta-analysis of effects on lipids and homeostatic factors. *Journal of the American Medical Association, 319,* 1523-1528.

Schober, R., & Annis, H. M. (1996). Barriers to help-seeking for change in drinking: A gender-focused review of the literature. *Addictive Behaviors, 21,* 81-92.

Serdula, M. K., Brewer, R. D., Gillespie, C., Denny, C. H., & Mokdad, A. (2004). Trends in alcohol use and binge drinking, 1985-1999: Results of a multi-state survey. *American Journal of Preventive Medicine, 26*(4), 294-298.

Shaper, A. G., & Wannamethee, S. G. (2000). Alcohol intake and mortality in middle aged men with diagnosed coronary heart disease. *Heart, 83,* 394-399.

Sobell, M. B., & Sobell, L. C. (1998). Guiding self-change. In W. R. Miller & N. Heather (Eds.), *Treating addictive behaviors* (2nd ed., pp. 189-202). NY: Plenum Press.

U. S. Department of Health and Human Services. (2006). *Smoking can kill in middle age.* Re-trieved April 26, 2007 from http://www.healthfinder.gov

U. S. Environmental Protection Agency. (1992). *Respiratory health effects of passive smoking: Lung cancer and other disorders.* Retrieved June 28, 2007 from http://www.cdc.gov/tobacco/data_statistics/Factsheets/SecondhandSmoke.htm

U. S. National Institutes of Health. (2004). National Cancer Institute Fact Sheet. Retrieved January 18, 2008 from http://www.cancer.gov

U. S. Public Health Service. (1964). *Smoking and health: Report of the advisory committee to the Surgeon General of the public health service.* (PHS Pub. No. 1103.) Rockville, MD: U. S. Department of Health, Education, and Welfare, Public Health Service, Centers for Disease Control.

U. S. Public Health Service. (2000). Treating tobacco use and dependence: A clinical practice guideline. (AHRQ Publication No. 00-0032.) Washington, DC: U. S. Department of Health and Human Services.

Wenzel, L., & Glanz, K. (2004). Behavioral aspects of genetic risk for disease: Cancer genetics as a prototype for complex issues in health psychology. In R. G. Frank, A. Baum, & J. L. Wallander (Eds.), *Handbook of clinical health psychology* (Vol. 3, pp. 115-142). Washington, DC: American Psychological Association.

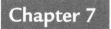

# Chapter 7

# The Concept of Stress

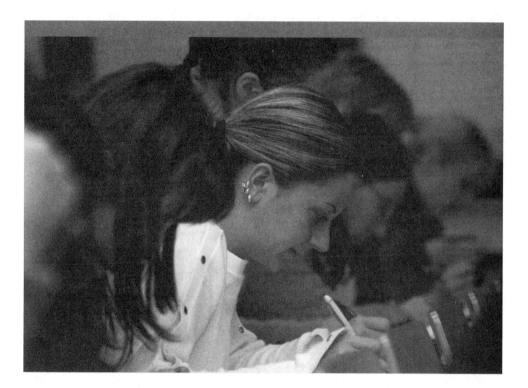

## Learning Objectives

After studying this chapter students will have the knowledge and skills to be able to:

1. Explain how the biopsychosocial approach relates to stress.

2. Clarify ways stress can be harmful to health.

3. Define the concept of stress as developed through the research of Cannon and Selye.

4. Describe the transactional stress appraisal process set forth by Lazarus and Folkman.

5. Discuss and evaluate ways of measuring stress.

## Introduction

Have you ever felt you were "stressed" or "burned out" at the end of a semester? Most college students answer this question with a resounding "yes!" **Stress** appears to be part of life whether we are taking college courses, trying to maintain good relationships with family members and friends, or attempting to get a job or advance in an occupation. A second question is, "How do you know you are under a lot of stress?" Evidence might include feeling worried and anxious, having difficulty sleeping, or feeling rushed, frustrated, and short tempered. A third question addresses how you manage stress in your life. Many people use alcohol or smoking to lessen stress (Park, Armeli, & Tennen, 2004).

The concept of stress is central to health psychology, so three chapters discuss this topic. Stress has biological, psychological, and sociocultural causes and consequences. It triggers physiological responses in the nervous and endocrine systems and can cause both immediate and long-term damage to health and well-being. The psychological component of experiencing stress is based in each individual's perception of a problem or trouble. Past social occurrences contribute to feeling vulnerable to stress. On the other hand, friends and family members often provide social support that improves our response to the stressors of life. Threats to our self-confidence and happiness can arise internally or from the environment. For example, poverty and discrimination are causes of stress for many people. Sources of stress can be cataclysmic events such as earthquakes, tsunamis, or raging fires. Stress also results from relatively minor events, such as the difficulty of finding a parking space or the unpleasant scent of a fellow student's perfume or cologne. In research, minor **stressors** are referred to as hassles. Reactions to stress are based on each individual. This means what is stressful for one person may not bother another at all. For example, some people are so accustomed to traffic noise they would lie awake at night if no horns were blaring or sirens screaming.

The purposes of this chapter and of the next two are to understand stress, its effects on health and safety, and ways to cope with stress. This initial chapter is about defining stress, including its biological and psychosocial aspects, and to consider how people react to threats of stressors. We will also explore different ways researchers in health psychology measure stress. Subsequent chapters examine illness and injury as outcomes of stress and ways to manage stress. We will also study the relationship of stress to disease and healing. Finally, pain is analyzed as a source of stress that can be managed in a variety of ways.

**stress** A physical and psychological reaction to a threat to physical, psychological, or social health.

**stressor** An event or situation perceived by persons to be a danger to their physical, psychological, or social health.

# Good Health and Wellness

Revisiting the wellness continuum found in Chapter 1 may lead to the discovery that stressful events move us away from wellness and toward illness and death. Many scientists believe stress kills us when there is great enough shock and damage to our physiological system. When people are in poor health due to chronic disease, their mental health is more vulnerable to stress. Health problems create stress for people, and stress aggravates health problems. We acknowledge this when we conceal bad news from sick or injured loved ones. We are afraid the stress of hearing negative news will delay their recovery. When people identify sources of stress and find ways to cope, they usually experience better physical, emotional, and social health.

## The Mind-Body Connection and Stress

The notion of stress includes biological, psychological, and social responses to events or situations perceived to be threatening. The perception of stressors is unique to each individual and based on past experiences and current situations. Stress illustrates the **mind-body connection**. Stressors do not even have to be real. Our minds can imagine threatening situations and our bodies will react as though they are actually occurring. These ideas may remind students of the placebo effect and the self-fulfilling prophecy. If we believe something to be true, it will be true in its effects. When our minds believe something bad is happening to us, our physiological, emotional, and behavioral responses are triggered.

For example, when driving down the street did you ever think you were going to run into a car or truck? Maybe the vehicle suddenly swerved in front of you, going slower than you. The perception of the threat triggered a biological response. Your eyes dilated and your vision sharpened, your blood thickened so you were less likely to bleed to death, and you braced yourself for the collision. When the threat was over you felt exhausted. Now imagine if you were threatened day after day by constant bombing or by fighting in a war in a jungle or on a desert. Given those situations you might develop a **panic disorder (PD)** or

---

**mind-body connection** The idea that emotions, personality, and culture affect physical health, and that the reverse is also true. One example is a belief in the power of positive attitudes on health outcomes, such as the effectiveness of cancer treatments. The idea is that mind–body illnesses and mind–body healing are possible.

**panic disorder (PD)** A tendency of humans to experience fear and anxiety in many situations where dangers are either imagined or real.

**post-traumatic stress disorder (PTSD)**, wherein you relive dangerous or harrowing experiences (Scherrer et al., 2000; Grinage, 2003). This is what happens to some war veterans, police officers, fire fighters, and victims of crimes such as rape. People report awakening in the night re-experiencing the dangerous situations. Perhaps when you were a child you watched a bloodcurdling movie or television show and you were bothered for a long time with creepy dreams. Stressful experiences have an enormous impact on our lives and our health.

## The Science of Stress and Stress Management

Scientists must agree on definitions of concepts such as stress before they can measure them or study their effects. Stress is a broad concept, and investigators usually define stress in one of three ways. They see stress as a stimulus, as a response to the stimulus, or as the interaction between the two (Martin & Brantley, 2004, p. 233–235). Once stress is defined and measured, researchers examine ways to manage stress in order to prevent damage to health. Most health psychologists agree that stress contributes directly and indirectly to illness and injury. The reverse is also true. Illness and injury are sources of stress for people who are sick or hurt, as well as for the people who take care of them. When we are sick or in pain, we feel stressed to a greater extent than when we are well or uninjured.

## Preventing Stress and Coping with Stress

There are many important questions about causes of stress and ways to prevent it, although some people contend that stress is an inevitable part of life. **Coping** refers to the way we handle or deal with stressors. In many cases, we can choose to avoid stressful situations or develop an avoidance-coping style that may result in depression (Cronkite, Moos, Twohey, Cohen, & Swindale, 1998). One special field of interest for many health psychologists is stress management. There are healthy and unhealthy ways to deal with stress. One example is abusing psychoactive substances to avoid feeling stress. Other people overeat, or eat almost nothing, saying they have no appetite. Still other people respond to stressors by grind-

---

**post-traumatic stress disorder (PTSD)** An anxiety disorder that occurs after having experienced a serious threat of death or injury to oneself or others as from an assault or from living in a war zone. It involves intense emotional reactions such as fear, helplessness, horror, and/or flashbacks of the trauma(s) and it may interfere with sleep and memory.

**coping** Strategies or processes used by individuals to deal with stressors or demands.

ing their teeth, tensing their neck and shoulder muscles, suffering with headaches, feeling tired all the time, or developing facial tics. There are healthier ways to respond to stressful situations. Adequate rest and sleep are beneficial and regular aerobic exercise makes us more resilient when faced with stressful situations. These are all important topics in health psychology.

## Theories of Stress

The word "stress" is used in fields other than social science. In music, stress marks indicate when to emphasize notes. In the study of languages, stress marks or accents tell us how to pronounce words. The same spelling of a word has different meanings depending on where the stress is placed in pronunciation. Stress in physics denotes pressure put upon materials such as those used in construction of buildings or bridges. A material's resistance to stress is measured in pounds of force per square inch. Stress may result in strain reaching a point when construction materials begin to break down. For example, if you put enough stress on both ends of a piece of chalk, it will break into two pieces. Rubber bands can be pulled apart or stretched to the point that they snap. The word *distress* indicates an unpleasant state of suffering. Airline pilots or ship captains put out distress calls or signals when their planes or ships are in danger.

### Development of the Concept of Stress

One of the most interesting things about the concept of stress is the way it developed over the years and each new idea broadened and built upon previous findings. Stress is an important field of research in health psychology, but there are disagreements about its definition. Some people refer to stress as what is felt by individuals; others use *stressor* to indicate causes of stress. The effects of stress on health are of major scientific concern to social scientists and health care professionals. Stress can be a cause, a stimulus, or a trigger for a variety of behaviors from yelling at your dog to committing suicide. Stress can contribute to injuries by distracting us and making us careless. Stress can be chronic or acute. We often say we are under a lot of pressure or some situation is causing strain in a relationship. Social and cultural conditions such as economic depressions and unemployment are sources of stress in the sociocultural environment. Events such as refinery explosions and declarations of war are stress-filled events for most citizens. Sometimes stress is defined as feelings of anxiety or a sense of doom. On the other hand, some people say they are more productive when they are under stress. For example, some students postpone studying for exams or writing papers until they are near the due date, which forces them into action. In the science literature, *stress* is used to refer to three different ideas: 1) the stimulus or stressor, 2) the person's response to the threat, or 3) interaction between the threat and the person.

## Walter Cannon and the Fight-or-Flight Response

One of the earliest scientific discussions of stress was **Walter Cannon**'s introduction of the notion of the **fight-or-flight response** (1929, 1939). Cannon suggested people become aroused and fearful when they perceive a threatening situation. He noted that people react differently to the same threat. They run away from danger (flight) or defend themselves (fight). The fight-or-flight response is very useful to any living thing dealing with danger. Stress triggers biological changes, making it possible to respond quickly and successfully to danger. Cannon defined stress as a stimulus of the flight-or-fight response (see **Figure 7.1**). After the danger is over our bodies return to a normal state, homeostasis.

## Hans Selye and the General Adaptation Syndrome

**Hans Selye**, a physiologist, was another early scientist who influenced the development of the concept of stress. His first book about the stress syndrome was published in 1936. Selye suggested stress was a general physical response of the body, triggered by many different things. In 1976, in *The Stress of Life*, Selye noted that he had published at least 1,500 articles on stress and more than 100,000 other books and articles had been written about stress by others. Selye's early research examined stress in laboratory rats that developed ulcers when injected with solutions. He discovered that the rats had the same response regardless of the type of fluid that was injected, and he concluded that responses to stress are not specific, but general physical reactions. He used the word stress to describe the reaction or response to threats or demands from the environment. The outcome of stress is strain, similar to the ways muscles are strained by overuse.

**Walter Cannon** Physiologist credited with naming the fight-or-flight response as a response to stressors. During the 1930s, Cannon experimented with cats and found that the adrenal glands secreted the hormone adrenaline or epinephrine when the animals were threatened, causing physiological changes.

**fight-or-flight response** The response of animals, including humans, when threatened with harm. It includes arousal by the sympathetic nervous and endocrine systems to attack or flee.

**Hans Selye** Physiologist who injected noxious agents into rats' bodies and put them under threatening conditions. Experimental animals developed hyperactivity, atrophy of lymph glands, and peptic ulcers. He believed that the response to stress was general and included three phases.

**Figure 7.1**
Humans react to real and imagined threats with physiological changes.

*Source:* Edlin, G. & Golanty, E. (2007). *Health and wellness* (9th ed.). Sudbury, MA: Jones and Bartlett Publishers.

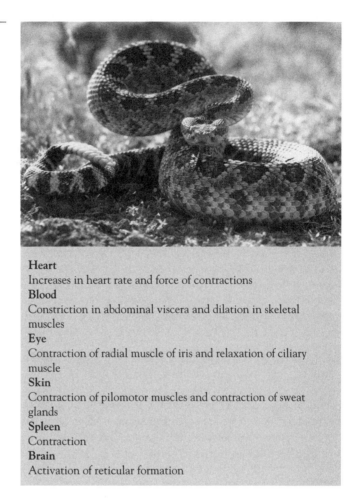

**Heart**
Increases in heart rate and force of contractions
**Blood**
Constriction in abdominal viscera and dilation in skeletal muscles
**Eye**
Contraction of radial muscle of iris and relaxation of ciliary muscle
**Skin**
Contraction of pilomotor muscles and contraction of sweat glands
**Spleen**
Contraction
**Brain**
Activation of reticular formation

Selye proposed three stages of reaction to stress or the **general adaptation syndrome (GAS)**. GAS is a defense mechanism occurring when living things are threatened. In the first stage, *alarm*, the body is mobilized by the nervous and endocrine systems, which trigger defensive and protective physical changes in the body. The second stage Selye named *resistance*. In this stage, the immune system is compromised and illness may be the result. For example, when exposed to stressors, people may have an asthma attack. The third and final

**general adaptation syndrome (GAS)**  Selye's conceptualization of three stages of stress, including the alarm stage (when an animal perceives a threat and prepares to fight or flee), the resistance stage (when the animal copes with stressful situations), and the exhaustion stage (when the body begins to deteriorate under stress).

**Figure 7.2**
Selye's general adaptation syndrome showing the three stages of alarm, resistance followed by exhaustion.

*Source:* Edlin, G. & Golanty, E. (2007). *Health and wellness* (9th ed.). Sudbury, MA: Jones and Bartlett Publishers.

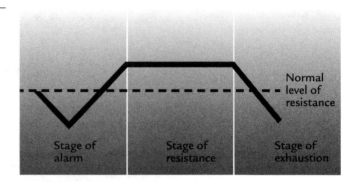

stage, *exhaustion*, refers to a low level of functioning following alarm and resistance. Exhaustion may result in depression or death. Selye's theory of stress emphasized a physical nonspecific response to something in the environment (see **Figure 7.2**).

Later researchers, such as Lazarus and Folkman, believe individual's perceptions of events are more important than what actually occurred (1984). Have you ever said to a friend, "Don't sweat the small stuff"? Then you understand that a situation that is stressful to one person may have no effect on another.

## The Biology of Stress: Physiological Reactions to Perceived Threats

An individual's perception of threats is important for another reason. We are not affected by threats of which we are unaware. Awareness, or conscious knowledge and understanding, is central to the stress reaction. Stress to the body may result in physical outcomes such as injuries, while emotional stress may damage immune systems.

### The Neuroendocrine Response to Stressors

The sympatho-adrenomedullary (SAM) and hypothalamo-pituitary-adrenocortical (HPA) systems are involved in the response to stress, and electrochemical changes in the brain stem mobilize the SAM axis to release catecholamines such as epinephrine and norepinephrine into the body (Martin & Brantley, 2004, p. 234). Cells of the central nervous system (CNS) transmit information controlling and coordinating all body functions. The **autonomic nervous system** affects involuntary action, such as lung expansion and digestion, so con-

**autonomic nervous system** Part of the nervous system that affects involuntary functions of the body such as blood vessels, the heart, smooth muscles, and glands. It includes the sympathetic and parasympathetic divisions.

scious control is not required. The **sympathetic nervous system** mobilizes the body to meet threats. Blood vessels constrict, raising blood pressure, and the heart rate increases. Pupils dilate and saliva production decreases. This is why your mouth feels dry when you have to make a report in class and why public speakers are provided with a glass of water. Blood flows to the muscles in arms and legs so you can fight or flee, and digestion slows because less blood is available. When the threat is resolved, the **parasympathetic nervous system** goes into effect, heart and breathing rates return to normal, intestines begin to churn again, and pupils contract. See **Figure 7.3** for a list of physical changes in response to stress.

The **endocrine system** is also involved in response to stressors. It is a network of glands that secrete hormones into the bloodstream. The endocrine system is slower to react than the nervous system. Some studies use levels of epinephrine in the body as a measure of stress or arousal. Some people like the rush produced by the nervous and endocrine systems and seek out risky or dangerous activities to trigger these effects. Over a period of time, damage to body organs may occur, due to the strength and frequency of the neuroendocrine response, leading to diseases such as high blood pressure, coronary occlusion, allergies, or asthma. Scientists also hypothesize that continual exposure to stressful situations produces long-term changes, resulting in deterioration of the immune system (Baum & Grunberg, 1995). When we are under stress, our wounds may be slower to mend and infections take longer to heal. Children under a great deal of stress may not grow and thrive as expected for their age group.

## Psychosocial Reactions to Stress

Many health psychology researchers and clinicians emphasize that people are not as simple as rats, and stress has emotional and social effects along with physical outcomes. There is enormous variation in the effects of stress on humans. Some people are more susceptible or vulnerable to damage from stress than others. Most agree that stress begins in the brain with the perception of a threat, but many believe that the stress response is interactional and mediates a person's response to a threat (Martin & Brantley, 2004, p. 235). See "Can You Diagnose Yourself?" on page 179 for warning signs of stress.

**sympathetic nervous system**  The part of the nervous system that mobilizes the body for action in response to stress by constricting blood vessels, raising blood pressure, and increasing the heart rate.

**parasympathetic system**  The part of the nervous system that slows the heart rate, dilates blood vessels, and relaxes sphincter muscles stimulating peristalsis and digestion.

**endocrine system**  A network of glands that produce and secrete hormones into the bloodstream, thereby regulating activities, including growth, digestion, metabolism, and reproduction.

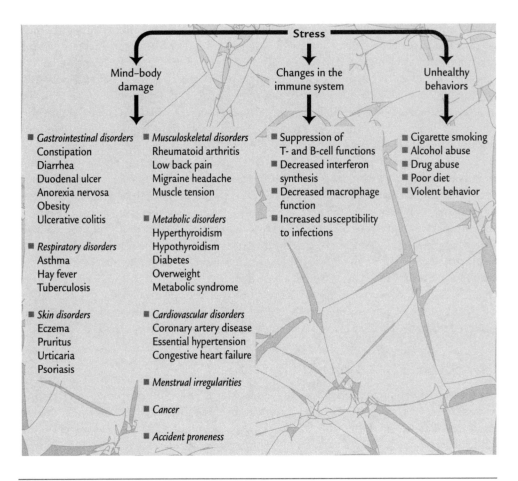

**Figure 7.3**   Our bodies go through many changes when we are challenged by stressful events.

*Source:* Edlin, G. & Golanty, E. (2007). *Health and wellness* (9th ed.). Sudbury, MA: Jones and Bartlett Publishers.

## Coping

Coping refers to the ways people respond to stressful situations. Richard Lazarus has studied stress for many years and published many books and articles on the relationship of stress to coping and health (1966, 1991, 1998, and 1999). He recognizes the effects of stress on the nervous and endocrine systems, but contends that stress is less damaging when people learn to cope effectively. Perceptions and interpretations of stressful events are more important than actual events. People are different and may evaluate identical situations in different ways. What seems stressful to one person is benign for others. Stress is the result of individual appraisals of situations. People think about the future, predict implications of their response to stressors, and consider how their behavior appears to others.

## Think About It!

### Can You Diagnose Yourself?

Although stress is pervasive in the life of a college student, it is not always easy to recognize when stress has become a threat to physical or mental health. If you experience any of these signs of stress, it's time to make some changes in your life, and perhaps seek professional help to reduce the stress.

- Trouble falling asleep
- Difficulty staying asleep
- Waking up tired and not well rested
- Changes in eating patterns
- Craving sweet/fatty/salty ("comfort") foods
- More headaches than usual
- Short temper or irritability
- Recurring colds and minor illness
- Muscle ache and/or tightness
- Trouble concentrating, remembering, or staying organized
- Depression

*Source:* Edlin, G., & Golanty, E. (2007). *Health and wellness* (9th ed.). Sudbury, MA: Jones and Bartlett Publishers.

## Transactional Analysis

Lazarus and a colleague, Susan Folkman, researched and wrote about stress, appraisal, and coping (1984). They use what they called a **transactional analysis** of stress, referring to a continuing exchange between people and their social and physical environments. Reactions

**transactional analysis** Lazarus and Folkman described stress as a continuing exchange between people and their environment. Reactions to stressors are based on an individual's cognitive processes or interpretations of the meaning of events and on their typical methods of coping or responding to stressors. Facing stressful situations involves a series of adjustments as people decide how to react. Lazarus and Folkman proposed that there are three steps in the transaction between an individual and a stressor.

to stressors are based on an individual's cognitive processes or interpretations of the meaning of events and on their typical methods of coping or responding to stressors. People react to stressors differently depending on past experiences and existing resources. Facing stressful situations involves a series of adjustments as people decide how to react. Lazarus and Folkman proposed that there are three steps in the transaction between an individual and a stressor.

### Primary Appraisal

The first stage of exposure to a possible source of stress results in different reactions. To some people a situation is no threat at all. It is harmless, or neutral, or even a positive and welcome event. For example, when confronted by a lion, most of us would run away. The same would not be true of lion tamers or zookeepers who understand how to deal with lions. Other stressors are not physical dangers, but threats to our self-esteem or sense of self-worth. The same biological reactions occur, but our **primary appraisal** may result in emotional reactions such as fear, anger, sadness, worry, or anxiety. Lazarus and Folkman suggest that, when faced with the exact same situations, some people will see a circumstance as stressful while others will view it as exciting and challenging. Some are glad to handle a situation, because it will facilitate their personal growth. Some people face stressors with eager anticipation and see it as an opportunity to star, to be a heroine or hero. Were you ever fired from a job, but rather than being upset, you decided it was good thing because it would force you to look for a better job? Folkman (2004) writes that the primary or opening appraisal focuses on significance and asks "Am I in trouble?" in relation to values, beliefs, and goals.

### Secondary Appraisal

The second stage of appraisal comes once a stressor is judged to be threatening and people think about their options and devise strategies to successfully meet the demand. This stage is influenced by beliefs about personal effectiveness or self-efficacy. Stress levels decline when people believe they have the ability to meet threats. A sense of vulnerability may also be part of the **secondary appraisal**. Some think about the worst thing that can happen and decide to ignore the situation because it is outside of their control. Vulnerability also depends on our resources. We feel more threatened if we have fewer resources to rely upon. Money, friends, and good health are resources. People consider their options and decide on the best way to cope.

---

**primary appraisal** In their first exposure to a potential stressor, people may decide there is a threat or that the stressor is harmless, neutral, or even a positive event in their life.

**secondary appraisal** The second stage of transactional analysis comes when a stressor is believed to be a threat. People think about their options and devise strategies to meet any demands being made upon them.

**Figure 7.4**
Arguments create stress
and disrupt emotional
well-being. Apply the
transactional model of
primary, secondary
appraisals, and reappraisal
to your last argument with
a friend or family member.

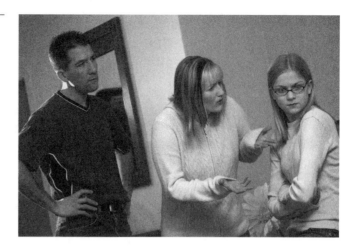

Reappraisal

The third stage in this transaction between individuals and stressors occurs when new and helpful information changes the original evaluation. **Reappraisal** can be a continuous process as people gain new perspectives and increase their understanding of important aspects of threats. Resources help us cope. Being healthy and energetic is more useful than being sick and tired. Self-efficacy, as exemplified by a belief that one can meet a challenge, is a very powerful resource. Problem-solving skills and support from other people are additional aids. People learn to organize their resources and control negative emotional reactions. On reappraisal, some people conclude that the stressor exceeds their resources, and they leave the scene. Processes for coping and options for stress management are explored in later chapters. College students often have conflicts with family and friends. Think back to the last argument you had with someone; did you go through the three stages suggested by Lazarus and Folkman? (See **Figure 7.4**.)

## Measurement of Stress

The physiological response to stress includes eye dilation; blood thickening; increases in oxygenated blood moving to major muscle groups; increases in blood pressure, heart rate, and respiration; along with the presence of stress-related hormones in the bloodstream. Research considers how to measure stress and how to determine the effects of stress on health.

---

**reappraisal** The third state of transactional analysis, when new information changes the original appraisal. People gain new perspectives and discover new resources.

## An Old Example of Measurement: Polygraph Tests

Measures of physiological parameters, such as heart rate and blood pressure, were among the first ways stress was measured. Students may have seen old movies in which people accused of crimes are strapped to polygraph machines or "lie-detectors." Theoretically, polygraphs measure stress or emotional reactions occurring when people tell lies. Technicians begin by asking simple questions like name, address, and age. Later questions concern the crime being investigated. The idea is that fear and anxiety provoked in guilty persons cause measurable increases in heart rates. One advantage of this test is that results are objective and quantifiable. Disadvantages are that detectors are unreliable, expensive, and somewhat invasive. You probably know polygraph evidence is not admissible in court as a proof of guilt or innocence. In movies, suspects often offer to take lie-detector tests to convince police officers not to arrest them. Some scientists believe that being hooked up to any machine causes enough stress to trigger reactions in the nervous system.

## Experiments to Assess Stress Using Performance Measures

Many researchers rely on laboratory experiments to measure stress. They look at heart rates or muscle tension under noxious conditions such as unpleasant odors or loud noises. Experimenters also investigate whether cold or heat will cause enough stress to interfere with people's ability to concentrate and complete math problems or difficult puzzles. Do you think you do better on tests in a quiet classroom or a noisy one? Do you learn better if the room temperature is normal or if it is very hot or very cold? Some scientists try to measure the amount and effect of stress by comparing subjects' performances under varying conditions.

## Self-Reports of Stress and the Social Readjustment Rating Scale

The most common way stress is measured is by self-report or asking people about their levels of stress. Researchers devise inventories or lists of stressful situations to discover links between stress levels and illness. The **social readjustment rating scale (SRRS)** is one of the earliest attempts to measure the effect of stressors on health. The scale, devised by Holmes and Rahe, was published in 1967 and included 43 life events ranging from "death of a spouse" to "minor violations of the law." "Death of spouse," the most stressful of all life events, was valued at 100 while "minor violations of the law" was valued at 11. Respondents are asked if any of the events occurred over the past 12 months. For example, if a person was divorced (73 points), fired from work (50 points), and revised personal habits (24 points), then the total for the year is between 150 and 300 life-change units. This person would have

---

**social readjustment rating scale (SRRS)**  An effort to assess the effect of stressors on health.

a 50% risk for stress-related illness. If scores exceed 300, then the risk of illness increases to 80%. The basic idea is that change, good or bad, is stressful. For example, whether you started or finished going to school, it is valued at 26 stress points. Taking a vacation counts 13 points toward stress-related illness. An advantage of this scale is it is easy to use and covers a wide range of events. A disadvantage was that over time, specific life events become out of date and meaningless. The life-change scale has been updated (Miller & Rahe, 1997). Another criticism of the scale is that injury and illness are included as items on the scale (53 points), so illness or injury is being used to predict additional illness or injury. Critics also suggest the degree of stress is not assessed (Martin & Brantley, 2004, p. 237).

In response to this objection, Cohen, Kamarck, and Mermelstein (1983) developed the perceived stress scale (PSS). In some instances, researchers found the SRRS predicted illness and aggravated chronic diseases. Life-event inventories continue to be the most widely used tools for stress measurement and are useful to practitioners and researchers (Scully, Tosi, & Banning, 2000). Later researchers assessed scales of minor life events or hassles. For example, Kanner, Coyne, Schaefer, and Lazarus (1981) devised a 117-item questionnaire measuring the severity and frequency of minor stressors and an uplifts scale to measure positive life events.

## Stress, Health, and the Immune System

A second approach to the relationship between stress and health is to study the effects of stress on chronic illnesses, such as diabetes, or on resistance to disease. Some studies find that obese individuals have stress-induced patterns of increases in glucose and insulin response when exposed to mental stress (Seematter et al., 2000). Stress may change metabolic activity in diabetics, causing pancreatic hormone stimulation (Surwit, Ross, & Feinglos, 1991).

The immune system helps protect against disease, so researchers explore effects of stress on the immune system, including cells in the blood that help disease resistance, such as antibodies and natural killer cells. Selye's rats developed tumors in reaction to the stress of being injected. It is believed that over a period of time negative emotional states suppress the immune system and reduce our resistance to disease (Cohen, Kessler, & Gordon, 1995). This area of study is called **psychoneuroimmunology (PNI)**, and a recent meta-analysis reported that negative emotions and stressful experiences intensify a variety of health threats (Kiecolt-Glaser, McGuire, Robles, & Glaser, 2002). For example, periods of high stress are followed by lowered resistance to respiratory illness (Cobb & Steptoe, 1996). Decreases in

**psychoneuroimmunology (PNI)** A science studying the bidirectional connections between behavior and the nervous, endocrine, and immune system. Research shows the brain influences immune reactivity. For example, depression may lower immune system resistance.

natural killer cell activity increase the incidence of cancer (Linn, Lin, & Jensen, 1982), and psychosocial factors are linked to risk of cardiovascular disease (Kop, 1997).

Have you ever gotten sick after final exams? Interestingly, exam stress in Canadian psychiatric residents lowered their resistance to disease (Dorian, Keystone, Garfinkel, & Brown, 1981). Scientists studying parachutists found changes in immune systems immediately following the first jump (Schedlowksi et al., 1993). Studies indicate resistance to disease is compromised by such diverse sources of stress as loneliness, marital conflicts, and caring for elderly parents or Alzheimer's patients (Glaser & Kiecolt-Glaser, 1994). Blood and urine tests are used to assess corticosteroid and catecholamine levels as reactions to stress but may be affected by caffeine and exercise (Martin & Brantley, 2004, p. 236).

## Stress and Gender Differences

Recent research and discussions about stress have expanded to focus on possible connections among stress, health, and gender. First, there is greater within-gender variability than gender difference in personality attributes. Health differences between women and men most often result from variations in behavior and psychosocial environments (Stanton and Courtenay, 2004, p. 106). Men and boys die earlier than women and girls when age is held constant (U.S. Department of Health and Human Services [USDHHS], 2000). This is partially due to men's attitudes and beliefs. More men than women believe they are not responsible for their health, and men respond to stress in less healthy ways than women by using denial, distraction, and alcohol consumption to cope with stressors (USDHHS, p. 107). At the same time, men consume more meat, fat, and salt, but less fiber, fruits, and vegetables than women. Men are less likely than women to exercise healthily, and are more likely to be overweight, drive while intoxicated, and engage in other risky behaviors (Courtenay, 2000). Many men have beliefs about being physically tough that lead to fighting, injuries, and death. Finally, men are more likely to delay getting medical help than women (Sandman, Simantov, & An, 2000).

Psychosocial factors, including role expectations, contribute to stress in women's lives. A meta-analysis of gender differences in stress revealed that women are more likely to express higher stress than men in both work and interpersonal roles (Davis, Matthews, & Twamley, 1999). Some examples are the occupational and caregiving roles assigned to women, including care of aging parents; women's lesser earning power; and the dearth of medical knowledge about women's health. For example, there is concern that the Food and Drug Administration oversight system fails to oversee gender-specific research on the effects of new medication (U.S. General Accounting Office, 2001). About 20% of women are victims of male partner violence (Koss, Ingram, & Pepper, 2001). Cardiovascular disease is the major killer of women, and yet less than a third of women say their physicians discussed the risks of this disease with them (Mosca et al., 2000).

Taylor and colleagues (2000) recently suggested that female stress response is less fight-or-flight than it is tend-and-befriend, and that gender bias excludes women from most stress research. They point out that females, both human and of other species, respond to stress by nurturing and protecting their offspring rather than by fighting or fleeing. They suggest a biobehavioral mechanism by which females befriend each other, forming social groups that provide members with resources and protection for tending offspring. Oxytocin and soothing endogenous opioid mechanisms associated with childbearing and nursing soothe both infants and their mothers. Even during adolescence, human females are more likely than males to mobilize social support in times of stress in an exchange of resources and responsibilities. Taylor and her colleagues further suggest that a down-regulated stress response in females may reduce vulnerability in women's health and partially explain the fact that women live longer than men.

## Summary

This chapter presents an initial look at stress, which is one of the most important concepts in health psychology. It is followed by three chapters focusing on the effects of stress on illness and injury, coping and stress management, and pain as a major source of stress. This introductory chapter explored theories, concepts, and definitions used in health psychology to describe the phenomenon of stress and its effect on human health.

Theories about the effects of stress began with Walter Cannon who wrote about the fight-or-flight response, which described a response of the nervous and endocrine systems to threats. Hans Selye defined the general adaptation syndrome and used the construct to explain the effects of stress on health. Immediate biological responses to stress are well researched and include increases in heart rate, blood pressure, coagulation of the blood, and blood flowing to large muscle groups. Scientists and health care professionals studying the effects of stress on the body often find that stress weakens our immune systems. This is the field of health psychology known as psychoneuroimmunology.

Psychological and sociocultural theories of stress call attention to people's intellectual and emotional responses to stressful situations. Lazarus and Folkman envisioned the appraisal of stressors as a transaction between the individual and their social environment. The initial or primary appraisal is a judgment about danger, which can be physical, social, psychological, or a combination of the three. Individuals respond to stress in terms of their resources. Reappraisal may continue as information and resources change. Polygraph tests, laboratory experiments, blood assays, and self-reports provide additional data about the effect of stress and negative emotions on biological processes such as heart rate and blood pressure.

## Review Questions

1. Explain why stress is an appropriate subject for the biopsychosocial approach to health.

2. Describe the biological reactions that occur when one is confronted with upsetting situations.

3. Explain ways exposure to stressors can be harmful to health.

4. What ideas did Walter Cannon and Hans Selye contribute to the study of stress?

5. Describe the stress appraisal process outlined by Lazarus and Folkman.

6. Summarize and evaluate different ways to measure the effects of stress on human activity and health.

7. What did Taylor and her colleagues add to the traditional approaches to the stress response?

## Student Activity

1. Describe an important stressor you faced over the last 4 weeks. Identify its origin as biological, psychological, sociocultural, or some combination of the three.

2. List any immediate physiological changes that occurred when you were first confronted with the stressor. For example, did your heart start beating more rapidly or did your rate of breathing increase? Did you feel hot or cold?

3. List any physiological changes that occurred somewhat later in time. For example, did you get a headache or wake up the next day with a sore throat?

4. Describe your initial reactions when faced with the stressor. Using the words of Lazarus and Folkman, describe your primary appraisal. Did you immediately see the situation as a source of stress to be dealt with or did you see it as an exciting challenge?

5. Write a description of your secondary appraisal. Describe the resources you thought you could use to deal with the stressor. For example, did you turn to others for social support or more tangible assistance? Who did you turn to for help?

6. Evaluate the situation you faced and list any additional resources you had but did not use at the time.

7. Based on your answers to the above questions explain how you would rate your response to the stressor. What grade would you give yourself?

8. Describe how you would act differently next time you face a similar stressor.

## References

Baum, A., & Grunberg, N. (1995). Measurement of stress hormones. In S. Cohen, R. C. Kessler, & L. U. Gordon (Eds.), *Measuring stress: A guide for health and social scientists* (pp. 175–192). New York: Oxford University Press.

Cannon, W. B. (1929). *Bodily changes in pain, hunger, fear and rage* (2nd ed.). New York: Appleton.

Cannon, W. B. (1939). *The wisdom of the body* (2nd ed.). New York: W. W. Norton.

Cobb, J. M., & Steptoe, A. (1996). Psychosocial stress and susceptibility to upper respiratory tract illness in an adult population sample. *Psychosomatic Medicine, 58*(5), 404–412.

Cohen, S., Kessler, R. C., & Gordon, L. U. (Eds.) (1995). *Measuring stress: A guide for health and social scientists*. New York: Oxford.

Cohen, S., Kamarck, T., & Mermelstein, R. (1983). A global measure of perceived stress. *Journal of Health and Social Behavior, 24*, 385–396.

Courtenay, W. H. (2000). Behavioral factors associated with disease, injury, and death among men: Evidence and implications for prevention. *Journal of Men's Studies, 9*(1), 81–142.

Cronkite, R. C., Moos, R. H., Twohey, J., Cohen, C., & Swindle, R., Jr. (1998). Life circumstances and personal resources as predictors of the ten-year course of depression. *American Journal of Community Psychology, 26*(2), 255–280.

Davis, M. C., Matthews, K. A., and Twamley, E. W. (1999). Is life more difficult on Mars or Venus? A meta-analytic review of sex differences in major and minor life events. *Annals of Behavioral Medicine, 21*, 83–97.

Dorian, B. J., Keystone, E., Garfinkel, P. E, & Brown, G. M. (1981). Immune mechanisms in acute psychological stress. *Psychosomatic Medicine, 43*, 84.

Folkman, S. (2004). Stress appraisal. In A. J. Christensen, R. Martin, & J. M. Smyth (Eds.), *Encyclopedia of health psychology* (pp. 296–297). New York: Kluwer Academic.

Glaser, R., & Kiecolt-Glaser, J. K. (Eds.). (1994). *Handbook of human stress and immunity.* New York: Academic Press.

Grinage, B. D. (2003). Diagnosis and management of post-traumatic stress disorder. *American Family Physician, 68*, 2401–2408.

Holmes, T. H., & Rahe, R. H. (1967). The social readjustment rating scale. *Journal of Psychosomatic Research, 11*, 213–218.

Kanner, A. D., Coyne, J. C., Schaefer, C., & Lazarus, R. S. (1981). Comparisons of two modes of measurement: Daily hassles and uplifts versus major life events. *Journal of Behavioral Medicine, 4*, 1–39.

Kiecolt-Glaser, J. K., McGuire, L., Robles, T. F., & Glaser, R. (2002). Emotions, morbidity and mortality: New perspectives from psychoneuroimmunology. *Annual Review of Psychology, 53*, 83–107.

Kop, W. J. (1997). Acute and chronic psychological risk factors for coronary syndromes: Moderating the effects of coronary artery disease severity. *Journal of Psychosomatic Research, 43*(2), 167–181.

Koss, M. P., Ingram, M., and Pepper, S. L. (2001). Male partner violence: Relevance to health care providers. In A. Baum, T. A. Revenson, & J. E. Singer (Eds.), *Handbook of health psychology.* Mahwah, NJ: Lawrence Erlbaum Associates.

Lazarus, R. S. (1966). *Psychological stress and the coping process.* New York: McGraw-Hill.

Lazarus, R. S., & Folkman, S. (1984). *Stress, appraisal, and coping.* New York: Springer.

Lazarus, R. S. (1991). *Emotion and adaptation.* New York: Oxford University Press.

Lazarus, R. S. (1998). *Fifty years of the research and theory of R. S. Lazarus: An analysis of historical and perennial issues.* Mahwah, NJ: Lawrence Erlbaum Associates.

Lazarus, R. S. (1999). *Stress and emotion: A new synthesis.* New York: Springer.

Linn, B. S., Linn, M. W., & Jensen, J. (1982). Degree of depression and immune responsiveness. *Psychosomatic Medicine, 44*, 128–129.

Martin, P. D., & Brantley, P. J. (2004). Stress, coping, and social support in health and behavior. In J. M. Raczynski & L. C. Leviton (Eds.), *Handbook of Clinical Health Psychology* (Vol. 2, pp. 233–267). Washington, DC: American Psychological Association.

Miller, M. A., & Rahe, R. H. (1997). Life changes scaling for the 1990's. *Journal of Psychosomatic Research, 43*(3), 279–292.

Mosca, L., Jones, W. K., King, K. B., Ouyang, P., Redberg, R. F., & Hill, M. N. (2000). Awareness, perception, and knowledge of heart disease risk and prevention among women in the United States. *Archives of Family Medicine, 9*, 506–515.

Park, C. L., Armeli, S., & Tennen, H. (2004). The daily stress and coping process and alcohol use among college students. *Journal of Studies of Alcohol, 65*, 126–135.

Sandman, D., Simantov, E., & An, C. (2000). *Out of touch: American men and the health care system.* New York: Commonwealth Fund.

Schedlowski, M., Jacobs, R., Stratmann, G., Richter, S., Hadicke, A., Tewew, U., et al. (1993). Changes in natural killer cells during acute psychological stress. *Journal of Clinical Immunology, 13*(2), 119–128.

Scherrer, J. F., True, W. R., Xian, H., Lyons, M. J., Eisen, S. A., Goldberg, J., et al. (2000). Evidence for genetic influences common and specific to symptoms of generalized anxiety and panic. *Journal of Affective Disorders, 57*, 25–35.

Scully, J., Tosi, H., & Banning, K. (2000). Life events checklists: revisiting the social readjustment rating scale after 30 years. *Educational and Psychological Measurement, 60*, 864–876.

Seematter, G., Guenat, E., Schneiter, P., Cayeux, C., Jequier, E., & Trappy, L. (2000). Effects of mental stress on insulin-mediated glucose metabolism and energy expenditure in lean and obese women. *American Journal of Physiology, Endocrinology and Metabolism, 279,* 799–805.

Selye, H. (1976). *The stress of life* (Rev. ed.). New York: McGraw-Hill.

Stanton, A. L., & Courtenay, W. (2004). Gender, stress, and health. In R. H. Rozensky, N. G. Johnson, C. D. Goodheart, & W. R. Hammond (Eds.), *Psychology builds a healthy world: Opportunities for research and practice.* Washington, DC: American Psychological Association.

Surwit, R. S., Ross, S. L., & Feinglos, M. N. (1991). Stress, behavior, and glucose control in diabetes mellitus. In P. M. McCabe & N. Schneiderman (Eds.), *Stress, coping and disease* (pp. 97–117). Hillsdale, NJ: Lawrence Erlbaum Associates.

Taylor, S. E., Klein, L. C., Lewis, B. P., Gruenewald, T. L., Gurung, R. A. R., & Updegraff, J. A. (2000). Biobehavioral responses to stress in females: Tend-and-befriend, not fight-or-flight. *Psychological Review, 107*(3), 411–420.

U. S. Department of Health and Human Services. (2000). Deaths: Final data for 1998 (DHHS Publication No. [PHS] 2000-1120). *National Vital Statistics Reports, 48*(11). Hyattsville, MD: National Center for Health Statistics.

U. S. General Accounting Office. (July, 2001). *Women's Health: Women sufficiently represented in new drug testing, but FDA oversight needs improvement* (GAO-01-754). Washington, DC: Author.

# Chapter 8

# The Reciprocal Effects of Stress on Illness and Injury

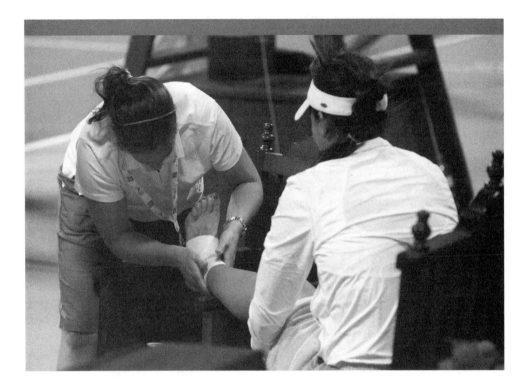

## Learning Objectives

After studying this chapter students will have the knowledge and skills to be able to:

1. Explain the bidirectional or mutual relationship of stress with illness and injury.

2. List and briefly describe some psychosocial indicators of stress.

3. Clarify the behaviors that make us less vulnerable to the damaging effects of stress on biopsychosocial health.

4. Explain the structural protection humans have against injury.

5. Explain the cellular protection humans have against illness.

6. Define psychoneuroimmunology and give two examples of the types of studies carried out in this field.

7. Provide research evidence that negative emotions contribute to illness and death.

8. Define post-traumatic stress disorder and describe situations in which it might occur.

9. Review research findings about the association between stress and injuries.

10. Describe styles of coaching that help prevent athletic injuries.

## Introduction

Stress is a condition of heightened alarm and awareness of danger. Stressors are events or situations that people perceive to be threatening to their physical, psychological, or social health. Perception of stressors and emotional reactions to stressors are highly individual. For example, different responses may occur when a woman hears she is pregnant. Similarly, her partner or husband may feel threatened or overjoyed by the news.

A stressor must be perceived and understood in order to be regarded as harmful, but stressors can be real or imagined. The previous chapter discussed reactions to stress at the biological level, beginning with protective responses by the autonomic nervous system that enable us to either defend ourselves or escape danger. Stressors are handled by a complex physiological network that includes the central nervous system, the adrenal system, the cardiovascular system, and the immune system.

Health psychology is a biobehavioral science, meaning people's physiology interacts with their behaviors, which in turn affect and are affected by psychological and sociocultural variables. These interactions can result in stress, illness, and injury. Human behaviors influence health, and health influences behavior.

Origins of stress can be biological, psychological, or social, or some combination of the three. Pathogens such as bacteria and physical injuries are examples of biological stressors. Humiliation is a psychological stressor, and being chased across campus by an angry mob is an example of a psychosocial stressor. Most of us have experienced the very common stressor of cars moving at high speed suddenly changing lanes in front of us on a freeway. In each case, our brain perceives the danger and defensive systems are activated. We feel physically threatened and emotionally upset. Stress also results if we fail to find employment and believe it to be because of our skin color, gender, or age. Frequent feelings of being under stress may be characteristic of the Type A personality, a person who tries to do more and more in limited periods of time and often ignores symptoms of physical illness, saying there is no time to stop and take a breath, much less see a doctor or submit to medical tests (Friedman & Rosenman, 1959).

Some stressors are acute, such as sudden job loss or an unexpected death in the family, while other stressors are chronic, including poverty or caring for a family member who is ill or disabled. In some instances, illness results because stress weakens our immune systems, allowing pathogens to thrive in our bodies. A stressor may cause distraction, making us more likely to make mistakes that lead to injury. The relationship of stress to illness and injuries is mutual or bidirectional. This means illness and injury both cause and result from stress. In addition, stress or its effects may cause additional stress, illness, or injury. Both illness and injury also create stress for family members, friends, and coworkers, because relationships are disrupted and normal functioning is restricted. Their stress causes further stress within us.

A second way stressors contribute to illness and injury is by triggering unhealthy and risky behaviors. For example, many people gravitate to comforting foods that are high in sugar, salt, or fat. People tend to smoke more and drink more alcohol when they are under stress. The nicotine in tobacco stimulates or speeds up metabolism, so smokers feel less fatigue even when they are very tired. Some people report they feel more relaxed after smoking, and this may also be due to relief from the craving for nicotine. Alcohol is a depressant on the central nervous system, so after drinking people are partially anesthetized and feel more relaxed. Being slightly anesthetized makes us more likely to be injured, especially in falls, car accidents, and during crimes. The biopsychosocial perspective of health psychology provides an ideal framework to study biological, psychological, and sociocultural causes of stress and biological, psychological, and sociocultural responses to stressors.

## Indicators of Stress

Immediate biological reactions to stressors include increases in heart rate, blood pressure, and drying of the mouth (Thompson & Van Loon, 2002, pp. 154–155), but prolonged

---

### Think About It!

#### Types of Stressors

**Acute Stressors: Catastrophic events or sudden aggravations in the environment involving extraordinary coping efforts**

Personal disasters: Death of a spouse, breakup of a marriage, intense arguments
Public disasters: Natural disasters (earthquakes) and human-made disasters (bombings)

#### Chronic Stressors: Aggravations that last months or years

Insufficient social support
Lack of socioeconomic resources
Neighborhood disorder and social incivility
Neighborhoods with high mobility, population density, and crime
Stressors from the home and family
Stressors from jobs: Women—low job control, unsupportive bosses, high family demands
                      Men—low job control and high job demands

*Source:* Suchday, S., Tucker, D. L., & Krantz, D. S. (2002). In S. B. Johnson, N. W. Perry, Jr., & R. H. Rozensky (Eds.), *Handbook of clinical health psychology* (Vol. 1, pp. 203–238). Washington, DC: American Psychological Association.

exposure to stressors contributes to exhaustion, sleeping difficulties, and repeated illnesses. Both acute and chronic illnesses reflect stress-related overeating, smoking, and drinking. In turn, drinking contributes to injuries sustained in automobile wrecks, assaults, and other crimes (National Institute on Drug Abuse [NIDA], 2008). Other outcomes of stress include infections and chronic diseases such as cancer, cardiovascular disease, diabetes, asthma, and gastrointestinal disorders (Martin & Brantley, 2004, pp. 238–239). Obese women may develop stress-induced glucose and insulin response while thin women do not (Seematter et al., 2000).

Social relationships and mental health suffer when we experience stress. Some people isolate themselves and withdraw from contact with family and friends. When dealing with stressors we may also be more argumentative with family members, friends, and coworkers, adding to their stress as well as our own. Some of the emotional indicators of stress are impatience, despair, fear, anger, and anxiety. Stress is related to depression, which contributes to suicides. Severe stress can cause illness, injury, and even death. See **Table 8.1** for ways that stress affects illness.

## Modifiers of Stress

Some people are stronger than others in resisting the effects of stress on their health, self-esteem, and social relationships. Sources of stress in one part of our lives are augmented by problems in other parts. For example, when elderly people are injured, they often feel greater stress than do younger persons, especially if they are more isolated and have chronic health problems. Physical health, emotional health, and social support all influence resistance to stress. Good nutritional practices and regular aerobic exercise help offset stressors. The following chapter on stress management discusses emotional health and social support. People who are typically serene, happy, and content are less bothered by stressors than people who usually feel, anxious, sad, or are dissatisfied with their lives. A person who has many close relationships with family and friends is less vulnerable than a person who is isolated and lacks meaningful relationships.

# Biological Defenses Against the Effects of Stressors

## Mechanical Protection Against Injury and Pain

The skeletal system is one form of protection for the body against painful physical damage. Thick skull bones and vertebrae and disks protect our brain and spinal cord. Cerebrospinal fluid fills and cushions cavities in the brain and spinal cord. The bones in the rib cage protect the heart and lungs, and to some extent the kidneys, liver, and spleen. Muscles and other soft tissue protect bones and joints. Skin and fat protect by insulating the body against extremes of heat and cold. The skin is also involved in keeping out pathogens such as bacteria and parasites. Even tears, ear wax, and nasal hairs and mucus are protective.

TABLE 8.1   Exacerbation of Specific Illness by Stressors

Coronary heart disease: Heart attack (myocardial infarction) and sudden cardiac death[1]

Chronic illness: Asthma and rheumatic diseases[2]

Poor antibody response to vaccine including flu, hepatitis, and tetanus[3]

Cancer progression[4]

Disease susceptibility: Cold symptoms, respiratory illness, and flu[3]

Dermatological conditions: Atopic dermatitis (eczema)[5]

Poor diabetic control: Change in hormones that block insulin and distractions from self-care[6]

Functional gastrointestinal disorders[7]

Elevations in blood pressure[1]

HIV progression[3]

Immune system[8]

[1]Suchday, S., Tucker, D. L., & Krantz, D. S. (2002). In S. B. Johnson, N. W. Perry, Jr., & R. H. Rozensky (Eds.), *Handbook of clinical health psychology* (Vol. 1, pp. 203–238). Washington, DC: American Psychological Association.

[2]Creer, T. L., Bender, B. G., & Lucas, D. O. (2002). In S. B. Johnson, N. W. Perry, Jr., & R. H. Rozensky (Eds.), *Handbook of clinical health psychology* (Vol. 1, pp. 239–282). Washington, DC: American Psychological Association.

[3]Ironson, G., Balbin, E., & Schneiderman, N. (2002). Health psychology and infectious diseases. In S. B. Johnson, N. W. Perry, Jr., & R. H. Rozensky (Eds.), *Handbook of clinical health psychology* (Vol. 1, pp. 5–36). Washington, DC: American Psychological Association.

[4]Henderson, R. N., & Baum, A. (2004). Neoplasms. In S. B. Johnson, N. W. Perry, Jr., & R. H. Rozensky (Eds.), *Handbook of clinical health psychology* (Vol. 1, pp. 37–64). Washington, DC: American Psychological Association.

[5]Tovian, S. M. (2004). Diseases of the skin and subcutaneous tissue. In S. B. Johnson, N. W. Perry, Jr., & R. H. Rozensky (Eds.), *Handbook of clinical health psychology* (Vol. 1, pp. 371–397). Washington, DC: American Psychological Association.

[6]Wysocki, T., & Buckloh, L. M. (2004). Endocrine, metabolic, nutritional, and immune disorders. In S. B. Johnson, N. W. Perry, Jr., & R. H. Rozensky (Eds.), *Handbook of clinical health psychology* (Vol. 1, pp. 65–99). Washington, DC: American Psychological Association.

[7]Toner, B. B., & Casati, J. (2004). Diseases of the digestive system. In S. B. Johnson, N. W. Perry, Jr., & R. H. Rozensky (Eds.), *Handbook of clinical health psychology* (Vol. 1, pp. 283–306). Washington, DC: American Psychological Association.

[8]Forlenza, M. J., & Baum, A. Psychoneuroimmunology. In R. J. Frank, A. Baum, & J. L. Wallander (Eds.), *Handbook of clinical health psychology* (Vol. 3, pp. 81–114). Washington, DC: American Psychological Association.

## Stressors and Bodily Injury

Many injuries are identified as accidents or unintentional, but predisposing factors may contribute to an accident. Have you ever played in a competitive game when you were worried about something and gotten hurt? Similarly, have you ever been driving and thinking about an important situation and caused a car wreck? Worry distracts our attention so we are more likely to be injured, and being in competitive situations like sports playoffs or other types of physical contests is stressful enough to cause errors in judgment and lead to injury.

Injury results in both inflammation and pain. Inflammation triggers cytokines, attracting immune cells to the site of injury in a beneficial reaction to help repair tissue damage, but also lowering immunity by binding other immune cells, making illness more likely (Forlenza & Baum, 2004, p. 90). Unfortunately inflammation is also linked to slower muscle repair and a decline in physical functioning, including frailty and disability (Kiecolt-Glaser, McGuire, Robles, & Glaser, 2002). Injury-related pain is a major additional cause of stress and may require medical solutions so patients can get adequate rest to promote healing.

## Cellular Protection Against Illness

Our immune system protects us from infections through the circulatory and lymphatic systems. **Immunology** is the study of the body's response to foreign invasion. Blood and lymph contain cells that help us resist viruses, bacteria, fungi, and parasites. This is why good hygiene, such as hand washing, helps prevent transmission of diseases such as colds and flu. We develop antibodies as we grow and we acquire immunity to some diseases by vaccination or by experiencing them. Commonly, we acquire immunity to measles, mumps, chicken pox, and polio. Antibodies in our immune systems seek out and destroy pathogens. Harmful pathogens are discovered by defensive cellular structures including phagocytes, T cells, and B cells, and by body chemicals, including a protein called interferon (Cruess, Schneiderman, Antoni, & Penedo, 2004).

Immune deficiencies can be life threatening. Some people are born with immune-system deficiencies. You have probably heard of children who must grow up in isolation in order to be protected from common pathogens in the environment. **Human immunodeficiency virus (HIV)** is a contagious, life-threatening deficiency of the immune system. Over time, HIV may progress to **acquired immune deficiency syndrome (AIDS)**. HIV/AIDS patients may fall victim to pathogens commonly found in the environment. In other instances, people's immune systems are overactive. For example, some people are highly allergic to insect stings, foods such as peanuts and seafood, or to medicines such as penicillin. Being exposed to very small amounts of these substances causes allergic persons to experience a sudden life-threatening illness called **anaphylactic shock**. Symptoms may include swelling of the throat and closure of the airway, a rash, itching, burning of the skin and eyes, nausea, vom-

**immunology** The study of the body's response to foreign invasion.

**human immunodeficiency virus/acquired immune deficiency syndrome (HIV/AIDS)** HIV is a contagious virus that causes a life-threatening deficiency of the immune system (AIDS), leading to vulnerability to opportunistic infection and disease.

**anaphylactic shock** A serious allergic response to insect stings, foods such as peanuts and seafood, or to medicines such as penicillin; being exposed to very small amounts of these substances causes allergic persons to experience this sudden life-threatening illness.

iting, dizziness, confusion, restlessness, rapid pulse, coughing or wheezing, and tightness in the chest (American National Red Cross, 2005). Sometimes the face, neck, and tongue swell so a person is unable to breathe. Anaphylaxis requires emergency treatment. Some people who are highly allergic carry kits containing a syringe with a dose of epinephrine to counter the allergic reaction. Lupus and rheumatoid arthritis are autoimmune disorders in which the immune system produces antibodies against its own body tissue (Huyser & Parker, 2002). See **Figure 8.1** for organs of the immune system.

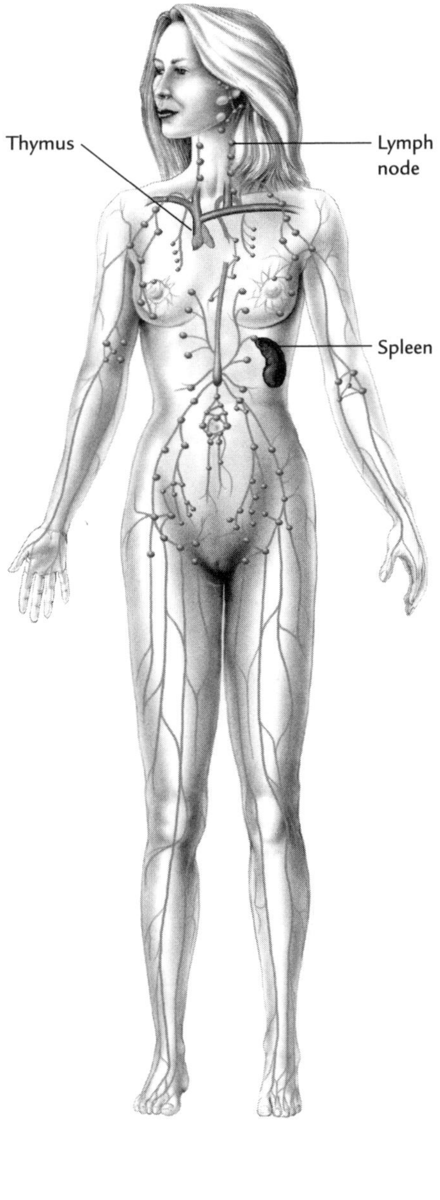

**Figure 8.1**
The immune system defends our body against disease-causing agents. Stress weakens the immune system, making us more vulnerable to disease.

# Psychoneuroimmunology (PNI)

Engel (1954), writing in the field of psychosomatic medicine, was among the first to suggest that diseases are rooted in many different causes, including psychological factors. Psychoneuroimmunology combines three areas of study that focus on the effects of stress on the body. *Psycho* refers to psychological factors, *neuro* to the nervous system's reaction to stressors, and *immunology* to cellular protection (Forlenza & Baum, 2004, p. 81). All three act together to combat development of disease. The field engages health psychologists and other researchers interested in the resistance of the immune system and the effects of physical, psychological, and sociocultural stressors on health. Stress directly lowers the resistance of the immune system, allowing invasion and infection by pathogens, resulting in illness. There are three less direct pathways between stress and health. First, negative emotions in response to stressors damage our health; second, stress contributes to poor health habits; and third, stress interferes with important social relationships. All three pathways put health at even greater risk. Psychoneuroimmunology is the study of the relationship between the nervous and immune systems. Many health psychologists are experts in this field of study.

## Negative Emotions Contribute to Illness and Death

Studies show that negative emotions intensify threats to health, affecting both the development of illness and the effectiveness of medical treatments on infections, cardiovascular disease, osteoporosis, arthritis, cancer, lupus, Alzheimer's disease, and periodontal disease (Kiecolt-Glaser et al., 2002). Depression, anxiety, anger, and hostility are just a few examples of negative emotions (Cruess et al., 2004). Depression is the most common psychiatric illness, and depression in turn increases the risk of experiencing a heart attack (Glassman & Shapiro, 1998). People with diabetes who are depressed are less likely to follow medical recommendations about controlling blood sugar levels (Katon, 1998). At the same time, many who experience serious illness become depressed as a result (Katon & Sullivan, 1990). Coronary heart disease is influenced by antagonistic behavior and hostility (Siegman, Townsend, Civelek, & Blumenthal, 2000). Hostility, including cynical attitudes and a tendency to respond to situations with anger, is linked to cardiovascular disease (Smith & Ruiz, 2002).

## Stress and Chronic Health Problems

Health psychology specialists in infectious diseases and PNI study the relationship of stress to susceptibility to disease, to vaccine effectiveness, and to reactivation of latent viruses. In their discussion of whether health psychologists can help prevent and treat diseases, Ironson, Balbin, and Schneiderman (2002) concluded that the answer to this question is "a qualified yes," because it is very difficult to measure stress responses related to psychosocial variables (pp. 23–24). For example, dealing with pediatric asthma is distressing for children and their families, and asthma attacks interfere with normal physical and social activity

(Creer, Bender, & Lucas, 2002, p. 255). **Atopic dermatitis (AD)**, or eczema, is a neuroder-matitis characterized by itching, redness, oozing, crusting, scratching, and thickening of the skin. It is often preceded and followed by shock, worry, and emotional upset (Tovian, 2002). Stress contributes to poor diabetic control by interfering with self-management and by in-creasing the intake of dietary sugar blocking insulin action (Wysocki & Buckloh, 2002; Cruess et al., 2004). HIV infection is a chronic disease, and its outcomes are influenced by psychosocial factors, including stress (Schneiderman, 1999). Students may believe that re-activation of the herpesvirus or fever blisters is often related to psychosocial stressors, which in turn causes more negative emotional reactions, exacerbating the problem. Herpes is a la-tent virus that may be reactivated. Studies investigating reactivation often measure increases in antibody titers to the virus, and numerous studies find that stress increases antibody titers. Results of studies on the stress-related recurrence of cold sores and genital herpes are mixed (Ironson, Balbin, & Schneiderman, 2004, pp. 13–14). In some studies, stressful life events are associated with cancer progression, but other studies do not report significant relationships. Stress-buffering factors such as social support may be more relevant than stressful life events (Henderson & Baum, 2004, pp. 46–47).

## Stress Influences Health Habits

Stressful psychosocial processes interact with biology, adversely affecting health. Stress con-tributes to deterioration in health-related practices, including failure to exercise, poor diet, smoking, and alcohol abuse. This puts people at greater risk of illness and injury (Cruess et al., 2004, p. 31). Poor health practices form the biobehavioral bases of common diseases such as cardiovascular disease and cancer. Stress increases the likelihood of starting and contin-uing substance abuse and to relapsing even after periods of abstinence (NIDA, 2008). Stress is a major contributor to relapses in smoking, contributing to both cancer and heart dis-ease. Stress often results in poorer sleep practices (Kiecolt-Glaser et al., 2002). Adverse envi-ronmental factors such as low socioeconomic status result in negative emotions, hostility, and belligerence, further aggravating behaviors detrimental to good health practices.

## Exam Stress

Have you noticed a tendency to get sick in the weeks following final exams? Both exam stress and academic stress negatively affect the immune system. This type of stress is considered

**atopic dermatitis (AD)** A neurodermatitis characterized by itching, redness, oozing, crusting, scratching, and thickening of the skin, also called eczema.

**naturalistic stress**, because taking exams is an actual experience for many (Forlenza & Baum, 2004, p. 94). Another study demonstrated that wound healing in students occurs more slowly during exam periods than during vacation periods (Kiecolt-Glaser, Marucha, Malarkey, Mercado, & Glaser, 1995). During exam periods, college students probably do not get enough rest, do not exercise, and do not sleep as much as at other times. Our immune systems and healing suffer when we do not take in adequate nutrients, exercise, or get enough rest.

## Laboratory Experiments and Stress

Research in PNI includes measurement of immune system response to various types of stressors generated under laboratory conditions. Experiments are designed to cause participants to feel threatened in some way. Some short-term experiments put participants through onerous tasks such as giving a speech or working mathematical problems and then test their blood for antibodies (Forlenza & Baum, 2004, pp. 97–98). (It is possible that taking multiple blood samples, even through in-dwelling catheters, increased participants' stress too.) In laboratory investigations of the effect of loud noises on immune response, participants given greater control experienced less immune suppression than those who had less control. This study lends credibility to the idea that resources that give one a sense of control over the environment may help offset the effects of stress. A sense of control reduces our stress levels and may help us maintain more competent immune systems.

## Experiencing Highly Traumatic Stressors

Facing highly stressful events threatening to our well-being or the well-being of others may trigger very serious physiological, psychological, social, and behavioral problems. One adaptive response to stress is the release of a neurotransmitter, **norepinephrine**, which is involved in memory. This may be one reason why people remember stressful events so clearly (NIDA, 2008). Experiencing a terrifying ordeal is often followed by recurring distress; because the event is so disturbing, the memory remains with us for a long time. Shell shock described the stress soldiers in World War I experienced. As many 20% of American soldiers who fought

---

**naturalistic stress**  A stressor faced outside of laboratory testing situations. One example is college students taking exams. When students take examinations their immune system may be weakened, resulting in illness.

**norepinephrine**  A hormone secreted by the adrenal medulla, and a neurotransmitter released at nerve endings that constricts small blood vessels, raises blood pressure, slows heart rate, increases breathing, and relaxes the smooth muscles of the intestinal tract.

in World War II experienced **combat stress reaction (CSR)**. Both shell shock and combat stress reaction were viewed as temporary or transient reactions to traumatic experiences in normal or nonpathological individuals (Bryant & Harvey, 2004, pp. 5–6).

The World Health Organization and the American Psychiatric Association define and include traumatic stress reactions in their classifications of diseases and mental disorders, emphasizing that these symptoms were persistent rather than transient. One outcome of the war in Vietnam was development of the concept of post-traumatic stress disorder (PTSD), an anxiety disorder defined by the American Psychiatric Association that results from experiencing a threat of death or injury to oneself or others, and very intense emotional reactions such as fear, helplessness, and horror (2004). Unlike other more transient anxiety reactions, PTSD persists through time. For example, soldiers returning home may continue to experience nightmares about danger. Even when awake they react to loud noises or sudden bright lights as though they were back in combat. Symptoms of PTSD and acute stress disorder (ASD) may include avoidance of people, places, and thoughts attached to a violent event. Other indicators are restlessness, sleeping difficulty or insomnia, irritability, hypervigilance, and increased startle response (Bryant & Harvey, 2004). Both PTSD and ASD impair normal functioning, and clinical psychologists and psychiatrists often treat victims of emotional trauma. The bombing of the federal building in Oklahoma City and terrorists' attacks in New York City and Washington, D.C., continue to haunt thousands of people. In one national survey, 17% of adults living outside of New York City continued to have PTSD symptoms 2 months after the attacks of September 11, 2001 (Silver, Holman, McIntosh, Poulin, and Gil-Rivas, 2002). Experiencing other disasters such as fires, hurricanes, and tornados also triggers these incapacitating disorders. Many victims of crime develop PTSD following assaults or rapes. Rates of PTSD are higher for women, the young, the less educated, and those with fewer socioeconomic resources (Cordova & Ruzek, 2004).

Some research indicates that many people exposed to severe trauma show only minor disruption in their ability to function. Bonanno (2004) suggests only about 10% to 15% of bereaved individuals exhibit chronic symptoms of PTSD. Many people are able to maintain healthy levels of biological and psychosocial adjustment in their lives in spite of severe stress. For example, some victims of childhood sexual abuse are able to disclose the abuse during therapy and then disassociate from their experiences, developing protective approaches to life (Bonanno, Noll, Putnam, O'Neil, & Tricket, 2003). **Resilience** refers to an

---

**combat stress reaction (CSR)** Name given to the reaction of some American soldiers to the stress of combat in World War II. It was viewed as a temporary or transient reaction to traumatic experiences in otherwise-normal individuals.

**resilience** Refers to an ability to maintain balance in the face of trauma and loss.

ability to maintain balance in the face of trauma and loss. Bonanno (2004) believes there are multiple pathways to resilience, including using positive emotions and laughter and avoiding unpleasant thoughts, emotions, and memories. The chapter on stress management includes a discussion of other ways to offset the effects of traumatic experiences.

## Stress and Relationships

Students will recall that death of a spouse received the highest score on the original social readjustment rating scale (SRSS) (Holmes & Rahe, 1967). Divorce, marital separation, death of a close family member, getting married, being fired at work, a marital reconciliation, retirement, pregnancy, sex difficulties, and similar items all appear on the SRSS scale. These items reflect changes and readjustments in social relationships at home and at work. In fact, the majority of the items on the SRSS were directly related to changes in relationships.

Pychoneuroimmunologists focusing on stress in married women found that the women who reported being less satisfied with their marriages had weaker immune function than those who reported greater marital satisfaction (Kiecolt-Glaser et al., 1987a). Stressful experiences in relationships may result when we are deprived of sleep, are responsible for relatives who are sick or disabled, or are separated from a spouse. All of these situations result in impaired immune function (Cruess et al., 2004, p. 44). There is poorer immune resistance in caregivers of people with Alzheimer's disease than among those caring for kin with acute injuries or illnesses such as a broken leg or the flu (Kiecolt-Glaser et al., 1987).

## Stress and Injuries

Injuries are the most common cause of emergency room visits and are more likely to happen to teens and young adults. Each year about 1 in 12 people seek medical treatment for injuries, and more than 150,000 people die from those injuries (American National Red Cross, 2005). Injuries are the leading cause of death for those aged 1 to 44 and are a significant public health issue (Dilillo, Peterson, & Farmer, 2002). There is less research in health psychology on the connections between stress and injury than about connections between stress and illness, but examples abound. **Rehabilitation psychology** focuses on the post-injury phase and centers on helping people with disabilities recover from injuries and disease. Treatment focuses on cognitive, emotional, behavioral, and social difficulties following disability (Dilillo et al., 2002, p. 570). Some solutions are found in the chapter on stress management. See **Figure 8.2** for the model of unintentional injuries (often called accidents).

---

**rehabilitation psychology** A specialty centering on helping people recover from injuries and disease. Treatment focuses on cognitive, emotional, behavioral, and social difficulties following disability.

**Figure 8.2**

Many automobile "accidents" are a result of stress and reflect biological and psychosocial causes.

*Source:* Edlin, G. & Golanty, E. (2007). *Health and wellness* (9th ed.). Sudbury, MA: Jones and Bartlett Publishers.

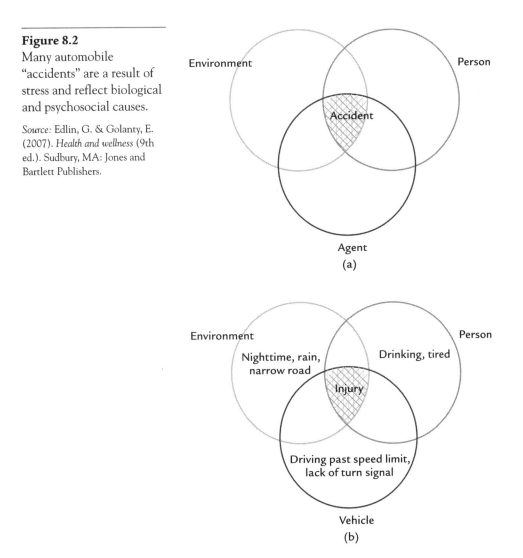

Stress associated with negative emotions such as depression, hostility, and anxiety plays a significant role in many injuries. For example, stress-induced alcohol abuse frequently results in automobile accidents. Substance abuse is discussed in an earlier chapter, but it is worth noting here that 13,952 alcohol-related vehicular fatalities were reported in 2004. This is equal to the occurrence of a traffic-related fatality every 31 minutes in the United States (National Highway Traffic Safety Administration, 2008). Alcohol usage is also a clear risk factor for drowning and traumatic brain injury (Dilillo et al., 2002, p. 561).

## Stress and Sports Injuries

There is evidence relating stress to sports-related injuries. These include injuries due to sports and to exercise. In competitive situations, injuries may be either intentional or unintentional. Injuries also result from poor training practices, improper equipment, lack of conditioning, or insufficient warmup and stretching (U.S. Department of Health and Human Services [DHHS], 2008). There may be some confusion, because the word stress is also applied to physical injuries resulting from repetitive impact on feet and legs. These are called **stress fractures** and are physiological rather than psychosocial. This section focuses on the connection between injuries and psychosocial stressors.

Millions of people are injured each year during sports events and recreational activities such as aerobic exercises and strength training. Psychosocial stress is one contributor to these injuries. At least two theories attempt to explain the relationship between stress and sports injuries, and both may be accurate. One theory suggests that stress interferes with concentration, making players less vigilant about danger so they miss warning cues and fail to protect themselves. Another possibility is that the physical arousal of stress combined with a competitive spirit increases muscle tension and reduces muscle coordination among players so they are more likely to get hurt.

Think about your own high school competitive experiences. Was your performance hurt or improved by the presence or absence of your parents or friends in the audience? Did you perform better or worse when you were worried about grades and exams? Athletes who have a history of playing under the influence of many stressors and who have few coping resources are more likely to experience injuries. Many times coaching decisions made in the hopes of winning a game also put players at risk. See **Figure 8.3** for cause of sports injuries among young males.

### Biological Approaches to Sports Injury Prevention
The chapter on exercise included discussion of ways to prevent exercise-related injuries. These recommendations also apply to athletes. Part of the physical preparation for sports events is maintaining a regular training program. Most professional and amateur athletes know to warm up their muscles and other soft tissue prior to both practices and events, to stretch for flexibility, to follow healthful nutritional practices, and to get adequate rest.

### Psychosocial Approaches to Sports Injury Prevention
From a psychological viewpoint, before participating in any competition, athletes typically clear their minds of negative emotions, including anxiety, anger, and fear, and visualize successful performances throughout the event. From a psychosocial viewpoint, team loyalty, mutual social support among players, and respect for coaching staffs contribute to injury-free experiences.

**stress fractures**  Physical injuries usually resulting from repetitive impact on limbs.

**Figure 8.3**

Emergency room admissions reflect sports and recreational injuries for males ages 10 to 19.

*Source:* CDC, National Center of Health Statistics, 2005, and Edlin, G. & Golanty, E. (2007). *Health and wellness* (9th ed.). Sudbury, MA: Jones and Bartlett Publishers.

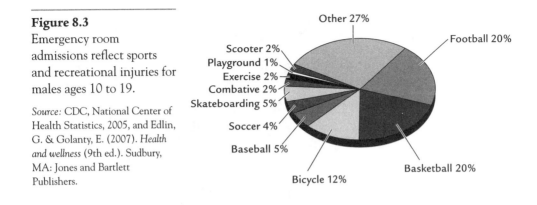

More than half of all sports injuries occur at practice, and about 3.5 million children ages 14 and younger receive medical treatment for sports injuries each year (National Center for Sports Safety, 2008, p. 1). Young athletes are often at greater risk of injury due to variety in size and physical maturity even at the same age. Some children try to perform at levels beyond their ability in order to keep up with their peers (DHHS, 2008, p. 10). Coaches and caregivers should understand that a child's self-esteem and enjoyment of sports are influenced by adults' reactions. It is important to acknowledge children's feelings of pain, fright, and anxiety. Caregivers should also provide emotional support, treat children with respect, and never ridicule or belittle them, especially in front of their peers. Children's mental health and development are as important as physical health (DHHS, 2008, pp. 17–18).

Major life events and the amount of change players have recently experienced contribute to injuries. Researchers altered the SRRS and gave it to high school football players (Bramwell, Masuda, Wagner, & Holmes, 1975). They discovered that high life-change scores correlated significantly with injuries on the playing field. Football players with low levels of change had an injury rate of about 30%. Players whose life-change scores were in the middle third of the players had a 50% chance of an injury. Players with high levels of life change had a 73% injury rate. When the SRRS was given to players in non-contact sports, similar results occurred.

Most other studies are based on football players, but some include baseball, skiing, skating, and women's collegiate gymnastics (Williams, Rotella, & Heyman, 1998). Social support and coping skills also play a role in injury prevention. Additional study found that injuries were higher among athletes with fewer coping skills and low levels of social support (Smith, Smoll, & Ptacek, 1990). An increase in the number of daily hassles also contributes to injuries (Fawkner, 1995). Knowledgeable coaches can use this information to screen players for life changes and hassles and avoid putting excessive pressure on vulnerable athletes (see **Figure 8.4**).

Professional athletes are highly visible and expected to be role models for younger athletes (Quick, Gavin, Cooper, & Quick, 2004). Athletics takes a great deal of time and even college athletes spend 30 to 60 hours a week on their sport (Miller, 1999). The primary psychosocial problems seen in athletes are anxiety, stress, depression, eating disorders, substance

**Figure 8.4**
Atheletes are under constant pressure to excel and win. Stress and distraction contribute to injuries.

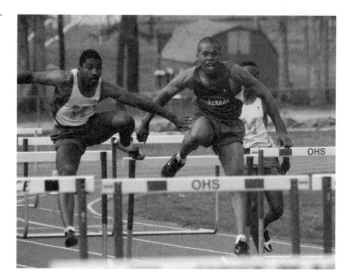

abuse, and relationship issues. The public's expectations and athletes' underdeveloped life skills may block realization that they need therapeutic counseling (Quick et al., 2004). Athletes often experience social isolation and interact only with team members, coaching staff members, agents, and family (Begel & Baum, 2000).

## Summary

There is a mutually reinforcing or bidirectional relationship between stress and illness or injury. Stress contributes to both, and both create additional stress in human lives. Biologically we are protected from injury by the skeletal structures of our body. The immune system and cellular structure protect us against pathogens. Health psychologists and other scientists in the field of psychoneuroimmunology discovered stressful situations can damage that immune function, leading to illness and death. Potentially health-damaging social situations include marital discord, caring for a parent with Alzheimer's disease or another disability, and taking examinations in school. Psychosocial indicators of stress include negative emotions such as fear, anxiety, depression, and anger. These negative emotions decrease the ability of immune systems to protect us against pathogens such as viruses. When we are under stress we are more likely to become ill. Further, people distracted by stress are more likely to be injured in accidents and while participating in competitive events.

Stress encourages some people to abuse alcohol and other substances, to overeat, to drive recklessly, and to get less sleep. Social relationships suffer when we are faced with stressors. Some people are more vulnerable to the effects of stressors on their physical and mental health due to sociocultural factors such as poverty. All of these practices and conditions negatively affect health. Behaviors that make us less vulnerable to stress include getting adequate rest, regular aerobic exercise, good nutritional practices, finding enjoyable ways to relax, and maintaining close social relationships. In extremely threatening situations such as war, abuse, and crime, some people develop post-traumatic stress disorders.

Research shows that stress also contributes to sports injuries. Good training practices and positive relationships with teammates and coaches help offset stressors associated with competition. Athletes going through many life changes are more likely to be injured than those experiencing less change. Coaches and parents of child athletes must be especially careful about what they say and do at games in order to maintain the child's self-esteem and the sense of fun associated with sports. Professional athletes are faced with special problems including performance pressures, public adulation and high expectations, few social relationships, and physical complaints.

## Review Questions

1. Explain the quote: "People get sick not only from what they eat but from what is 'eating' them."

2. Give examples of how stress may cause problems in physical health, psychological health, and social relationships.

3. Describe how stress causes illness and how illness causes stress.

4. List some common indicators that people are dealing with stressors in their lives.

5. Clarify the relationship between vulnerability to stressors and the effects of stress on our health.

6. Define post-traumatic stress disorder and cite three examples of situations that may cause it.

7. Explain mechanical and cellular protection humans have against the effects of stressors.

8. What is the basis of the science of psychoneuroimmunology and how does it relate to stress?

9. From the research, cite three different examples of the effects of psychosocial stressors on immune function.

10. Describe the ways stress is related to sports injuries.

11. Describe recommended approaches to sports injury prevention.

## Student Activity

Choose and describe an illness or injury that occurred in your life over the past few years. Think and then hypothesize about the physical, psychological, and sociocultural factors that contributed to the illness or injury. Summarize the physical, emotional, and social difficulties that developed as a result of the injury or illness. This includes your own difficulties and those of your family, friends, fellow students, teachers, and coworkers. In retrospect explain what you could have done to prevent or avoid the illness or injury and what you might have done to speed recovery.

# References

American Psychiatric Association. (2004). *Diagnostic and statistical manual of mental disorders* (4th ed.). Washington, DC: Author.

American National Red Cross. (2005). *First aid, responding to emergencies* (4th ed.). Yardley, PA: StayWell.

Begel, D., & Baum, A. L. (2000). The athlete's role. In D. Begel & R. W. Burton (Eds.), *Sports psychiatry* (pp. 55–56). New York: W.W. Norton & Company.

Bonanno, G. A. (2004). Loss, trauma, and human resilience. *American Psychologist, 59*(1), 20–28.

Bonanno, G. A., Noll, J., Putnam, F. W., O'Neill, M., & Tricket, P. (2003). Predicting the willingness to disclose childhood sexual abuse from measures of repressive coping and disassociated experiences. *Child Maltreatment, 8,* 1–17.

Bramwell, S. T, Masuda, M., Wagner, N. N., & Holmes, T. H. (1975). Psychosocial factors in athletic injuries. *Journal of Human Stress, 2,* 6–20.

Bryant, R. A., & Harvey, A. G. (2004). *Acute stress disorder: A handbook of theory, assessment, and treatment.* Washington, DC: American Psychological Association.

Cordova, M. J., & Ruzek, J. I. (2004). Posttraumatic stress disorder. In A. J. Christensen, R. Martin, & J. M. Smyth (Eds.), *Encyclopedia of health psychology* (pp. 215–218). New York: Kluwer Academic/Plenum.

Creer, T. L., Bender, B. G., & Lucas, D. O. (2002). Diseases of the respiratory system. In S. B. Johnson, N. W. Perry, Jr., & R. H. Rozensky (Eds.), *Handbook of clinical health psychology* (Vol. 1, pp. 239–282). Washington, D.C.: American Psychological Association.

Cruess, D. G., Schneiderman, N., Antoni, M. H., & Penedo, F. (2004). In R. G. Frank, A. Baum, & J. L. Wallander (Eds.), *Handbook of clinical health psychology* (Vol. 3, pp. 31–79). Washington, DC: American Psychological Association.

Dilillo, D., Peterson, L., & Farmer, J. E., (2002). Injury and poisoning. In S. B. Johnson, N. W. Perry, Jr., & R. H. Rozensky (Eds.), *Handbook of clinical health psychology* (Vol. 1, pp. 555–582). Washington, DC: American Psychological Association.

Engel, G. L. (1954). Selection of clinical material in psychosomatic medicine. *Psycho-Somatic Medicine, 16,* 368–378.

Fawkner, H. J. (1995). *Predisposition to injury in athletes: The role of psychosocial factors.* Unpublished master's thesis, University of Melbourne, Melbourne, Australia.

Forlenza, M. J., & Baum, A. (2004). Psychoneuroimmunology. In R. G. Frank, A. Baum, & J. L. Wallander (Eds.), *Handbook of clinical health psychology* (Vol. 3, pp. 81–114). Washington, DC: American Psychological Association.

Friedman, M., & Rosenman, R. H. (1959). Association of a specific overt behavior pattern with increases in blood cholesterol, blood clotting time, incidence of arcus senilis, and clinical coronary artery disease. *Journal of the American Medical Association, 169,* 1286–1296.

Glassman, A. H., & Shapiro, P. A. (1998). Depression and the course of coronary artery disease. *American Journal of Psychiatry, 155,* 4–11.

Henderson, B. N., & Baum, A. (2004). Neoplasms. In S. B. Johnson, N. W. Perry, Jr., & R. H. Rozensky (Eds.), *Handbook of clinical health psychology* (Vol. 1, pp. 37–64). Washington, DC: American Psychological Association.

Holmes, T. H., & Rahe, R. H. (1967). The social readjustment rating scale. *Journal of Psychosomatic Research, 11,* 213–218.

Huyser, B. A., & Parker, J. C., (2002). Rheumatic diseases. In S. B. Johnson, N. W. Perry, Jr., & R. H. Rozensky (Eds.), *Handbook of clinical health psychology* (Vol. 1, pp. 399–441). Washington, DC: American Psychological Association.

Ironson, G., Balbin, E., & Schneiderman, N. (2002), Health psychology and infectious diseases. In S. B. Johnson, N. W. Perry, Jr., & R. H. Rozensky (Eds.), *Handbook of clinical health psychology* (Vol. 1, pp. 5–36). Washington, DC: American Psychological Association.

Katon, W., & Sullivan, M. D. (1990). Depression and chronic medical illness. *Journal of Clinical Psychiatry, 51,* 3–11.

Katon, W. (1998). The effect of major depression on chronic medical illness. *Seminar in Clinical Neuropsychiatry, 3,* 82–86.

Kiecolt-Glaser, J., Fisher, L., Ogrocki, P., Stout, J., Speicher, C., & Glaser, R. (1987a). Marital quality, marital disruption, and immune function. *Psychosomatic Medicine, 49,* 13–34.

Kiecolt-Glaser, J. K., Glaser, R., Shuttleworth, E. C., et al. (1987b). Chronic stress and immunity in family caregivers of Alzheimer's-disease victims. *Psychosomatic Medicine, 49,* 523–535.

Kiecolt-Glaser, J. K., Marucha, P. T., Malarkey, W. B., Mercado, A. M., & Glaser, R. (1995). Slowing of wound-healing by psychological stress. *Lancet, 346,* 1194–1196.

Kiecolt-Glaser, J. K., McGuire, L., Robles, T. F., & Glaser, R. (2002). Emotions, morbidity, and mortality: New perspectives from psychoneuroimmunology. *Annual Review of Psychology, 53,* 83–107.

Martin, P. D., & Brantley, P. J. (2004). Stress, coping, and social support. In J. M. Raczynski & L. C. Leviton (Eds.), *Handbook of clinical health psychology* (Vol. 2, pp. 233–268). Washington, DC: American Psychological Association.

Miller, P. (1999). *Life skills development in high-level sport.* Paper presented at the 7th International Post-Graduate Seminar on Olympic Studies. Olympia, Greece.

National Center for Sports Safety. (2008). The rate and severity of sports-related injuries increases with a child's age. Retrieved February 12, 2008 from http://www.sportssafety.org

National Highway Traffic Safety Administration. Counter Measures That Work. Retrieved February 2, 2008 at http://www.nhtsa.dot.gov

National Institute on Drug Abuse. (2008). NIDA Community Drug Alert Bulletin—Stress & Substance Abuse. Retrieved February 8, 2008 from http://www.drugabuse.gov/StressAlert/StressAlert.html

Quick, J. C., Gavin, J. H., Cooper, C. L., & Quick, J. D. (2004). Working together: Balancing head and heart. In R. H. Rozensky, N. G. Johnson, C. D. Goodheart, & W. R. Hammong (Eds.), *Psychology builds a healthy world: Opportunities for research and practice* (pp. 219–273). Washington, DC: American Psychological Association.

Schneiderman, N. (1999). Behavioral medicine and the management of HIV/AIDS. *International Journal of Behavioral Medicine, 6,* 3–12.

Seematter, G., Guenat, E., Schneiter, P., Cayoeux, C., Jequier, E., & Trappy, L. (2000). Effects of mental stress on insulin-mediated glucose metabolism and energy expenditure in lean and obese women. *American Journal of Physiology, Endocrinology and Metabolism, 279,* 799–805.

Siegman, A. W., Townsend, S. T., Civelek, A. C., & Blumental, R. S. (2000). Antagonistic behavior, dominance, hostility, and coronary heart disease. *Psychosomatic Medicine, 62,* 248–257.

Silver, R. C., Holman, E. A., McIntosh, D. N., Poulin, M., & Gil-Rivas, V. (2002). Nationwide longitudinal study of psychological responses to September 11. *Journal of the American Medical Association, 288,* 1235–1244.

Smith, R. E., Smoll, F. L., & Ptacek, J. T. (1990). Conjunctive moderator variables in vulnerability and resiliency research: Life stress, social support and coping skills and adolescent sport injuries. *Journal of Personality and Social Psychology, 58,* 360–369.

Smith, T. W., & Ruiz, J. M. (2002). Psychosocial influences on the development and course of coronary heart disease: Current status and implications for research and practice. *Journal of Consulting and Clinical Psychology, 70,* 548–568.

Thompson, R. J., Jr., & Van Loon, K. J. (2002). Mental disorders. In S. B. Johnson, N. W. Perry, Jr., & R. H. Rozensky (Eds.), *Handbook of clinical health psychology* (Vol. 1, pp. 143–172). Washington, DC: American Psychological Association.

Tovian, S. M. (2002). Diseases of the skin and subcutaneous tissue. In S. B. Johnson, N. W. Perry, Jr., & R. H. Rozensky (Eds.), *Handbook of clinical health psychology* (Vol. 1, pp. 371–397). Washington, DC: American Psychological Association,

U.S. Department of Health and Human Services. (2008). Sports Injuries. Retrieved February 12, 2008 from http://www.pueblo.gsa.gov

Williams, J. M., Rotella, R. J. & Heyman, S. R. (1998). Stress, injury and the psychological rehabilitation of athletes. In J. M. Williams (Ed.), *Applied sport psychology* (pp. 409–428). Mountain View, CA: Mayfield Publishing Company.

Wysocki, T. & Buckloh, L. M. (2002). Endocrine, metabolic, nutritional, and immune disorders. In S. B. Johnson, N. W. Perry, Jr., & R. H. Rozensky (Eds.), *Handbook of clinical health psychology* (Vol. 1, pp. 65–99). Washington, DC: American Psychological Association.

# Chapter 9

# Coping and Stress Management

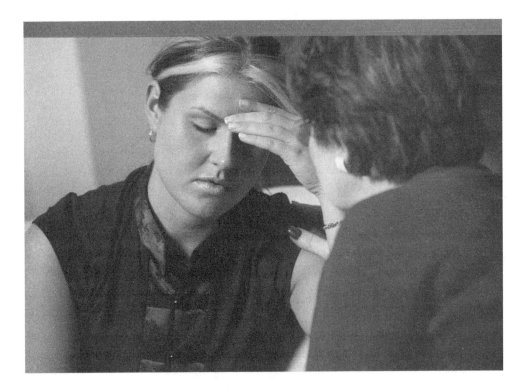

## Learning Objectives

After studying this chapter students will have the knowledge and skills to be able to:

1. Explain what is meant by coping and stress management.
2. Identify ways coping is linked to physical and emotional health.
3. Describe the transactional process of coping.
4. Explain how coping styles are measured.
5. Distinguish between emotion-focused and problem-focused coping, giving examples of each.
6. List and explain three cognitive coping strategies.
7. Summarize the benefits of developing social support.

8. Explain the various ways personality is related to stress.

9. Define resilience and explain how it helps in responding to stressors.

10. Briefly describe biological approaches to stress management.

11. Summarize and evaluate three stress management methods that can be accomplished alone or with the help of trained personnel.

## Introduction

At this point in the course, students understand that stress is an important research topic in health psychology. Stress contributes to emotional and physical illnesses and to injuries, and interferes with recovery from both. You already know that many humans respond to stressors at the physiological level with arousal of the nervous system and subsequent jeopardy to their immune systems. When threatened, some people respond at the behavioral level by smoking more, overeating, and abusing substances such as alcohol. This further endangers their health and safety. Emotional responses to stress include depression and negative emotions such as anger, helplessness, and shame. At the cognitive level we respond to stressors by worry, flashbacks of trauma, and even memory loss (Martin & Brantly, 2004). The biopsychosocial approach of health psychology is ideal for discussions of interactions among biopsychosocial pathways.

This chapter summarizes research about **coping** and **stress management**. Both skills are useful in life, so this chapter can help students live healthier lives. Many stressors are individual problems based in unique personal perceptions of situations that cause stress. Nevertheless, everyone's health benefits from developing good coping and stress management skills.

Coping refers to people's efforts or behaviors to meet the challenges of stressors in their lives and to alleviate residual distress. Common stressors include physical and psychological problems; troubles with relationships at home, school, work, or play; monumental disasters such as fires, wars, explosions, and hurricanes; and minor stressors or hassles. Stress management refers to interventions or programs designed to improve the ability to cope by increasing knowledge and skills. As students, you are currently coping each semester with the chronic stressors involved in taking courses required to earn a college degree.

The ability to cope is a learned skill. Coping skills do improve with practice and usually with age. You realize this fact when you compare your current coping skills with those you used in elementary and high school. You may now handle difficulties in more productive

**coping**  People's efforts or behaviors to meet the challenges of stressors in their lives and to alleviate distress.

**stress management**  Interventions or programs designed to improve people's ability to cope by increasing their knowledge and skills.

and effective ways. As we grow older, we even discover what types of coping mechanisms are more effective for us and what types are not.

Competent coping contributes to biological, psychological, and sociocultural health. There is an entire array of physiological problems you might face as college students. For example, if you break a leg, you learn to get around with a cast until the bone heals. When you contract a bacterial infection, you go to the campus health center for an antibiotic and take it correctly. When a physical health issue such as arthritis becomes chronic, people develop new skills and become adept at handling the pain, limitations, and inconvenience. Psychological problems can range from severe mental illness requiring long-term psychiatric care to comparatively less complicated problems like anger control, depression, or phobias such as fear of flying. Relationship problems requiring coping include serious disagreements with parents, siblings, spouses, peers, coworkers, and professors. Very serious relationship stressors include the loss of loved ones through divorce or death. New situations present opportunities to develop new proficiencies in coping.

**Proactive coping** refers to actions to prevent exposure to known stressors (Aspinwall, 1997). There are positive ways to accomplish even preemptive coping. Exercise, good nutritional practices, and getting adequate amounts of sleep improve our physical and emotional health, making us more resistant when facing stressors. Unhealthy coping includes becoming so enraged over problems we put our fist through a door, get drunk, or drive recklessly. These methods often produce additional problems, causing additional stress. Students realize that "fighting or fleeing" is rarely the most efficient or healthiest way to respond to stress. Many times our response to stressors puts at risk our physical, emotional, and social health.

Learning stress management techniques also contributes to better health. Therapies used in health psychology include both cognitive and behavioral interventions designed for stress management. Pain is a stressor, and many of the methods taught for managing pain, such as **biofeedback**, are also useful in managing other types of stressors. Other stress management techniques include **stress inoculation training (SIT)**,

**proactive coping** Taking actions to prevent exposure to known stressors.

**biofeedback** A cognitive-behavioral instructional process combining talk therapy with technology to teach individuals to gain control over anxiety, tension, or pain. Sensors placed on the body feed back information to a receiver that emits sound or light depending on muscle tension. Individuals learn to control and relax tense areas of the body to such an extent that the sound or light fades and disappears. The success of biofeedback-facilitated relaxation training (BFRT) depends on the individual following up on training sessions by frequently practicing going into relaxed states of mind and body.

**stress inoculation training (SIT)** A form of cognitive-behavioral therapy designed to immunize people against stress. SIT consists of three stages: conceptualization, skills development and application, and coping skills, including relaxation, distraction, and redefinition.

**guided imagery**, meditation, **deep breathing**, and **progressive muscle relaxation (PMR)**. The last refers to the skill of intentionally relaxing our bodies when faced with stressors. In most situations, stress management techniques will be better for our health than fighting or fleeing. Mediators of stress include our physical condition or state of wellness, our psychological emotional states, our personalities, our coping abilities, the level of social support we receive from others, and our ability to learn and use stress management practices. Three of the most heavily researched moderators of stress in health psychology are coping, social support, and stress management interventions.

## Defining Coping

Coping refers to ways of handling or dealing with stressors in our physical, psychological, and sociocultural environments. Coping is a complex process and it requires effort. Coping includes using thoughts or cognitions, emotions, and behaviors to adapt successfully to stress. One purpose of coping is to intervene during stressful events and prevent the occurrence of negative outcomes such as illness or injury. Coping includes behaviors used when directly facing stressful situations and strategies to alleviate the resulting distress. We can choose from a wide range of thoughts and behaviors to cope with threats or demands made upon us. See the Think About It! feature for examples of college student stressors.

Sometimes we have no reaction to common stressors. When faced with demands, we may decide to tolerate or ignore a threat. On the other hand, we may take drastic, far-reaching efforts to reduce or eliminate threats to well-being. There are many choices in between these two extremes. Because stress is based in each individual's perception of a situation, identical situations trigger different responses in different people. For example, in response to threats, some people react emotionally and become angry, while others become depressed. Still others view threats in a positive light and see stressors as exciting new challenges with opportunities for self-improvement.

Here is an extreme and unlikely example of the range of reactions to a serious stressor. Imagine a lion leaping into your bedroom one night. You could turn over and go back to

---

**guided imagery** A therapist guides patients' thinking so they visualize or imagine a pleasant relaxing situation. Individuals learn to use their own imaginations whenever they feel stressed.

**deep breathing** A stress management/relaxation technique that encourages one to give attention only to one's breathing rather than thinking about anything else.

**progressive muscle relaxation (PMR)** A stress management/relaxation technique based on first tensing and then relaxing muscle groups to gain an understanding about the way a muscle or limb feels when relaxed.

## Think About It!

### Does This Describe You?

**Academic**
Competition
Schoolwork (difficult, low motivation)
Exams and grades
Poor resources (library, computers)
Oral presentations/public speaking
Professors/coaches (unfair, demanding, unavailable)
Choosing and registering for classes
Choosing a major/career

**Time**
Deadlines
Procrastination
Waiting for appointments and in lines
No time to exercise
Late for appointments or class

**Environment**
Others' behavior (rude, inconsiderate, sexist/racist)
Injustice: seeing examples or being a victim of
Crowds/large social groups
Fears of violence/terrorism
Weather (snow, heat/humidity, storms)
Noise
Lack of privacy

**Social**
Obligations, annoyances (family/friends/girl-/boyfriend)
Not dating
Roommate(s)/housemate(s) problems
Concerns about STDs

**Self**
Behavior (habits, temper)
Appearance (unattractive features, grooming)
Ill health/physical symptoms
Forgetting, misplacing, or losing things
Weight/dietary management
Self-confidence/self-esteem
Boredom

**Money**
Not enough
Bills/overspending
Job: searching for or interviews
Job/work issues (demanding, annoying)

**Tasks of Daily Living**
Tedious chores (shopping, cleaning)
Traffic and parking problems
Car problems (breaking down, repairs)
Housing (finding/getting or moving)
Food (unappealing or unhealthful meals)

*Source:* Edlin, G., & Golanty, E. (2007). *Health and wellness* (9th ed.). Sudbury, MA: Jones and Bartlett Publishers.

sleep, assuming it is a bad dream. You could escape by jumping out of the window. You could pick up a gun and shoot the lion. There are many other options that fall between ignoring a threat and taking extreme action. For example, you could call for help and fend off the lion with a chair as you saw lion tamers do on television or at a circus. You have many choices about coping with this threat.

## Coping Is a Process

Coping is a response to stressful situations in life. Coping is shaped by many factors including our emotional state, our personality, our previous experiences, our social relationships, our sociocultural backgrounds, and especially by resources available to us. Students will recall from a previous chapter that Lazarus (1966) and Lazarus and Folkman (1984) suggested that when faced with a demand or stressor we will go through a cognitive process or think about the threat. This is a transactional process between the demands made by stressors upon us and the resources we have available for coping. **Appraisal** is an intellectual activity in response to a specific demand. People evaluate threatening situations and think about possible responses. The process is dynamic or changeable, because people often alter their reaction when they gain new insight into a situation or after they try a few methods of coping.

### A Review of the Transactional Process of Coping

People first think about whether an event is irrelevant and neutral, positive and good, or negative and threatening. Vulnerable people may decide they are helpless in the face of a threat and give up. Others who have a greater sense of self-efficacy and control rise to meet challenges. For example, when hearing the diagnosis of a life-threatening cancer, some people give up, deciding they are powerless in the face of the illness and the situation is hopeless. Others seek additional medical advice and explore different treatment options. They join support groups and adopt healthier lifestyles to offset the effects of the cancer. There are support groups for many different stressors of college students. These are organized by campus counseling centers. **Reappraisal** of a stressful situation is often a continuous process as people gain new perspectives and increase their understanding of important factors associated with a source of stress. After appraisal and reappraisal comes coping. Coping may take different forms and includes a variety of strategies to manage both the stressors and our emotions or feelings about the stressors.

Imagine your professor announcing that students who earned below a score of 50 on the last exam must attend tutoring sessions. You scored more than 50, so you are unaffected. You do not feel personally threatened by the announcement. Affected students continue to the next stage of coping by thinking about their options. They move into secondary appraisal to decide what can be done in response to the stressor. Anxiety interferes with academic performance and is affected by coping ability (see **Figure 9.1**).

**appraisal** The first stage of the coping process in which persons think about a stressor or demand made upon them. People evaluate threatening situations and think about possible responses.

**reappraisal** Another stage in the coping process following the initial appraisal of a stressful situation.

**Figure 9.1**
Being too anxious distracts the mind and reduces academic performance. Many students have test anxiety.

*Source:* Edlin, G. & Golanty, E. (2007). *Health and wellness* (9th ed.). Sudbury, MA: Jones and Bartlett Publishers.

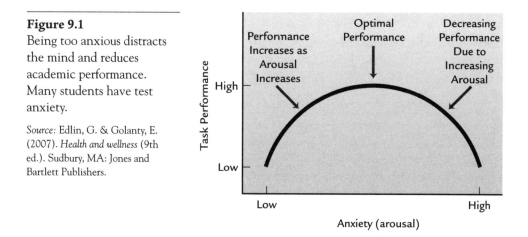

## Measuring Coping Styles

Students will recall that stressors can be labeled as chronic or acute, major or minor, and be associated with specific situations such as jobs, conflicting role expectations, illness, or injury. As mentioned earlier, Holmes and Rahe (1967) devised the social readjustment rating scale to predict illness by assigning points to reflect the amount of stress generated by 43 events. Other researchers try to assess coping using other measures, such as Folkman and Lazarus's (1988) ways of coping questionnaire, which assesses a variety of cognitive and behavioral coping responses to stressors. Using a Likert-type 4-point scale ranging from "most likely to use" to "least likely to use," respondents report their preferred coping techniques. The statistical technique of multiple factor analysis produced varying results. In a concise description and evaluation, Martin and Brantley (2004) report no current consensus in research and contradictory findings with regard to the ways of coping questionnaire.

## Two General Types of Coping

Health psychology research suggests two general ways of coping. It is possible to use either or both in a given situation (Lazarus & Folkman, 1984). There are alternatives within each general type. **Problem-focused coping** aims at managing a stressor. **Emotion-focused coping** is directed toward managing feelings aroused by a stressor.

**problem-focused coping**  Coping aimed toward managing a stressor.

**emotion-focused coping**  Coping directed toward managing the emotions or feelings aroused by a stressor.

## Emotion-Focused Coping

Emotion-focused coping addresses managing feelings when facing stressors. This type of coping is more useful when there is not a great deal a person can do about a stressor. There are positive and healthful ways to cope emotionally. Some people simply laugh the threat off by finding humor in the situation. Another option is to seek comfort from others. We can be consoled by family members and friends. Hugs and other kinds of reassuring touching are used during childhood to soothe and comfort. Spiritual, religious, or philosophical approaches may be part of emotion-based responses to stressors. Prayer and meditation are examples of this approach. Maladaptive or unhealthy ways of emotional coping include abusing alcohol or other mood-altering substances that numb our emotions. Some smokers cope with stressors by lighting up more cigarettes than usual (National Institute on Drug Abuse [NIDA], 2008).

Crying can be a useful emotion-focused coping technique, because it expresses or gives vent to distress. Adolescent girls and adult women are more likely to be encouraged to cry than boys or men, because in this culture it is less acceptable for boys and men to cry (William & Best, 1990). From youth, boys are teased if they shed tears when confronted by stressful situations. This eliminates crying in public as an option to relieve tension by boys. In most communities, it is acceptable for boys and adult males to cry at funerals of close family members or friends. Other examples of emotion-focused coping are yelling, hitting, slamming a book on a table, or angrily walking away. These are currently more acceptable ways for males to show disappointment or frustration. This is unfortunate for the health of males, because anger is associated with higher pain levels in some studies (Burns, 1997).

## Emotional Disclosure

Students will remember from the previous chapter that fears, anxiety, and depression have negative effects on the immune system. Talking with a professional counselor or other **emotional disclosure** often helps in dealing with stress (see **Figure 9.2**).

Research also indicates that writing or journaling about stressful events can be a healthful response to stressors. A great deal of research suggests that both emotional and physical health is at risk when we avoid expressing our thoughts and feelings (Pennebaker, 1995, 1997). Some people develop symptoms of a biological illness following a traumatic event and are relieved by emotional disclosure that even improves their immune function (Petrie, Booth, Pennebaker, Davison, & Thomas, 1995). Keeping a journal or diary can be done in conjunction with other coping methods such as joining a support group or talking to a therapist. In a study of the stressors involved in going through genetic testing for adult-

**emotional disclosure** Relieving stress from a traumatic event by talking with someone or writing or journaling it.

**Figure 9.2**
Professional counselors are usually available at
college counseling centers.

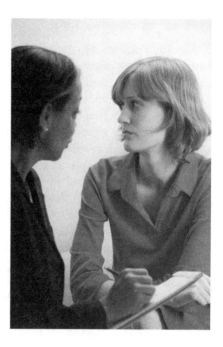

onset diseases, health psychologists designed a psychosocial telephone counseling intervention to identify changeable and unchangeable aspects of stressors, problem solving, decision making, and thought changing (Wenzel & Glanz, 2004). The study also incorporated
coping effectiveness training, including problem management, and emotional regulation
(Chesney, Folkman, & Chambers, 1996).

   Avoidant Coping
Distracting ourselves and postponing stressful situations are other examples of emotion-
focused coping. If we do not want to think about problems right away, we can read or watch
television. Later, new and different options may occur to us. Studies often refer to this temporary solution as **avoidant coping** (Suls & Fletcher, 1985). In some situations, denial and
disengagement are damaging. For example, people who suspect a serious illness or injury
may delay seeking medical care rather than face negative diagnoses. Delay is detrimental for
most diseases and injuries (Cruess, Schneiderman, Antoni, & Penedo, 2004). Research
shows that an active coping style is associated with a lower likelihood of symptom development in HIV-infected gay men, while denial about the disease predicts a greater number of
symptoms and poorer immune response (Cruess et al., 2004).

**avoidant coping**  Reacting to a stressor by denial or minimizing a threat rather than
taking some kind of action to resolve the issue.

## Problem-Focused Coping

Problem-focused coping meets and reduces demands being made on us by threatening situations. As adults, our problem-focused coping skills include planning and setting goals to find practical solutions to stressors. As you would expect, people who are optimistic are more likely to experience less distress when dealing with psychosocial issues than pessimistic people. People may be able to view some stressors as opportunities for learning new things, making it more likely they will reach important long-term goals. When facing stressors as educated adults, we can expand our coping repertoire by seeking new viewpoints, knowledge, and resources. For example, librarians can point students directly to useful sources of information, yet many college students use the library only for study or to check out required books and articles. We can also talk with friends who faced similar stressors, or we can consult clinical professionals to help us find solutions to stressors. College counseling centers help with both personal and academic problems.

Crying is an emotional expression, but under some circumstance it may generate access to more resources. Crying is problem-focused coping when it is used to move others to act to relieve our distress. When you were an infant, you coped with stressors by crying to communicate with your caregivers. This behavior or action told them you were hungry, wet, hot, cold, or anxious. Some adults use crying to manipulate others, and crying sometimes stops aggressive behavior in others (Vingerhoets, 2004).

## Cognitive Coping Strategies

**Cognition** refers to ways of thinking about things. There are many sayings that encourage cognitive change about stressors or that suggest one's perspective may change over time. If you tend to view every stressful event as catastrophic, then others may encourage you to remember other situations that improved with time. Some people analyze, intellectualize, and then postpone facing stressful situations until they have a better perspective for addressing them.

## Take Direct Action

One way to deal with stressors is to take direct action. This style of coping is fairly straightforward, but taking direct action sometimes seems too obvious and simple, and so many think of it last when considering their options. For example, if you do not like a course you are taking or if you are failing and see no hope for a better grade, you can drop the course. The same approach holds true for jobs we dislike.

**cognition** Thinking, learning, or the process of knowing or interpreting.

## Acquire More Knowledge and Skills

Increasing knowledge and skills is always an excellent way to cope with aversive conditions in our lives. Perhaps you are seeking a college degree because you want to improve your standing in the job market. If you want to improve technical skills, you can take courses specific to that purpose. Training courses are available in many cities and at junior colleges. Books and the Internet provide information and help develop abilities—and there are hundreds of books about stress management. Assertiveness training, conflict management, and effective communication can help minimize stress.

## Improve One's Sense of Control over Life

"Time management skills, focusing on establishing priorities, maintaining leisure and enjoyable activities, and scheduling time effectively, are especially useful strategies for managing stress overload" (Martin & Brantley, 2004, p. 241). Research demonstrates that increasing our inner sources of control and emotional strength are very beneficial in dealing with stressors. Self-efficacy refers to the belief that one can gain control over situations (Bandura, 1997). People develop the ability to solve problems and become more capable of controlling stressors. One way to improve control over our lives is to become more efficient and organized. People improve control by making lists of things they need or want to do. They gain satisfaction and a sense of accomplishment by checking off each item as it is accomplished. Once you have a list of things to do, you can even reorder the list by prioritizing items according to importance and due dates. For example, exam dates and due dates for papers are strict deadlines. It is more stressful to leave academic work to the last minute, so even daily and weekly time schedules can be beneficial. Writing up a time schedule to prevent conflicts can provide a sense of control.

## Seek and Develop Social Support

**Social support** makes an enormous difference in our physical and emotional health. Social support is a broad concept referring to the many ways social relationships promote well-being and success when facing stressful situations. Most of us have several sources of social support including friends, family members, coworkers, and neighbors, as well as groups of people based on religious preference, recreational choices, and other activities such as hobbies. At home and in kindergarten you learned to share and take turns. You were taught basic politeness such as saying "please" and "thank you." Standard politeness is

**social support** Efforts by others to make us feel loved and valuable, including providing tangible help and encouragement during sad times.

essential to gaining and maintaining social support. Relationships and social support from others provide us with a sense of value and self-worth and are resources in times of trouble.

In most studies, isolated people are not as healthy as people with supportive social relationships (Berkman & Syme, 1979; Berkman & Breslow, 1983). Turning to others for help is an effective way to deal with stressors. Close social relationships act as barriers or buffers against stressors. Social support also provides resources from others, including information and consolation. For example, you probably have friends and family members who provide emotional comfort in times of stress, but also offer practical suggestions, referrals, or recommendations. Additionally, they may offer material assistance such as money, food, clothing, and shelter. Social relationships even encourage health-related behaviors, including adherence to medical treatment.

If you are employed, coworkers may be good sources of additional support and ideas. Your college advisor and professors are added sources of support and knowledge. Most campuses have resources to provide academic advice as well as affective or emotional counseling. Many hospitals organize support groups for patients dealing with specific illnesses or injuries. There are support groups for parents whose children are dealing with such diverse issues as disabilities, cancer, and being a twin or triplet. Sources of social support can improve our sense of self-worth and personal control (Cohen, Underwood, & Gottlieb, 2000).

Researchers assess social support in a variety of ways. For example, there are quantitative measures of the extent of social networks, as well as measures of the quality of support received in the past. Researchers sometimes differentiate between social networks and social relationships, while other studies distinguish between **structural support**, including social ties and connections such as marital status, and **functional support**, which focuses on what the relationships provide, such as financial help or affection. In still other cases, the focus is perceptions of one's social support rather than actual indices quantifying social support (Martin & Brantley, 2004, p. 250-251).

Social isolation is damaging to health and makes life more difficult for everyone. We should make every effort to avoid isolating ourselves from others. At the same time, some people in our social networks can be detrimental to our health. Parents, spouses, children, and friends who abuse us, physically or emotionally, are sources of stress and very harmful. They contribute to poorer, not better, outcomes. When trapped in such relationships, we can seek help outside the family from mental health professionals or agencies.

**structural support** That part of social support that includes networks of close social ties and connections such as marital status.

**functional support** That part of social support that provides resources such as financial help or other aids to help us to cope with stressors.

## Personality, Stress, and Health

Personality differences influence people's reactions to stressors. **Personality** is a broad and complex concept reflecting individual biological, psychological, and sociocultural circumstances. Genetic background, conditions in the mother's uterus, and early experiences as infants and children contributed to the development of our personality. Personality can change as people age, although the term generally refers to fairly stable characteristics (Twenge, 2002). Personality traits influence risk-taking behaviors such as reckless driving, smoking, overeating, and substance abuse. Personal characteristics even affect people's response to symptoms and their adherence or cooperation with medical treatment.

Freud (1952) described patients who used defensive measures such as repression to avoid facing stressful thoughts and discovered that the extent of stress in his patients affected the course of their disease. Distraction, denial, and re-interpretation are other strategies used to blunt effects of stressors (Myers, Newman, & Enomoto, 2004). Early in the 20th century, physicians identified a coronary-prone type of person, or the **Type A personality**. Health psychologists also note that personality traits, such as hostility, predict illness, while others, such as conscientiousness, moderate the likelihood of serious illness (Smith & Gallo, 2001).

Do you have a tendency to feel anxious, fearful, or sad? Would you describe yourself as friendly or hostile, dominant or submissive, extroverted or introverted? Some studies show that optimistic and pessimistic people deal with illness differently, and the differences influence outcomes of heart disease and breast cancer. Prospective studies find that optimism and pessimism may predict health outcomes. For example, optimism predicted lower incidence of complications in bypass surgery patients, and pessimism predicted decreased survival probabilities in breast cancer patients (Smith & Ruiz, 2004, p. 171). Lobel and DeVincent (2000) found that optimism in expectant mothers predicted the delivery of healthier newborns. In other studies, the trait of hopelessness diminished longevity (Stern, Dhanda, & Hazuda, 2001). Research considers both personality characteristics and responses to illness, reflecting individual social environments. For example, cancer patients with unsupportive spouses made poorer emotional adjustments to their illnesses than patients married

**personality** Attributes or aspects of an individual that may be revealed through conversation and other activities. Personality is indicated by perceptions or cognitions, through emotional responses or affect, and through behaviors or actions.

**Type A personality** A behavioral and emotional pattern of responding to experiences in life with a chronic sense of time urgency and free-floating hostility. It may include a competitive attitude and anger; this type of personality may be a response to insufficient self-esteem or self-confidence.

to supportive partners (Manne & Glassman, 2000). Smith and Ruiz (2004) propose a trans-actional stress moderation model that includes stressors relating to appraisal, to personality, and to coping responses connected to physiological arousal and illness. Personality traits are re-lated to health behaviors, to risk factors including negative emotions and stress, and also affect people's responses to illness (Smith & Ruiz, 2004).

## Resilience in Responding to Stressors

Do you remain healthy in the face of setbacks in your life or are you easily overwhelmed by negative events? Most college students overcome many stressors and will continue to do so into old age. **Resilience** refers to the capacity to recover quickly from adversity regardless of the source. Some researchers use the terms *resistance* and *vulnerability* when referring to individual characteristics involved in withstanding severe difficulties or dangerous situations (Vingerhoets, 2004). Feeling in control of your life, being logical when under pressure, and adapting to changing situations are all indicators of resilience.

We know that many people face horrifying stressors, recover from those experiences, and go on to lead healthy, happy, and successful lives. In the face of catastrophic natural events such as hurricanes and manmade events such as wars, some people develop serious physical or emotional illnesses, while others facing similar situations remain healthy. Researchers in health psychology and related fields conduct studies to discover what characteristics and conditions are helpful when coping with highly stressful situations. Some personality char-acteristics related to resilience are **hardiness**, optimism, a sense of coherence, an internal locus of control, and learned resourcefulness.

### Hardiness

Kobasa (now Ouellette) (1979) uses the term *hardiness* to describe the ability to withstand stressful events by taking decisive action. She studied people who faced stressors but did not develop physical or mental health problems. "Resistance resources" or "buffers" protected these people. The quality of being hardy can become part of one's personality. It consists of three characteristics: commitment, control, and challenge. Kobasa found that development of these qualities resulted in people making optimistic appraisals of stress and viewing sit-uations as changeable or manageable. A committed person has a sense of purpose in life. Individuals with an internal locus of control believe they influence what occurs in life. When people have low levels of hardiness they react by feeling alienated and powerless. People tend to feel threatened by events they pessimistically see as unchangeable. Maddi and Kobasa

---

**resilience** The capacity to recover quickly from adversity regardless of the source.

**hardiness** Ability to withstand stressful events and take appropriate and decisive action.

(1984) tested the hardiness theory in a study of executives at Illinois Bell. The results supported the idea that hardiness protects health by changing stressful events into a less stressful form or by altering perceptions of stressors. Social support from others and regular aerobic exercise combined with personal hardiness protected the health of the executives in the study.

This study led Maddi and Kobasa to believe that hardiness begins early in life when children are encouraged to finish moderately difficult tasks and view change as an opportunity. Children develop hardiness by assuming life's experiences are purposeful and interesting events over which they have some control. They also suggest that children also benefit from the realization that changes during life are inevitable. Successfully meeting the challenges of change is a learning experience.

## A Sense of Coherence

Antonovsky (1987), a medical sociologist teaching in Israel, began his research by focusing on origins of good mental and physical health rather than on origins of pathology or disease. He studied the ways people coped and managed severe tension and were able to prevent it from turning into harmful stress. His early research included women born in central Europe who were between 16 and 25 years old in 1939, who had survived the concentration camps before and during World War II, and who lived for years as displaced persons before finally reestablishing lives in the new, but wartorn country of Israel. Antonovsky concluded that about 29% of the women who survived these traumatic experiences were mentally and physically healthy. In developing his theory, he considered a variety of resources, including money, ego strength, cultural stability, and social support. He came to believe that resources do give people a stronger sense of coherence. A sense of coherence includes an enduring feeling of confidence that life has meaning and an optimism that events will work out well. He believed that childrearing patterns build up our resistance resources, resulting in a strong sense of coherence and consistency that carries into adulthood.

## Learned Resourcefulness

Rosenbaum (1980) also focused on qualities that help people deal with stress. He developed a 36-item scale to measure the characteristic of **learned resourcefulness** that includes items on coping skills, self-control, and adaptive behaviors. The concept of learned resourcefulness includes both skills and intellectual qualities. Resourceful individuals learn to anticipate, plan, self-regulate, cope with failure, and change coping strategies. Failures in

**learned resourcefulness**  Skills and intellectual qualities of persons who learn to anticipate, plan, self-regulate, cope with failure, and change coping strategies.

managing stressors were redefined as learning opportunities. Rosenbaum suggests that some conditions in modern life promote illness-related behaviors, such as smoking, unhealthy eating patterns, and spending spare time in activities that require no physical exercise. He believes that health-related changes are learned and maintained through a process of self-control. This process occurs when people observe themselves in response to stressors, make conscious efforts to confront disruptive changes, and believe they are capable of rising to a challenge. People develop repertoires or collections of thoughts, emotions, and behaviors that make an effective response to stressors more likely. This repertoire is learned resourcefulness and includes beliefs, behaviors, and self-control skills. In many studies learned resourcefulness has been applied to the treatment of depression, abnormal fears of open or public places (agoraphobia), severe trauma, and the performance of hazardous duties. For example, studies of bomb-disposal operators and military parachute jumpers reveal that all experienced fear, but most performed competently despite severe danger (Rachman, 1990).

## Stress Management Techniques

The purpose of stress management is to improve our coping and decrease the likelihood of stressors taking a negative toll or damaging our physical, emotional, and social health. It is worthwhile to learn to reduce the potential for stress before a stressful crisis occurs in our lives. There are biological, psychological, and sociocultural ways to accomplish this. Stress management skills have been shown to be effective in patients with HIV, diabetes, cancer, and asthma (Martin & Brantley, 2004, pp. 241–242).

### Biological Approaches to Stress Management

Habitual health and safety practices prevent stress. Following recommendations for exercise and nutrition discussed in earlier chapters are biological ways to reduce the impact of stressors. Obesity, muscle weakness, stiffness in joints, and poor aerobic capacity are sources of frustration. From a stress management viewpoint, it makes sense to stay physically fit throughout our lives. Research reviewed in previous chapters showed that regular aerobic exercise reduces negative emotions, tension, and stress. Freedom from serious and chronic diseases such as heart disease, diabetes, and cancer makes it more likely we will successfully handle other stressors in our lives. When we are aerobically fit, we sleep better and are more serene. Being well rested increases our ability to deal with problems. When we are in good health, we are less likely to be seriously affected by stress.

Habitually making good decisions from a safety viewpoint also limits the effect of stress. For example, taking the time to put on a seat belt and avoiding driving under the influence of substances such as alcohol can prevent the enormous stresses brought on by car wrecks, medical costs, pain, court appearances, and traffic fines. For those who are unable to obtain relief through healthy and safe lifestyles, there are medications and counseling. Medications for depression may have unwanted side effects and medications should be combined with counseling or talk therapy. Cognitive techniques are the least invasive of stress management methods, because they involve changing our thinking processes, but they may not be effective in all situations.

### Control of Body Tension

You already know you can consciously slow or speed up your rate of breathing by inhaling more deeply and exhaling very slowly. The breathing rate is one biological indicator of stress in the body. People who practice body-control systems such as yoga can slow their heartbeats and lower their blood pressure. Clinical psychologists employ biofeedback to treat stress-related chronic health problems such as stomachaches, high blood pressure, diabetes, and asthma. Tension awareness and control can be a stress management teaching tool for stress-related problems such as insomnia, depression, anxiety disorders, motion sickness, and phobias. Research has shown that people can be taught to control their body's reactions.

## Progressive Muscle Relaxation

We may be tense but unaware of the tension in our muscles because we are tense all day long. For example, many people have tension in their shoulders and walk around all day with their shoulders up around their ears. Progressive muscle relaxation (PRT) uses intentional tensing and relaxing of muscle groups to increase understanding of what it feels like to be relaxed. "Relaxation techniques are a well-established treatment for over arousal and muscular tension" (Martin & Brantley, 2004, p. 241). See the Think About It! feature "Try This Before or After Your Next Test" for step-by-step instructions for PMR.

### Massage Therapy

Massage therapists are trained, but not in medical or psychologically based training programs. Massage practitioners typically use their hands to rub and knead soft tissues of the body. They may apply oils and provide music and a darkened room to enhance patient relaxation. Massage helps in relaxation and may even result in pain relief. Massage is the act of treating discomfort by rubbing, stroking, or kneading parts of the body. This action may relax a person and improve circulation. Cardiac massage to restore heartbeats is part of cardiopulmonary resuscitation (CPR). Other types of massage are discussed in Chapter 10.

## Therapeutic Psychosocial Approaches to Stress Management

A great deal of research in health psychology focuses upon effective methods of reducing sources of stress and improving mental health. If we are happy and satisfied with our lives, then we are more focused and organized about our important goals. Being mentally fit means we have less worry and anxiety. Better psychological health contributes to better physical health, and vice versa. When people respond to stress by becoming hostile and bitter, they often lose their bases of social support, because hostility and bitterness tend to isolate us from other people.

## Think About It!

### Try This Before or After Your Next Test

A Technique for Progressive Muscular Relaxation

1. Choose a quiet location and sit in a comfortable position, hands down at your sides, and both feet flat on the floor.

2. Close your eyes and take a few deep breaths; concentrate on becoming as relaxed as possible.

3. With your arms at your sides, make a fist with one of your hands. Hold your clenched fist for about 5 seconds, release your hand from this position, and concentrate on the feeling as the muscular tension "drains" out of your hand.

   This basic exercise is repeated as you tense muscles, hold the tensed position for 5 seconds, and then relax the major muscle groups in your body. It is important to focus on recognizing the difference between muscular tension and relaxation sensations. Continue breathing normally as the activity progresses. Begin with your head.

4. Tense your forehead and scalp muscles; feel the tight muscular sensations as you hold this position for 5 seconds; relax these muscles.

5. Tense your facial muscles; hold this position for 5 seconds; relax.

6. Tense the muscles of your neck and jaw; hold this position; relax.

7. Tense your back muscles—but not too tight; hold this position; relax.

8. Tense your right arm; hold; relax.

9. Tense your left arm; hold; relax.

10. Tense your chest muscles; hold; relax.

11. Tense your stomach muscles; hold; relax.

12. Tense your buttocks; hold; relax.

13. Tense your right leg—but not too tight; hold; relax.

14. Tense your left leg—but not too tight; hold; relax.

Now, imagine traveling back through your body searching for muscles that are not relaxed. As you find tense muscles, relax them. Maintain this position for several minutes, concentrating on your breathing. In this relaxed state, you may practice tranquil imagery and positive self-talk. To regain your normal physical activity, open your eyes, stand, and stretch your muscles.

*Source:* Alters, S., & Schiff, W. (2009). *Essential concepts for healthy living* (5th ed.). Sudbury, MA: Jones and Bartlett Publishers, LLC.

Self-Help and Professional Help with Stress Management
There are many books available to help people create closer connections between their minds and bodies. This is accomplished through **meditation**, reading, or by therapy sessions with trained clinicians about relief from stressors. This section examines methods for stress relief that can be accomplished by effort on the part of a person with or without the help of trained personnel. Some techniques can be used both for general stressors and for the specific stressor of pain. Relaxation is an important part of stress management. Relaxation of the body helps because tension in the body focuses attention on discomfort and pain. People who learn to manage stressful thoughts can learn to concentrate and reduce tension.

Religious and Spiritual Orientations to Stress Management
Religion and/or spirituality is sometimes a daunting topic for scholars but encompasses an emerging area in health psychology research and practice related to stress and coping (Baumeister, 2002; Thoresen & Harris, 2004). In some instances religion and spirituality are approached as ethnic or cultural factors influencing health practices (American Psychological Association, 2002). Religion and spirituality are related to beliefs, values, goals, behaviors, and experiences, which in some studies correlate with improved mortality, morbidity, and reduced disability (Thoreson & Harris, 2004, pp. 273–374). There is evidence that religious and spiritual perspectives result in less disease and better health, although the effects may be most related to positive emotions (McCullough, Hoyt, Larson, Koenig, & Thoresen, 2000). A meta-analysis of these issues by a National Institutes of Health panel concluded that attending religious services weekly or more often was associated with lower mortality, less disability, and better recovery from acute illness (George, Ellison, & Larson, 2002). Consider setting aside time each day to relax (see **Figure 9.3**).

People use a variety of focusing techniques in a variety of settings for many purposes. Early descriptions of religious practices included times during the day specifically set aside for meditation, relaxation, and prayer. Monks and nuns might meditate on the goodness of a deity, the mysteries of their faith, or on ways to perfect their lives. In contemporary times, meditation may include avoiding specific thoughts and staying in the present moment. This means not allowing any thoughts to enter the mind. Thought control takes considerable practice. Research suggests that yoga, **transcendental meditation (TM)**, and similar practices may be beneficial in clinical settings to manage stress (Carlson, Speca, Patel, & Goodey,

---

**meditation** A process of using the mind-body connections to improve health, including contemplation, thinking, and concentration of thoughts that may produce positive outcomes including relaxation.

**transcendental meditation (TM)** A form of reflection that instructs people to choose a mantra or secret word to be repeated over and over in order to focus thoughts away from distressful ideas or pain.

**Figure 9.3**
Yoga includes exercise, meditation, and breathing techniques. It also helps people feel relaxed and refreshed.

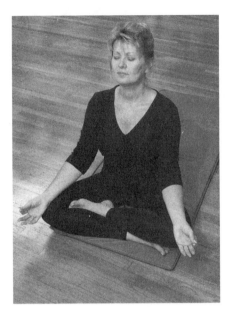

2003). Jon Kabat-Zinn has offered **mindfulness meditation** at stress reduction clinics to relieve people from physical suffering; patients are taught to focus on the present moment (Moyers, 1993). Assessing effectiveness of these techniques is difficult, but over a 3-year period, TM was more effective than both mindfulness meditation and training in relaxation techniques (Alexander, Langer, Newman, & Chandler, 1989). The TM group was most improved on cognitive and behavioral flexibility, mental health, blood pressure, and survival rate.

Stress Inoculation Training (SIT)
Stress inoculation training is another stress management technique. As children, you were immunized against some diseases, and each fall adults are inoculated to avoid the flu. Meichenbaum (1985) devised and tested a form of cognitive therapy designed to immunize people against stress. SIT consists of three stages: conceptualization, skills development, and application. Following a discussion of previous coping attempts, the patient is taught new coping skills, including relaxation, distraction, and **redefinition**. Patients practice using

**mindfulness meditation** An effort to relieve people from physical suffering by teaching them to focus on the present moment and on nothing else, including the past or future.

**redefinition** A stress management technique that substitutes positive constructive thoughts for frightening ones or devises positive statements about the likelihood of tolerating a stressor.

these skills while imagining a dreaded situation. Eventually they are able to actually participate in some previously terrifying activity.

### Biofeedback

Biofeedback training combines counseling or talk therapy with technology to learn relaxation. Through instruments that measure and feed back information about muscle tension, people learn to control anxiety in the body through notification by sounds or flashing lights. Feedback from sensors placed on the body teaches individuals to relax to such an extent that they receive relief from frightening factors interfering with their lives. The success of biofeedback-facilitated relaxation training (BFRT) depends on individuals following up on training sessions by frequently practicing going into relaxed states of mind and body.

For example, if a person is afraid of flying, but wants to fly, then several biofeedback sessions may enable the person to get on a plane without extraordinary stress. The process is very gradual. The therapist suggests patients think about or imagine buying an airline ticket. During the next session the patient may learn to control body tension to the extent that no sound is made through the biofeedback machine. In other sessions patient and therapist may talk about actually going through the security check at the airport and then sitting waiting for the flight to be called. Eventually the patient is able to actually make a plane trip.

### Redefinition

Therapists teach this method to change the ways we think about stressors. We are encouraged to substitute constructive thoughts to replace threatening ones. The method also includes devising positive statements about the likelihood of tolerating a stressor through coping statements such as, "I can put up with this because I have tolerated things before now that were a great deal worse, and so have millions of other people before me," or "This is not so bad." **Affirmations** are statements about one's ability to overcome adversity and go through life free of stress or pain. Patients are also encouraged to examine the logic of their beliefs.

### Guided Imagery

This approach is similar to the talk therapy used in biofeedback, but there are no electrodes or flashing lights. Guided imagery is also linked to distraction. A trained therapist guides your thinking so you visualize pleasant scenes or situations. One example might be to visualize the seashore. You would be encouraged to use all of your senses to imagine the sea and the beach. The therapist might tell you to listen to the seagulls and see them wheel through the air, smell the briny water, taste the saltiness of the sea, and feel the grains of warm sand sifting through your fingers. Patients learn to use their imagination whenever they feel

---

**affirmations** Statements about one's ability to overcome adversity and go through life free of stress or pain.

stressed. Some therapists provide patients with tape recordings that combine several approaches to relaxation. Commercially produced tapes are also available.

## Summary

Researchers in health psychology and related fields of medical sociology, psychiatry, and pain management study ways to cope or manage stressors. Stress management is important for both physical and mental health. Lazarus and Folkman developed the idea that people go through three stages in their effort to cope with stressors. In their primary appraisal or encounter with a stressor, people decide if the situation is stressful or challenging. In their secondary appraisal, people make judgments about coping or meeting a threat or challenge. A third stage, reappraisal, occurs if there is new information that changes a person's original assessment of stressful situations.

When facing stress, people often react both emotionally and intellectually while focusing on solutions to the challenge. Both emotion-focused coping and problem-focused coping can be beneficial. Some general coping strategies available to us are taking direct action, acquiring more skills or knowledge, seeking support from others, changing our thinking, and improving our sense of control. Three important theories about coping include the ideas of hardiness, having a sense of coherence, and learned resourcefulness. People can also reduce the likelihood of stress due to illness and injury by following good health and safety practices. Sociocultural approaches to stress include developing good social support from family, friends, and associates.

Stress management includes techniques for relaxing the mind and body. These include stress inoculation training, meditation, breathing exercises, progressive muscle relaxation, guided imagery, redefinition, control of body tension, and massage therapy.

## Review Questions

1. Differentiate between the concepts of coping and stress management.

2. Explain how stress management is related to physical and mental health.

3. Describe the three stages of coping from the viewpoint of the transactional approach.

4. Distinguish between emotion-focused coping and problem-focused coping. Explain the circumstances under which each may be useful.

5. Describe four general coping strategies, giving one example of each.

6. Explain three theories of developing resistance to stress and give examples from health psychology illustrating each.

7. Describe in detail some biological approaches to reducing stress in our lives.

8. Summarize psychosocial ways to help people face stressors. Relate each to a specific stressor you have faced.

9. Differentiate three different ways of managing stressors that can be aided by the help of trained personnel.

## Student Activity

Try to remember the details of one stressful event from your own or someone else's life, or analyze a news article about a stressful situation. Write a brief description of the situation. Using information provided in the chapter and taught by your professor, write about all of the different coping mechanisms that were or could be applied. Evaluate the helpfulness of each for this situation. Based on your new knowledge from this and other chapters, write a paragraph about what recommendations you would make to someone faced with a similar situation. List any stress management techniques that were used or could be used to handle the situation. As a group the entire class can list coping and stress management efforts to determine what are most commonly used or suggested by class members.

## References

Alexander, C. N., Langer, E. J., Newman, R. I., & Chandler, H. M. (1989). Transcendental meditation, mindfulness and longevity: An experimental study with the elderly. *Journal of Personality and Social Psychology, 57*, 950–964.

American Psychological Association. (2002). *Guidelines on multicultural education, training, research, practice, and organizational change for psychologists*. Washington, DC: Author.

Antonovsky, A. (1987). *Unraveling the mystery of health: How people manage stress and stay well*. San Francisco: Jossey-Bass.

Aspinwall, L. G. (1997). Where planning meets coping: Proactive coping and the detection and management of potential stressors. In S. L. Freidman & E. K. Scholnick (Eds.), *The developmental psychology of planning: Why, how and when do we plan?* (pp. 283–320). Mahwah, NJ: Lawrence Erlbaum Associates.

Bandura, A. (1997). *Self-efficacy: The exercise of control*. New York: W. H. Freeman.

Baumeister, R. F. (2002). Religion and psychology: Introduction to the special issue. *Psychological Inquiry, 13*, 165–247.

Berkman, L., & Syme, S. (1979). Social networks, host resistance, and mortality: A nine-year follow up study of Alameda County residents. *American Journal of Epidemiology, 109*, 186–204.

Berkman, L., & Breslow, L. (1983). *Health and ways of living: The Alameda County study*. NY: Oxford University Press.

Burns, J. W. (1997). Anger management style and hostility: Predicting symptom-specific physiological reactivity among chronic low back pain patients. *Journal of Behavioral Medicine, 20*, 505–522.

Carlson, L. E., Speca, M., Patel, K. D., & Goodey, E. (2003). Mindfulness-based stress reduction in relation to quality of life, mood, symptoms of stress and immune parameters in breast and prostate cancer outpatients. *Psychosomatic Medicine, 5*, 571–581.

Chesney, M. A., Folkman, S., & Chambers, D. (1996). Coping effectiveness training for men living with HIV disease: Preliminary findings. *International Journal of STD and AIDS, 7*, 75–82.

Cohen, S., Underwood, L. G., & Gottlieb, B. H. (Eds.). (2000). *Social support measurement and intervention: A guide for health and social scientists*. New York: Oxford University Press.

Cruess, D. G., Schneiderman, N., Antoni, M. H., & Penedo, F. (2004). In R. G. Frank, A. Baum, & J. L. Wallander (Eds.), *Handbook of clinical health psychology* (Vol. 3, pp. 31–79). Washington, DC: American Psychological Association.

Folkman, S., & Lazarus, R. S. (1988). *Manual for Ways of Coping Questionnaire*. Palo Alto, CA: Consulting Psychologists Press.

Freud, S. (1952). Selected papers on hysteria. The major works of Sigmund Freud. In C. M.

Baines (Trans.), *Great books of the western world* (Vol. 54, pp. 422–427). Chicago: Encyclopedia Britannica.

George, L. K., Ellison, C. G., & Larson, D. (2002). Explaining the relationship between religious involvement and health. *Psychological Inquiry, 13,* 190–200.

Kobasa, S. C. (1979). Stressful life events, personality, and health: An inquiry into hardiness. *Journal of Personality and Social Psychology, 37,* 1–11.

Lazarus, R. S. (1966). *Psychological stress and the coping process.* New York: McGraw Hill Book Company.

Lazarus, R. S., & Folkman, S. (1984). *Stress, appraisal, and coping.* New York: Springer.

Lobel, M., & DeVincent, C. J. (2000). The impact of prenatal maternal stress and optimistic disposition on birth outcomes in medically high-risk women. *Health Psychology, 19,* 544–553.

Maddi, S. R., & Kobasa, S. C. (1984). *The hardy executive: Health under stress.* Chicago: Dow Jones-Irwin.

Manne, S., & Glassman, M. (2000). Perceived control, coping efficacy, and avoidance coping as mediators between spouses unsupportive behaviors and cancer patients' psychological distress. *Health Psychology, 19,* 155–164.

Martin, P. D., & Brantley, P. J. (2004). Stress, coping, and social support in health and behavior. In J. M. Raczynski & L. C. Leviton (Eds.), *Handbook of clinical health psychology* (Vol. 2, pp. 233–268). Washington, DC: American Psychological Association.

McCullough, M. E., Hoyt, W. T., Larson, D. B., Koenig, H. G., & Thoresen, C. (2000). Religious involvement and mortality: A meta-analytic review. *Health Psychology, 19,* 211–222.

Meichenbaum, D. (1985). *Stress inoculation training.* Elmsford, NY: Pergamon.

Moyers, B. (1993). *Healing and the mind.* New York: Doubleday.

Myers, L. B., Newman, S. P., & Enomoto, K. (2004). Coping. In A. A. Kaptein & J. Weinman (Eds.), *Health psychology* (pp. 141–157). Malden, MA: Blackwell Publishing.

National Institute on Drug Abuse (2008). NIDA Community Drug Alert Bulletin-Stress & Substance Abuse. Retrieved February 8, 2008 at http://www.drugabuse.gov/StressAlert/StressAlert.html

Pennebaker, J. W. (1995). *Emotion, disclosure and health.* Washington, DC: American Psychological Association.

Pennebaker, J. W. (1997). *Opening up: The healing power of expressing emotions.* New York: Guilford.

Petrie, K. J., Booth, R. J., Pennebaker, J. W., Davison, K. P., & Thomas, M. G. (1995). Disclosure of trauma and immune response to hepatitis B vaccination programs. *Journal of Consulting and Clinical Psychology, 63,* 787–792.

Rachman, S. (1990). Learned resourcefulness in the performance of hazardous tasks. In Rosenbaum, M. (Ed.), *Learned resourcefulness: On coping skills, self-control, and adaptive behavior* (pp. 166–181). New York: Springer.

Rosenbaum, M. (1980). A schedule for assessing self-control behaviors and tolerance of painful stimulation: Preliminary findings. *Behavior Therapy, 11,* 109–121.

Smith, T. W., & Gallo, L. C. (2001). Personality traits as risk factors for physical illness. In A. Baum, T. Revenson, & J. Singer (Eds.), *Handbook of health psychology* (pp. 139–172). Hillsdale, NJ: Lawrence Erlbaum Associates.

Smith, T. W., & Ruiz, J. M. (2004). Personality theory and health behavior. In R. G. Frank, A. Baum, & J. L. Wallander (Eds.), *Handbook of clinical health psychology* (Vol. 3, pp. 143–199). Washington, DC: American Psychological Association.

Stern, S. L., Dhanda, R., & Hazuda, H. P. (2001). Hopelessness predicts mortality in older Mexican and European Americans. *Psychosomatic Medicine, 63,* 344–351.

Suls, J., & Fletcher, D. (1985). The relative efficacy of avoidant and non-avoidant coping strategies: A meta-analysis. *Health Psychology, 4,* 249–288.

Thoresen, C. E., & Harris, A. H. S. (2004). Spirituality, religion, and health: A scientific perspective. In J. M. Raczynski & L. C. Leviton (Eds.), *Handbook of clinical health psychology*, (Vol. 2, pp. 269-298). Washington, DC: American Psychological Association.

Twenge, J. M. (2002). Birth cohort, social change, and personality: The interplay of dysphoria and individualism in the 20th century. In D. Cervone & W. Mischel (Eds.), *Advances in personality science* (pp. 196-218). New York: Guilford.

Vingerhoets, A. (2004). Stress. In A. A. Kaptein & J. Weinman (Eds.), *Health Psychology* (pp. 113-140). Malden, MA: Blackwell Publishing.

Wenzel, L., & Glanz, K. (2004). Behavioral aspects of genetic risk for disease: Cancer genetics as a prototype for complex issues in health psychology. In R. G. Frank, A. Baum, & J. L. Wallander (Eds.), *Handbook of clinical health psychology* (Vol. 3, pp. 115-142). Washington, DC: American Psychological Association.

Williams, J. E., & Best, D. L. (1990). *Measuring sex stereotypes: A multination study*. Newbury Park, CA: Sage.

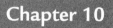

# Chapter 10

# Pain: A Serious Health Problem and Source of Stress

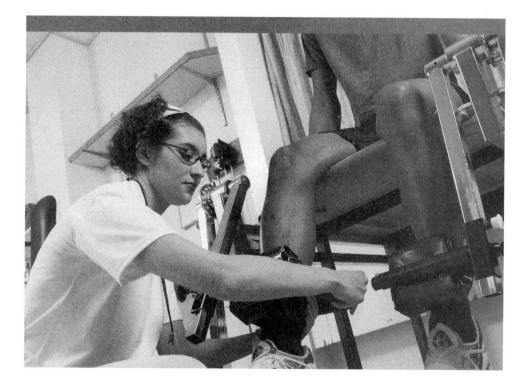

## Learning Objectives

After studying this chapter students will have the knowledge and skills to be able to:

1. Define pain and give examples of pain-related behaviors.

2. Using data, justify the idea that pain is a major health problem.

3. Explain why pain is best studied from the biopsychosocial perspective used in health psychology.

4. Describe the biological and psychosocial aspects of pain.

5. Summarize sociocultural factors influencing acknowledgement and expressions of pain.

6. Explain the gate control theory and the neuromatrix model of pain.

7. Define types of pain and give examples.

8. Summarize various ways to measure pain.

9. List and evaluate invasive and noninvasive pain management techniques.

## Introduction

In medical textbooks, **pain** is defined as an unpleasant sensory experience due to stimulation of nerve endings. It is a symptom and may warn us of injury or disease. Pain causes suffering and interferes with day-to-day activities, including sleep. Pain is distracting, and persons experiencing pain may be so disturbed by the pain that they fail to protect themselves from danger. Sensitivity to pain varies from person to person, reflecting physiological, psychological, and sociocultural differences. Acknowledgement of pain by individuals reflects their experiences with pain during childhood and any past dealings with medical personnel, including school nurses. Headaches and backaches are the most common types of pain in adults. You probably experienced pain before you were a year old.

Pain is a common and serious health problem. It causes people to miss school and work, making it costly to both organizations and individuals. Billions of dollars are spent each year on analgesics or pain treatments (Gatchel & Mayer, 2000). Millions of people use over-the-counter (OTC) analgesics such as non-steroidal anti-inflammatory drugs (NSAIDs) every day. These include aspirin, acetaminophen, and ibuprofen. There are hundreds of prescription pain medications. Pain is a global health problem. The International Association for the Study of Pain (1979) studies pain, including terms, definitions, and their usage (see **Table 10.1**).

Pain is a major research interest in health psychology, and many clinical health psychologists are on medical teams helping patients with pain management. One example of interdisciplinary pain care is treatment of serious burns. Burns over wide areas of the body usually involve long, painful hospitalization, risk of infections, and significant disfigurement. Biological, psychological, and sociocultural factors are involved in recovery from serious burns. Clinical health psychologists help patients manage pain in a variety of ways, including biofeedback, relaxation therapy, distraction, and redefinition of the situation. Other treatments for pain include hypnosis, acupuncture, massage therapy, **transcutaneous electrical nerve stimulation (TENS)**, and chiropractic adjustment.

The biopsychosocial approach of health psychology provides more complete analyses of pain than traditional biomedical practices, because pain has psychological and sociocultural causes and effects. Biological factors are involved in the transmission of pain to a conscious level in the brain and in the medical management of pain. Reactions, meanings, interpretations, and expressions of pain fall within the scope of psychological issues, including emotional or affective responses to pain such as fear and depression. Psychosocial ap-

**pain**  A sense of discomfort and distress due to a sensation in the body.

**transcutaneous electrical nerve stimulation (TENS)**  A process by which electrodes are placed on the skin near the site of pain and the area is given a mild electrical shock. The theory is that the electrical shock will interfere with the transmission of the pain signal from the injury site to the brain.

TABLE 10.1   The 20 Most Common Reasons for Doctor Visits

One in eight persons goes to the doctor without any complaint or symptom.

| Rank | Reason | Rank | Reason |
|---|---|---|---|
| 1 | Progress visits | 11 | Gynecological exam |
| 2 | Physical exam | 12 | Visit for medication |
| 3 | Pain, etc.—lower extremity | 13 | No medical reason |
| 4 | Pregnancy exam | 14 | Headache |
| 5 | Throat soreness | 15 | Fatigue |
| 6 | Pain, etc.—upper extremity | 16 | Pain in chest |
| 7 | Pain, etc.—back region | 17 | Well-baby exam |
| 8 | Cough | 18 | Fever |
| 9 | Abdominal pain | 19 | Allergic skin reaction |
| 10 | Cold | 20 | All other symptoms |

*Source:* Edlin, G. & Golanty, E. (2007). *Health and wellness* (9th ed.). Sudbury, MA: Jones and Bartlett Publishers.

proaches to pain management include improvement in self-efficacy along with changes in attitudes, emotions, and pain-related behaviors. Social and cultural factors, including national origin, ethnicity, educational level, and socioeconomic status, affect treatment and recovery from painful conditions (Zborowski, 1969). Social support includes friends and family members who are willing to assist patients in reducing stress, fear, pain, and discomfort. There are also pain support groups led by professional counselors that provide an opportunity for therapeutic discussions with fellow patients. It is important to understand that pain is a very personal experience, but our pain also affects family members and friends. Similarly, it is worrisome to us when a family member, friend, or our pet is in pain.

## Defining Pain

The word *pain* is widely used in reference to emotional or psychological distress. Emotional pain or heartache appears in conversations, literature, and songs. Grieving parents feel enormous emotional pain on the death of a child. There are also sayings in our culture connected to pain (e.g., describing someone as a "pain in the neck"). From a biological standpoint, pain is an unpleasant sensation resulting from stimulation of nerve endings by injury, disease, or other harmful factors (Rothenberg & Chapman, 1989). Reaction to pain usually includes using medications and seeking medical care for an injury or disease.

There are many different words for pain. For example, *anguish* may refer to severe pain that continues for long periods of time. Pain may also be described as overwhelming or intolerable. Sometimes people faint from pain. Severe pain may cause people to go into shock and die

(American National Red Cross, 2005). Students can make connections to earlier chapters by recalling that pain is an important cause of stress, and stress can also cause pain. One example of possible stress-related pain is a headache. Migraines are severe headaches that often result from a combination of biological, psychological, and social factors, including stress.

Back pain, joint pain, arthritis, and rheumatism are leading causes of chronic pain and disability that result in absenteeism from work. Other people, including insurance companies, may not understand the intensity and frequency of our pain. For example, the Social Security Act includes instructions about how pain should be evaluated for purposes of determining eligibility for disability benefits, but administrators often deny claims, triggering many appeals and court cases (Osterweiss, 1987).

## Biopsychosocial Aspects of Pain

### The Biology of Pain

Some researchers distinguish between pain and **nociception**. The latter refers to nervous system information about tissue damage. Acknowledgement of pain by individuals reflects their perceptions and interpretations of stimulation in the nervous system (Gatchel & Maddrey, 2004, p. 361). Pain results when sensory nerve fibers are irritated by injury or disease. The pain sensation moves from the site of the injury or disease through the spinal cord to the brain and consciousness. The brain processes and interprets pain signals. For example, some nerve fibers are receptive to pressure, while others respond to temperature, such as heat and cold. These sensations may eventually become painful. Other nerve fibers transmit information telling us pain characteristics such as whether a pain is sharp or dull.

Body chemicals also affect perception of pain. For example, when we cut ourselves, neurochemicals are released that inflame nerve endings, making the cut painful. Other neurochemicals, such as endorphins, help block the sensation of pain. The site and type of pain also have physiological associations. **Visceral pain** results from injury or disease to an organ in the thoracic or abdominal cavities. **Somatic pain** originates in the skin, ligaments, muscles, bones, and joints. Other sensations such as numbness, tingling, or burning are sometimes described as painful. The term **tenderness** refers to a slight but unusual pain. Physicians may palpate or feel an area of the body asking if the area is tender.

---

**nociception**  The perception of pain produced when body tissue is damaged; nociceptors are nerve endings that respond to painful stimuli causing the sensation of pain.

**visceral pain**  Pain sensations resulting from injury or disease to an organ in the thoracic or abdominal cavities.

**somatic pain**  Pain sensations originating in the skin, ligaments, muscles, bones, or joints.

**tenderness**  Pain perceived when the affected area is touched or pressed.

The Purpose of Pain

The biological usefulness of pain is that it warns us of damage to our bodies. It may even force us to stop what we are doing and prevent further damage. For example, the sensation of pain notifies us when we strain a muscle, tear a ligament, dislocate a joint, or break a bone. Interestingly, some people experience great pain with no discernible tissue damage, while others experience severe tissue damage from diseases such as cancer and yet experience no pain. Pain behaviors such as limping may also elicit aid and sympathy from friends and family.

Pain Behaviors

Because we cannot see other people's pain, we only know they are in pain if they tell us or if we notice pain-related behaviors or obvious changes in their appearance. We assume others are in pain if we see them grimace, hear them groan, or if they grasp some part of their body. If we hear people crying, moaning, or whimpering, we assume they are hurt and in pain. If someone has difficulty walking, we suspect pain in a foot, ankle, leg, or hip. This behavior is called **distorted ambulation**. Wrinkled facial expressions or frowns also tell us someone is in pain. We know when close friends or family members have headaches just by the expression on their faces. Another pain behavior is called **guarding**. People try to avoid pain by guarding the hurt area. For example, children with broken arms often hold the arm against their body, because any movement causes greater pain (American National Red Cross, 2005).

## Psychological Aspects of Pain

There is enormous variation in how people react to pain. It is sometimes difficult to separate the psychological from the sociocultural, because attitudes about pain reflect social factors such as childrearing practices as well as individual differences. Pain may indicate serious harm or disease, so worry and fear add stress to pain perception. People are less likely to be bothered by pain if a knowledgeable and sympathetic person can relieve their anxiety and fear about it. People with different cognitive styles may be identified as either blunting or monitoring pain (Skevington & Mason, 2004).

Researchers distinguish between individual pain thresholds and levels of pain tolerance. The **pain threshold** is the point at which an individual describes a sensation as being painful

---

**distorted ambulation**  An abnormal walking behavior indicating pain in some area of the body.

**guarding**  A protective behavior that may indicate a painful injury. For example, when someone breaks a bone in his arm he may hold that arm against his body with the undamaged hand to diminish movement and pain.

**pain threshold**  The point of perception of a pain that results in people describing a sensation as painful. Thresholds vary from person to person.

rather than describing it as some other sensation. Thresholds for pain vary from person to person. **Tolerance** for pain refers to the point at which people want the sensation to stop. In general, the older a person is, the greater the tolerance for pain (Skevington, 2004, pp. 199–200). This may reflect biological, psychological, or sociocultural differences. Emotions influence our perception of pain, and pain influences our emotional state. In general, pain causes us to be unhappy. **Psychogenic pain** is a source of frustration, because it refers to chronic pain with no currently identifiable physical basis. Pain, especially chronic pain, often results in depression. Stress and depression make sensitivity to pain much more likely.

Individual expectations about pain, anticipation of pain, and beliefs about the likelihood of pain influence our perception and reaction to pain. If we read or hear that childbirth, surgery, or chemotherapy will be a painful experience, then we tend to focus on that likelihood. On the other hand, if we are told some event will not be painful, then we may not even notice discomfort. Many physicians and hospital employees try to help people cope with pain using distraction or descriptions, but do not tell anyone, especially a child, that a medical treatment will not hurt if it may cause pain (see **Figure 10.1**).

There is great variability in the way people experience pain. Sociocultural factors such as ethnicity, age, gender, past experiences, and socioeconomic situations are sources of differences in the ways people experience and acknowledge pain.

## Sociocultural Aspects of Pain and Pain Experiences

Cultural factors influence the experience of pain (Baum, Gatchel, & Krantz, 1997). One component of cultures and subcultures is the acceptability of acknowledging or calling attention to one's own pain. This means cultures, and families within those cultures, may encourage, discourage, or even ignore pain (Skevington, 2004). For example, **stoic** refers to a philosophy of enduring whatever occurs during one's lifetime without complaint, including pain. History and anthropology textbooks contain discussions of groups that require painful initiation rites for young people. Some cultures praise those who tolerate pain as being brave.

Most cultures and subcultures have different norms for girls and boys with regard to pain acknowledgement. In the United States, young boys are often mocked if they cry when they are hurt or complain about pain. Athletes learn to ignore pain unless it interferes with their team winning a game. Different viewpoints in neighborhoods, schools, and the mass

---

**tolerance** Tolerance for pain refers to the amount of pain individuals will put up with before they ask for something to stop the sensation.

**psychogenic pain** A chronic pain with no currently identifiable physical basis.

**stoic** A person who is patient and who endures adversity including pain.

**Figure 10.1**
Telling children that an
injection for immunization
will prevent serious illness
may help them tolerate the
pain of injections.

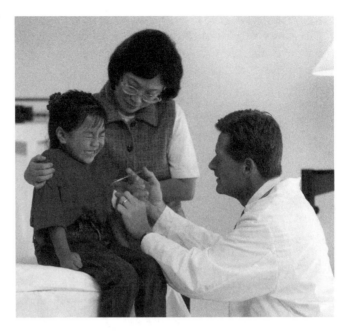

media also influence attitudes about pain. Think about your own attitude toward people who mention their pain. Have you ever made fun of friends who grumble about pain? Pain is socially disruptive. It isolates people by keeping them at home or in hospitals, and away from school, work, social, and recreational activities. When we are in pain, we find it difficult to be nice to other people. This negatively affects our social relationships. Pain can be so persistent it dominates people's lives. Early childhood experiences also affect our reaction to pain and our pain behaviors.

Parental Viewpoints and Early Childhood Experiences
Pain perception and expression reflect childrearing practices. A study of more than 7,000 adolescents found attitudes of parents heavily influenced the likelihood that a teen would want to visit a physician about a symptom (Quadrel & Lau, 1990). These attitudes continue to influence our response to pain even when we become adults. **Socialization** is the process of teaching or learning what behavior is acceptable. Attitudes about pain are learned in the family.

Beginning in infancy, many children are ignored or told to be quiet when they cry, especially in public situations such as at a church or temple, mall, or restaurant. How did your

**socialization**  The process of teaching young persons what is acceptable behavior within a society.

caregivers react when you were growing up and reported that something hurt? Did your family allow both girls and boys to cry, or was crying only permissible for females? Was crying allowed only if there was a serious physical injury with blood or broken bones showing? Did a parent, coach, or teacher ever tell you that you were more afraid than hurt? When you cried from pain, were you offered a cookie or candy to distract you? This can influence future eating patterns to the extent that when we face the stress of being in pain from any source, physical or emotional, we eat comforting foods with sweets and fats. Distraction is sometimes helpful during painful medical experiences, especially with children. Children may also hide pain if it resulted from their doing something they were forbidden to do, such as climbing a fence or sneaking over to a friend's house. Research reveals that family feelings about dental treatment affected children's anxiety about dental visits (Milgrom, Mand, King, & Weinstein, 1995).

Gender and Age Differences

Until recently, researchers assumed women and men experienced pain in similar ways. It is still not known if differences are based in physiology or social factors such as role expectations (Gatchel & Maddrey, 2004). Analgesics may be more effective for women than men, but this is also related to body size. In experiments there are differences in pain thresholds and tolerance, with females having lower thresholds and tolerance than males (Miaskowski, 1999). Women and men are similar in reactions to chronic pain. Reactions include frequent physician visits, narcotics dependence, and an inability to respond to standard primary treatments (Rosenfeld, 2001, p. 295). In the United States, social norms generally allow women more than men to acknowledge pain.

Pain is prevalent among the very old, and yet pain is understudied and undertreated in the elderly (Ratcliff, 2002, p. 176). Elderly people may hide pain to keep from being put into nursing homes. Some people use pain complaints and behaviors to avoid some task or to draw attention to themselves when they feel neglected. This is referred to as a **secondary gain of pain**.

Meanings of Pain

The significance of social situations and incidents influences pain experiences. For example, soldiers who want to leave a combat zone may be grateful for painful and serious wounds (Beecher, 1959). Combat wounds often mean extra medical attention, time out from battle, transfer to a military hospital, and eventually returning home as a hero. **Malingering** is the medical term for patient exaggeration about symptoms of a disease or injury to gain some end

**secondary gain of pain**  Any benefit of pain used by persons to avoid some task or to draw attention to themselves.

**malingering**  A deliberate feigning of symptoms such as pain or illness to try to gain some end such as attention, sympathy, or release from obligations.

such as attention, sympathy, or release from obligations. On the other hand, some people deny pain because they want to continue their current activity. This often happens in the middle of important athletic events. Organized religions also shape attitudes toward pain. Throughout history some people wanted to experience pain due to remorse over past behaviors or to show their love for a deity.

## Headache Pain: A Biopsychosocial Analysis of a Specific Pain Category

Headaches highlight the benefits of using the biopsychosocial approach, because headache pain may reflect biological, psychological, or social origins or some combination of all three. Some biological bases of headaches are sinus infections, flu, dehydration, tumors, allergies, and changes in air pressure or barometric pressure. Psychological origins of headaches are difficult to separate from the social, because most stressors include both components. Stress-related headaches are often caused by anxiety or worry, but the origins of anxiety may stem from troubled relationships within the family, at work, or at school. Anticipation of visits from unpleasant relatives or concerns about grades on upcoming final exams may cause headaches.

## Theories About the Origins of Pain

Theories and models help clarify biological and psychosocial aspects of pain. History provides multiple theories about pain and its origins. For example, some people believed pain was sent as a divine gift or as a satanic punishment. Most early theories of pain were biomedical in emphasis. Physicians wrote about pain systems, pain receptors, and pain centers in the brain. Some suggested there was one sense for pain, similar to unique organ systems for hearing, seeing, and tasting. Others thought the sensation of pain was a simple mechanical process or that pain resulted from excessive stimulation of nerves in some area of the body that the brain then interpreted as pain.

Most early theories failed to incorporate all of what is now known about pain, including individual variations in pain perception. Even when people have identical injuries, they report different types of pain or no pain at all. The specificity theory of pain suggested that sensory receptors in the skin were specific to pain sensation, and the pattern theory of pain proposed that the pattern and quantity of nerve fiber discharge produced differences in pain sensations (Gatchel & Maddrey, 2004). In health psychology, the most widely accepted pain theory is a biopsychosocial one, the **gate control theory of pain**, introduced in 1965 by Melzack and Wall.

> **gate control theory of pain** A theory of pain perception that explains pain as a sensation that can be blocked by a neural gate in the spinal cord that modifies pain signals.

## The Gate Control Theory of Pain

Wall commented on 30 years of scientific progress based on this theory, which posits that pain is a response to stimulation of nerve endings, but sensations can be modified or changed by "gating actions" or "control mechanisms" in the spinal cord (Wall, 1996). This theory incorporates biological, psychological, and sociocultural factors. From this perspective the sensation of pain does not follow a simple single circuit or flow along a line between an injury or disease and the brain. Many factors affect or modify pain perception, including social situations, emotions, thought patterns or cognitions, ideas, interpretations, and beliefs. Messages from the site of injury or disease are transferred to the brain through the spinal cord, but information also moves in the opposite direction. Messages descending from the brain may include suggestions to relax or some other thought distracting people from the pain sensation. For example, the application of heating pads, cold packs, or massage to a painful area may "close the gate" and the patient feels relief from pain. Positive emotions also change pain sensations. For example, happiness due to impending childbirth may put a different connotation on labor pains to a pregnant woman. Even concentrating and reflecting on pain may be soothing as a person records the rise and fall in the intensity of pain. Some analgesics and cultural practices allow people to disassociate from the pain, making it less bothersome.

## The Neuromatrix Model of Pain

The **neuromatrix model of pain** merges the gate control theory with the concept of stress. Melzack (1999) proposes that pain is a unique experience for each individual, because it reflects distinctive psychological states and social experiences along with biological components. For example, symptom descriptions and the extent of disability associated with pain vary from person to person, even when patients appear to have identical injuries. Symptoms vary among people with the same injury who are receiving identical treatment. In discussions of this model, Turk and Monarch (2002) remind us that the term *disease* should be used in reference to objective biological conditions resulting from physiological changes, while the word *illness* reflects people's subjective experiences, including their distress, pain, and disability. They continue with the idea that any medical treatment should take into consideration the unique biology, psychology, and sociocultural context of each patient. This theory explains the variations in patients' responses to identical treatments and variations in ability to cope with pain. Acknowledgement of pain sensation may also reflect genetic background and current health status. When you tell a friend, "I feel your pain," it

---

**neuromatrix model of pain** An extension of the gate control theory that integrates the concept of stress. This explanation of pain emphasizes the biopsychosocial model of pain that is more helpful in understanding and treating pain disorders.

is a way of being supportive about a stressor the person is facing, but it is never true that we can feel another person's pain.

## Specific Types of Pain

Discussions of pain make distinctions about the duration of the pain. In medicine, **acute pain** comes on suddenly and is severe. Acute pain usually indicates tissue damage and compels us to seek relief. **Chronic pain** persists for a very long period of time, usually more than 6 months. Causes of chronic pain include arthritis and back injuries. **Recurrent pain** and **chronic intermittent pain** go away and return. All types of pain are distressing and may result in depression, frustration, and even anger.

### Acute Pain

Almost everyone experiences acute pain at some time in their lives. Pain signals the brain that body tissue is injured. Acute pain has survival value because it prevents further damage. For example, when hot grease splashes on your skin, you jerk your hand away. Acute pain is often severe, especially when it results from burns, cuts or tears in the skin, dental work, and surgery. If you have ever cut your finger or hand you experienced acute pain. This is partly because there are many nerve endings in the skin on your hands. The damaged cells get your attention, so you stop what you are doing and care for the injury. Following safe practices to prevent accidents is the best approach to avoiding acute pain. Acute pain may become chronic.

Gatchel and Maddrey (2004, p. 366–367) propose a three-stage diathesis-stress model, during which patients become increasingly demoralized due to the stress of coping with pain, and the pain becomes chronic or lasting. In stage 1 there is fear, anxiety, and worry about the pain and its cause. Stage 2 is characterized by negative affect or emotions such as helplessness, depression, anxiety, and anger. Substance abuse to relieve the pain may begin in this stage. In stage 3, patients accept that a pain is chronic and adopt a maladaptive sick role behavior and begin to avoid responsibility for social or occupational obligations, using the pain as the justification. Patients then suffer physical deterioration due to disuse. Their strength and mobility diminish along with their self-esteem and social well-being.

**acute pain**  Pain that usually indicates tissue damage sending a signal of physical harm and causing enough anxiety that a person will seek medical care.

**chronic pain**  Pain lasting 6 months or longer; normal healing should have occurred and there should be no residual pain. One example of chronic pain is the pain of arthritis.

**recurrent pain** and **chronic intermittent pain**  Brief but acute pain episodes repeated over and over and distressing to patients.

## Chronic Pain

Chronic pain is pain that persists even after body tissue appears to have healed. In fact medical personnel cannot always detect the extent of damage to body tissue and must rely on patients to accurately report pain. Chronic pain is rarely cured, but can be managed. Management should be tailored for each individual (Gatchel & Maddrey, 2004, p. 366; Turk & Okifuji, 2001). Chronic pain is often accompanied by depression and frustration. Both are barriers to full recovery. Pain disturbs sleep and slows healing. Chronic pain disrupts social relationships, because it means continued suffering for patients and their family members and friends. No one wants to see their loved ones suffer.

Lower back pain is a common chronic pain. It is difficult to determine the cause, so treatments are complex. Many patients try pain-deadening medications, heat, cold, acupuncture, bed rest, biofeedback, massage, posture analysis, and stretching and strengthening exercises. Self-management of chronic pain includes training individuals to assume responsibility for managing the pain and pain-related stress. See **Table 10.2** for ideas about how to manage chronic back pain.

---

**Table 10.2   Caring for and Preventing Back Pain**

Back pain, especially acute pain in the lower back, is one of the most common complaints for which people seek help from physicians, chiropractors, massage therapists, or other healers. Diagnosing the cause of back pain is crucial for proper treatment. If no injury or disease of the spine is detected by x-rays or other medical tests, muscle strain and/or tension is the probable cause of the pain.

For back pain caused by strain, poor posture, or muscle tension, the accepted medical treatments are bed rest or back extension exercises. In general, studies comparing bed rest, exercises, and continuing with one's daily activities as much as possible show that continuing with normal activities is the best choice, as long as one is careful not to worsen the condition. Most back pain caused by strain or tension clears up without treatment, although many sufferers get relief from chiropractic manipulation or massage. However, lifting heavy objects, including children, is not advised while recovering from back pain. Sleeping on a firm, flat surface can help.

Simple back care exercises can help prevent tension, strain, and pain in the back. One helpful exercise involves standing flat against a wall. Try to press your head, heels, shoulders, and butt flat against the wall. If there is a space between the small of your back and the wall big enough to insert your hand, your back is overarched. To correct this, slide your feet forward, bend your knees slightly, and try to press the small of your back against the wall. Try to hold this posture as you slide your back up the wall. Make sure the small of your back is as close to the wall as possible. Slowly walk away from the wall holding your back in this new position. Repeat the exercise several times each day until your posture improves and your back feels stronger.

*Source:* Edlin, G., & Golanty, E. (2007). *Health and wellness* (9th ed.). Sudbury, MA: Jones and Bartlett Publishers.

Some researchers focus on chronic intermittent pain such as arthritis, migraines, and sinus headache pain. Chronic intermittent pain comes and goes and is often unpredictable. Some people who suffer from arthritic pain say the weather exacerbates their pain. Those who suffer from migraines can sometimes predict social situations that will trigger an attack, although this may be a self-fulfilling prophecy. Sometimes when we dread doing something we feel obligated to do, our pain becomes an acceptable excuse to avoid the odious task. **Chronic intractable pain** is severe and constant, like lower back pain or headaches. These are often triggered by sociopsychological events, and there is no discernible tissue damage. Another type of chronic pain is progressive pain, which gets worse over time.

People may also have **referred pain** due to confusion of sensations within the nervous system. Referred pain is felt in one part of the body, but the injury or disease is actually in another part. Referred pain is difficult to diagnose, but experienced physicians who specialize in pain control are aware of connections among various parts of the body. **Phantom limb pain** is the name given by S. W. Mitchell (1871) to a "persistent sensory awareness" that is perceived to be located in a part of the body that was removed or amputated. For example, people who have had an injured or diseased arm or leg removed may still report pain in the missing limb. They may also experience tingling, discomfort, itching, or other sensations (Katz, 1999).

**Pain syndrome** refers to a combination of **signs** and **symptoms**. Physicians and clinical psychologists have identified and studied more than 14 pain syndromes (Block, Kremer, &

**chronic intractable pain**  Persistent pain that is not relieved by medications or medical procedures.

**referred pain**  Pain due to confusion of sensations within the nervous system. Referred pain is felt in one part of the body, but the injury or disease is actually in another part. Referred pain is difficult to diagnose, but experienced physicians who specialize in pain control are aware of connections among various parts of the body.

**phantom limb pain**  Persistent pain perceived to be located in a part of the body that was removed or amputated. Some people experience tingling, discomfort, itching, or other sensations.

**pain syndrome**  A combination of signs and symptoms. More than 14 pain syndromes have been identified including whiplash injuries, back pain, headaches, cancer pain, and pain from muscular dystrophy, multiple sclerosis, herpes zoster, rheumatic disease, and sickle-cell disease.

**signs**  Objective indicators of an injury or illness that can be observed by medical personnel. Examples are shortness of breath, vomiting, bleeding, and bones protruding from patients' arms.

**symptoms**  Subjective indicators of pain that must be reported by patients. Pain is a symptom.

Fernandez, 1999). These diverse syndromes include whiplash injuries, back pain, headaches, cancer pain, and pain from muscular dystrophy, multiple sclerosis, herpes zoster, rheumatic disease, and sickle-cell disease.

## Assessing Pain

One of the first questions asked in medical care is about a patient's pain. Some aspects of pain are so complex that they are not yet well understood. There is enormous individual variation in pain perception and pain-related behavior. Health psychologists and medical care professionals have developed different ways to assess pain and continue to study causes, effects, and treatments. Health psychologists especially study the interplay among physiological, cognitive, affective, behavioral, and social factors in the assessment of pain (Gatchel & Maddrey, 2004, p. 363). There are many methods of pain measurement, and none is more valid or reliable than others (Gatchel, 2001). The Joint Commission on Accreditation of Healthcare Organizations (JCAHO) requires the use of scales to document pain severity (2008). Questions include the location, duration, and amount of pain, any aggravating factors, what relief has been tried, and what was effective, if anything.

### Descriptors of Pain

Signs are objective indicators of an injury or illness that medical personnel can observe (American National Red Cross, 2005), such as shortness of breath, vomiting, bleeding, and bones protruding from a patient's limb. Symptoms, such as nausea or dizziness, are subjective and must be reported by patients. Pain is an important symptom, and accurate descriptions are essential for a timely and accurate diagnosis. For example, when someone is having a heart attack, pain may be located in the center of the chest, but it could also radiate into the arm, up into the jaw, or even be perceived as coming from the middle of the back. Medical personnel inquire about the location and duration of pain, and the nature of the pain, such as aching, throbbing, or stabbing.

### Measurement of Pain

Probably all students have experienced pain and have even described their pain to emergency room personnel or physicians. For intermittent chronic pain, such as migraine headaches or arthritis, it may even be useful to keep a pain diary. Diaries make it possible to identify foods, odors, weather changes, and people or social situations that trigger pain. Health psychologists and other researchers have developed scales to measure and judge pain. Most scales rely on patient reports, are systematic, and very specific. Students will recall from previous chapters that accurate scales must be both valid and reliable. For a pain scale, this means researchers have tested the scale and found it measures pain accurately and consistently. Scales are also used to compare pain levels from one medical visit to another or to compare the effectiveness of one treatment or another.

Visual Analogue Scales
**Visual analogue scales** usually ask about the amount of pain from a range of 1 to 10. Ten indicates "the worst pain possible" or "pain as bad as it can be." In hospitals and doctors' offices you may see posters with a sequence of faces showing increasing degrees of frowning and grimacing to indicate the extent and intensity of pain. This type of scale is very useful for children and others who may not have the vocabulary to accurately describe their pain.

The McGill-Melzack Pain Questionnaire
**The McGill-Melzack pain questionnaire (MMPQ)** allows patients to select words that fit their pain. It assesses both amount of pain and qualities of the pain (Melzack, 1975). The scale includes different kinds of pain from a sensory viewpoint, the affective meaning of pain or how fearful a person becomes when experiencing the pain, and an evaluation of the intensity of the pain. It includes questions about patients' negative moods, the amount of social support from family and friends, levels of dissatisfaction with pain treatments, and the extent to which pain interferes with their lives. Melzack identified 3 classes of pain descriptions, 20 subclasses, and over 100 adjectives. Patients score their pain ranging from 1 to 7. This scale is useful for adults with good reading and verbal skills. It is also useful in pain control clinics to help medical personnel determine if a certain pain management program is effective.

Physiological Measures
There are other ways to measure pain. One approach is assessment of movement. Trained analysts can observe patients performing various activities and record limitations likely due to pain. Students will recall that pain itself is not observable, but limitations in movement and changes in facial expressions can be used as indicators of pain. Biofeedback specialists infer pain by measuring muscle tension, skin temperatures, rates of breathing, and heartbeats. Once pain is assessed, treatment and management efforts can begin.

## Biopsychosocial Approaches to Pain Management

The purpose of pain management is to provide symptom relief and improve quality of life by advancing a person's ability to function. It is easy to underestimate another person's pain, because pain is only discernible through pain-related behaviors or descriptions by patients. Physicians are very interested in patients' complaints about pain, because the

**visual analogue scale** A series of pictures of faces from happy to grimacing. The scale is used to determine the amount of pain in patients with limited verbal ability such as children.

**McGill-Melzack pain questionnaire (MMPQ)** A complex and detailed set of questions used to assess people's pain.

information helps them make accurate diagnoses of injury or disease. Unfortunately, the word *complaint* has taken on a negative connotation in general conversation. Many people hesitate to "complain," even to physicians. Students of health psychology can understand that patient-physician discussions are a different type of information exchange than casual conversation, and discussions about pain are very important diagnostic aids.

One approach to pain management is based on three separate stages or steps: primary, secondary, and tertiary pain management (Gatchel & Maddrey, 2004, pp. 368–370; Von Korff, 1999). **Primary pain management** is appropriate for short-lived and less severe acute pain. It includes information and encouragement so patients can return to the same activity level that existed prior to the injury or disease. Analgesics relieve pain and allow healing. Patients are reassured that their condition is temporary and treatment will be effective. Physicians once treated chronic pain by cutting nerves, but the practice left people with permanent numbness (Skevington, 2004).

If patients do not heal as expected, then **secondary pain management** continues treatment. More intensive psychosocial interventions promote a return to pre-pain productivity levels and to prevent further deterioration in the patient's biological and psychosocial well-being. **Tertiary pain management** involves intense interdisciplinary treatments to offset physical deterioration and prevent permanent disability. Legal and work-related issues become significant. This is a stage of concentrated psychosocial and disability management team efforts. It includes using objective criteria to monitor and evaluate physical deficits, cognitive-behavioral approaches to disability management, psychosocial and socioeconomic assessments, and pharmacological detoxification. Studies indicate that interdisciplinary biopsychosocial treatment programs are cost-effective and successful (Mayer & Polatin, 2000).

## Biological Approaches to Pain Management

The placebo effect discussed in the earlier chapter on research methods is relevant in pharmacological pain management. When people believe a medication is effective it often is.

---

**primary pain management**  Pain management for short-lived and less severe acute pain. It includes information and encouragement so patients can return to the same activity level that existed prior to the injury or disease. Pain is relieved with analgesics and this treatment allows healing.

**secondary pain management**  Psychosocial interventions used to promote a return to pre-pain productivity levels and to prevent further deterioration in a patient's biological and psychosocial well-being. It is used if primary pain management does not succeed.

**tertiary pain management**  Intense interdisciplinary treatments to offset physical deterioration and prevent permanent disability due to pain. Psychosocial and disability management team efforts are combined.

There are many pharmacological treatments for pain. Many people self-medicate daily with OTC medications for pain relief. In addition to OTC medications, there is a plethora of different types of pain relievers available by prescription. Anesthesia refers to the absence of sensation, especially pain. It ranges from general anesthesia, which results in unconsciousness for surgery, to local anesthesia, in which numbness is limited to specific nerves, such as for setting broken bones. Epidural anesthesia prevents pain below a certain point on the body, such as below the waist to prevent pain during childbirth. In most cases there is no sensitivity to pain even when patients remain conscious. Anesthetics can be injected or inhaled. OTC treatments for skin surfaces can numb pain from burns or cuts and itching from insect bites or exposures to plants like poison ivy and oak. All result in temporary loss of sensation.

## Pain Management in Hospital and Home Settings

The availability of drugs, drug legislation that varies from state to state, and legal restraints on hospitals influence medical treatment of patient pain. Some physicians focus more on good medical treatment for the illness or injury than with the issue of pain management, because they believe pain will disappear when medical treatment is complete. Medical personnel often find it difficult to estimate patient pain, so they rely on descriptions by the patient to judge how much pain medication to provide. Other obstacles to pain relief for patients are medical personnel's beliefs about acceptance of pain, and physicians' knowledge about the effects of medications. Some physicians worry that patients will develop a tolerance for a medication or that patients will become addicted to a controlled substance. Tolerance occurs when an administered dose is no longer sufficient to suppress pain and the dosage must be increased. Two solutions to these problems are patient-controlled analgesia and continuous infusion. Most pain treatments contain sedatives that relieve anxiety, calm patients, and decrease activity levels. Pain must also be relieved when it interferes with healing. For example, pleurisy in the chest cavity may result in extreme pain with every breath. The pain must be relieved so a patient will take in sufficient oxygen to maintain life. Pain often interferes with rest and sleeping, which in turn hinders healing. Pain relief can reduce stress and anxiety, speed recovery, and ensure medical procedures go more smoothly.

### Patient-Controlled Analgesia

It is often difficult to keep patients free of pain without sedation, and many medications are effective only for a few hours. When patients awaken, they notice pain and ask for more medication. The nurse or aide responds to the call, checks patient records for doctor's orders to find out the recommended time interval between doses, and then unlocks medication cabinets or puts in an order to the hospital pharmacy. All of this takes more time, during which the patient's pain is increasing. Even after the correct dose is delivered to the patient, an hour or so may pass before the medication takes effect. The patient returns to sleep but awakens when pain returns, and the time-consuming process begins again. For this reason some physicians and hospitals have gone to patient-controlled analgesia, which allows patients to activate doses of medicine for their pain. The doses are controlled, in the sense that patients cannot give themselves dangerous amounts. Intermittent administration by patients avoids the problems associated with undertreatment of pain following surgery, childbirth, and some cancers (Bruera & Schoeller, 1992).

The most common medical treatment for pain in terminally ill patients is opiate analgesics. This includes drugs derived from opium or produced synthetically with opiate-like characteristics (Rothenberg & Chapman, 1989). Opiates such as morphine and codeine relieve pain by suppressing the central nervous system. Lower doses of opiates can be tolerated when patients have satisfactory social support, but excessive optimism and cheerfulness may contribute to distress if patients are not allowed to talk honestly about their pain and fears. One important concern of patients who experience a change in the sensation of sudden pain is the fear that a disease has returned or reinjury has occurred. This fear causes patients to be hypervigilant about symptoms (Fordyce, 1976). Health care providers are trained to teach new pain control strategies to patients and their significant others.

## Interdisciplinary Pain Management Centers for Chronic Pain

Students may be interested in careers as members of interdisciplinary teams for the management of chronic pain (Wright & Gatchel, 2002). The Commission on Accreditation of Rehabilitation Facilities (CARF) requires that a pain management team include a physician who acts as director of the treatment plan, a specialized nurse familiar with pain management medical procedures, patient education, and physical and occupational therapists among others. Clinical psychologists do the important work of psychosocial evaluation followed by cognitive-behavioral treatment approaches (CARF, 2008). This interdisciplinary treatment team must meet at least once a week to review patient progress and make changes. Functional restoration is the goal, but pain has survival value and warns about tissue damage, so treatment teams must be very cautious about stopping pain before the extent of an illness or injury is correctly diagnosed and treated. There is no survival value to pains triggered when a dentist drills and fills a tooth, so it makes sense to prevent pain during that procedure. Patients with unrelieved chronic pain become discouraged, angry, and depressed. A major focus in rehabilitation is to preserve remaining functioning and prevent further biopsychosocial complications.

Coping with pain involves professional assessment of patients' pain experiences. Clinical health psychologists and medical personnel work together in pain evaluation and treatment to discover the most effective and least invasive strategies to use with patients. Psychological approaches include enhancement of each patient's sense of control and self-efficacy, along with reduction in anxiety and pessimism. Fear avoidance is an important part of overcoming chronic pain, and multimodal pain control includes educating patients about this problem, because pain avoidance interferes with movement, including rehabilitative exercises (Vlaeyen & Linton, 2000).

# Psychosocial Approaches to Pain Management
## Complementary Health Care for Pain Management

**Complementary health care** or **alternative medicine** refers to therapeutic interventions developed outside of traditional Western medical practice that may be used in combination within traditional medical treatments (Gardea, Gatchel, & Robinson, 2004). Some examples are acupuncture, massage, relaxation therapy, self-help groups, herbal medicine, megavitamins, chiropractics, and self-hypnosis. This section examines methods for relief of pain and stress accomplished through patient effort with the help of trained personnel. The techniques can be used both for treatment of stress and for specific stressors such as pain. These are more complex than simply talking with a therapist or meditating on ways to ignore pain. These approaches are generally less invasive than injections or pills. Several types of pain relief and relaxation may be used at the same time.

### Biofeedback

Biofeedback was briefly discussed in the chapter on stress management, and it is also used in pain management. Biofeedback requires special training, equipment, and time on the part of both the therapist and patient. It is used in behavioral medicine and clinical psychology to treat pain and stress expressed in muscle tension. Some examples of pain treated with biofeedback are persistent back pain, muscle aches, headaches, pain in the jaw, menstrual pain (dysmenorrhea), and phantom limb pain. Research demonstrates that people can be taught to control tension in the body to such an extent that they achieve relief from pain (Green & Shellenberger, 1999). Electronic monitors placed on patients' skin are connected to lights, sounds, or computer graphics. The monitors provide feedback to patients and teach them to relax and control tension in the muscles of the jaw, neck, shoulders, abdomen, and even in blood vessels in the brain.

Patients are taught with monitors, with the expectation that eventually they will be able to relax and stop pain by themselves without a feedback device. Electromyography (EMG) is also used to give patients feedback on muscle tension.

### Relaxation Training

Progressive muscle relaxation is described in the chapter on coping with stress and is also appropriate for pain management. Relaxation training means developing the ability to relax

---

**complementary health care** or **alternative medicine**  Therapeutic pain treatment interventions developed outside of traditional Western medical practice. Examples are acupuncture, massage, relaxation therapy, self-help groups, herbal medicine, megavitamins, chiropractics, and self-hypnosis.

## Think About It!

### See if Any of the Psychology Staff Does This

Dan was a first-year graduate student who experienced frequent headaches, for which he sought help from the Student Health Center. Medical tests showed no brain pathology, such as a tumor, or brain infection or injury. Diagnosis: Dan's headaches were related to the stress and anxiety about doing well in graduate school.

Dan's therapy involved meeting with a counselor to discuss ways to manage the stress of graduate school and biofeedback training to deal specifically with his headaches. In biofeedback sessions, three small sensing devices, which monitored the activity of the forehead's frontalis muscle, were attached to Dan's forehead (see figure). The frontalis and certain muscles in the neck involuntarily contract during times of stress, which impedes blood flow to the head, resulting in a headache. Wires from the three sensors were connected to a biofeedback unit, which was placed on a table directly in Dan's view. Whenever Dan's frontalis muscle contracted, the biofeedback unit produced audible clicks. A very tense frontalis produced rapid clicks. A relaxed frontalis produced infrequent, irregular clicks.

Dan was instructed by his biofeedback therapist to try to reduce the number of clicks, a skill that required several training sessions to attain. Paradoxically, not trying to relax his frontalis produced the best results. The therapy proved successful. Dan seldom got headaches. And when he did, he could relieve them by relaxing the muscles in his forehead.

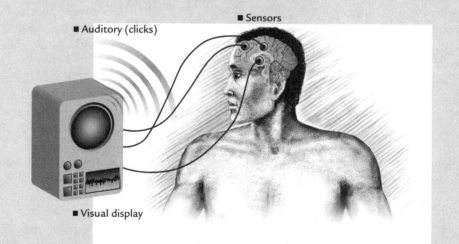

The biofeedback device measures muscle tension. A speaker produces loud clicks when muscles are tense. People learn to control muscle tension, stop the sound, and they eventually learn to stop pain without the device.

*Source:* Edlin, G., & Golanty, E. (2007). *Health and wellness* (9th ed.). Sudbury, MA: Jones and Bartlett Publishers.

without the electrodes of biofeedback. There is empirical evidence that focusing on deep diaphragmatic breathing and muscle relaxation will reduce muscle tension that contributes to pain (Belar & Deardorff, 1995).

### Hypnosis

You may have seen demonstrations of hypnosis. The hypnotist usually asks volunteer members from the audience to do silly things after being hypnotized. This is an old technique dating from at least the 19th century. Hypnosis is similar to relaxation training and biofeedback and puts individuals in a highly focused state (Gardea et al., 2004). A person choosing to cooperate with hypnosis concentrates and relaxes into an altered state of consciousness and becomes prone to suggestions by the hypnotist. Hypnosis may be used for those suffering from pain. Some people are not susceptible to hypnosis and it does not work for everyone. Hypnosis does not hasten healing, but is used for relaxation and to treat some types of pain, especially chronic pain following surgery or childbirth.

### Physical Therapy, TENS, and Massage

Physical therapy is used in addition to traditional medical approaches for injury and pain. It is accomplished by trained physical therapists working from prescriptions written by physicians. For example, physical therapists may use cold or heat treatments, salves or ointments, and closely supervised exercise to ease pain while increasing the range of motion in injured or painful joints.

TENS is transcutaneous electrical nerve stimulation. In this process, electrodes are placed on the skin near the site of pain and the area is given a mild electrical shock. The shock interferes with the transmission of the pain signal from the injury site to the brain.

Massage consists of manipulation of soft tissue to reduce pain and stress (Gardea et al., 2004, p. 372). Three types of massage are Swedish massage, in which tissue is kneaded, shiatsu, which manipulates pressure points, and rolfing, which is a type of deep muscle massage. Research indicates massage increases blood circulation, reduces stress, and may improve moods and immune systems (Field, 1999).

### Chiropractic

Chiropractors ease pain and suffering through manipulation of joints and other parts of the body. After medical doctors and dentists, they are the third largest group of health care providers (Gardea et al., 2004, p. 358). The field began in the United States in 1895 and is based on the theory that mechanical problems associated with poor posture and overuse injuries cause pain by obstructing blood flow and affecting nerves. Spinal manipulation is a common technique used to solve pain problems. According to its web site, the American Chiropractic Association (ACA) provides lobbying, public relations, funds for research regarding chiropractic issues, and offers leadership for the advancement of the profession (2008). ACA states that 7.4% of the population used chiropractic care in 2002, exceeding the use of yoga, massage, acupuncture, and diet-based therapies.

Acupuncture

This is an ancient traditional healing and pain-control technique practiced for over 2,500 years in China. It is also used in Japan, Korea, and other countries. Acupuncture is based on the theory that health problems arise from an imbalance of energy in the body. The imbalance is corrected by inserting thin needles into the skin, based on patients' descriptions of their discomfort or pain. Needles are placed at strategic points along pathways called meridians. There are about 400 possible entry points. The needles may be twirled, warmed, or energized with electricity. In 1997 the National Institute of Health published a summary of experiments and trials using acupuncture. The report now contains a warning that its statement is more than 5 years old, so the report is provided solely for historical purposes and may be inaccurate (2007). Acupuncture has been used to encourage relaxation, as an analgesic for headaches, muscle aches, postoperative pain, and to reduce nausea due to chemotherapy (see **Figure 10.2**). Some states have developed rules for training and certifying acupuncturists and there is a national accrediting agency, the Accreditation Commission for Acupuncture and Oriental Medicine.

Herbal Therapy or Botanical Medicine

In many parts of the world, plant-based or botanical medicines are used to relieve pain. For example, in Mexico a *curandero* (*herbalista*) uses herbal mixtures to alleviate pain and other difficulties. In the United States most herbs are not considered medicine, so they are not regulated by the Food and Drug Administration. Safety and effectiveness are questionable, and there is potential for abuse (Gardea et al., 2004, p. 353).

**Figure 10.2**
One example of pain management through complementary medicine is the ancient Asian technique of acupuncture.

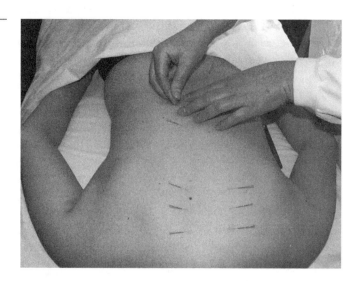

## Cognitive Techniques for Coping with Pain

Some pain-control techniques are cognitive rather than physical and teach patients how to control their own physiology. Cognitive techniques are the least invasive of pain control methods, because they involve changing thinking about pain or pain perspectives. Techniques include meditation, deep breathing, progressive muscle relaxation, and guided imagery. Many methods encourage patients to focus attention on positive things rather than on their pain. For example, transcendental meditation reduces oxygen consumption, blood pressure, and lowers metabolism (Gardea et al., 2004, p. 349). Sometimes patients are given tape recordings of a therapist's voice suggesting pleasant scenes proven to have a relaxing effect.

### Distraction
The **distraction** technique is used for both pain control and stress management. The basis of this approach is the belief that the mind can give full attention to only one thought or idea at a time. You have probably tried to distract yourself from pain or stressful thoughts by watching television, singing a song, or reading a book. Your parents may have used distraction when pulling bandages off. You anticipated pain, became tense, and so they distracted your attention before removing the bandage. You may have decided fairly early in life that it helps to look away from a wound being treated or an injection site when the needle goes into your body. While sitting in a dentist's chair to get a cavity filled, you could look up and count ceiling tiles to distract yourself from the noise of the drill, and from fears of pain and discomfort. Distraction works best with mild to moderate pain. Avoidance thinking or distraction is useful for short-term pain relief of about 3 days, while redefining or reinterpreting pain such as by saying the pain is just warmth is more enduring (Skevington, 2004, pp. 189–190).

Norman Cousins (1981) is generally credited with "laugh therapy," which is related to distraction, relaxation, and pain control. This is probably the most fun of all pain control and relaxation techniques. It can be completely self-directed. Cousins was hospitalized with a very painful health condition. For therapeutic relief he watched comedies and read books he thought were hilarious. A good laugh kept his pain under control for hours. His approach is related to all of the techniques discussed above, but particularly to distraction and taking an optimistic outlook.

### Redefinition
**Redefinition** is a method related to distraction and is used by therapists to change the ways we think about chronic stressors like pain. Patients are expected to substitute constructive

**distraction** Avoidance thinking or diversion that may be useful for short-term pain relief.

**redefinition** The re-interpretation of pain such as saying a pain is just a sensation such as "warmth."

thoughts to replace their fears. They are encouraged to make positive statements about the likelihood of their tolerating pain by using coping statements. Patients are also encouraged to look at the logic of their beliefs, so they feel less stress when pain begins. For example, people are more relaxed and less tense when they can tell themselves that not all headaches mean a malignant tumor in their brain. Affirmations can be part of redefinitions. Affirmations are statements about one's ability to overcome adversity and go through life with a stress- and pain-free existence.

## Summary

Pain is a common occurrence and defined as an unpleasant sensation often related to injury or illness. Pain helps us survive, because it warns us that what is happening is a danger to our health. Pain is a major health problem and best understood using the biopsychosocial approach of health psychology. The biological aspect of pain is the tissue damage plus the reaction of our neurological system, resulting in our perception of pain. We can have tissue damage with no pain. We can also have pain with no obvious tissue damage, such as a pain in a healed but scarred area of the body or phantom limb pain. Psychological and sociocultural aspects of pain include variations in thresholds, tolerance, and personality. Sociocultural aspects of pain reflect societal and family viewpoints and our early childhood experiences such as differential learning patterns. We respond to pain depending on its meaning and our expectations.

The physiology of pain is complex but one current theory is that a gating system in our spinal cord can either obstruct or open us to a pain sensation. The gate control theory of pain suggests that psychological factors, such as attention distraction, and sociocultural factors, such as feeling protective toward endangered loved ones, may block the pain sensation. We cannot see other people's pain, but we can recognize signs or behaviors that indicate others are experiencing pain. Pain is a health problem, because it interferes with the activities of life and often requires medical attention, including using analgesics. Health care providers often respond to patient pain with medications including narcotics. Pain can be acute or chronic and referred from body parts unconnected to the pain sensation. Pain can be evaluated using visual or verbal scales. There are a variety of nonpharmaceutical methods for controlling pain, including biofeedback, hypnosis, physical therapy, and acupuncture. Cognitive approaches include distraction and redefinition.

## Review Questions

1. Define pain and explain its purpose for health.
2. Define and give examples of pain-related behaviors.
3. Explain biological aspects of pain.
4. Review the main points of psychological aspects of pain.
5. Discuss the social and cultural aspects of pain.

6. How is pain studied using the biopsychosocial approach of health psychology?

7. Define and use examples to discuss types of pain.

8. Contrast early theories of pain with the gate control theory of pain and the neuromatrix model.

9. Describe three ways of measuring pain. Explain why this is important in pain management.

10. List, compare, and evaluate medical approaches to pain with nonpharmaceutical options for pain management.

11. Describe cognitive techniques for pain control and explain why they are helpful.

## Student Activity

Almost everyone has experienced back pain or headache pain at one time or another.

1. Students should develop and agree upon a short questionnaire about one of these pains.

2. Each student is responsible for interviewing one person about their pain experiences including:

    a. Beliefs about the causes or triggers of the pain.

    b. The extent of the pain.

    c. The nature of the pain, for example, whether it is acute, chronic, intermittent, etc.

    d. How do they exhibit pain behaviors.

    e. How others react to their pain behaviors.

    f. The various techniques they have used to stop or control the pain.

3. Students should then discuss all the different answers.

4. Each student should write an individual summary of findings and his or her interpretation of the data.

5. Students should individually evaluate whether the survey results verify the information about pain provided in class discussions and the textbook.

## References

American Chiropractic Association. ACA Fact Sheet. Retrieved March 18, 2008 from http://www.amerchiro.org

American National Red Cross. (2005). *First aid: Responding to emergencies.* Yardley, PA: StayWell.

Baum, A., Gatchel, R. J., & Krantz, D. (1997). *An introduction to health psychology* (3rd ed.). New York: McGraw-Hill.

Beecher, H. K. (1959). *The measurement of subjective response-quantitative measurement of drugs.* Oxford, UK: Oxford University Press.

Belar, C. D., & Deardorff, W. W. (1995). *Clinical health psychology in health settings: A practitioner's guidebook.* Washington, DC: American Psychological Association.

Block, A. R., Kremer, E. F., & Fernandez, E. (Eds.). (1999). *Handbook of pain syndromes: Biopsychosocial perspectives.* Mahwah, NJ: Lawrence Erlbaum.

Bruera, E., & Schoeller, T. (1992). Patient-controlled analgesia in cancer pain. *Principles and Practice of Oncology Updates, 6*(4), 1–7.

Cousins, N. (1981). *Human options.* New York: W. W. Norton.

Commission on Accreditation of Rehabilitation Facilities. (2008). CARF-accredited Service Providers Standards for Quality. Retrieved March 17, 2008 from http://www.carf.org

Field, T. (1999). Massage therapy. In W. B. Jones & J. S. Levin (Eds.), *Essentials of complementary and alternative medicine* (pp. 383–391). Philadelphia: Lippincott, Williams and Wilkins.

Fordyce, W. E. (1976). *Behavioral methods for chronic pain and illness.* St. Louis, MO: Mosby.

Gardea, M. A., Gatchel, R. J., & Robinson, R. C. (2004). Complementary health care. In R. G. Frank, A. Baum, & J. L. Wallander (Eds.), *Handbook of clinical health psychology* (Vol. 3, pp. 341–375). Washington, DC: American Psychological Association.

Gatchel, R. J. (2001). *Compendium of outcome instruments for assessment and researchers spinal disorders.* La Grange, IL: North American Spine Society.

Gatchel, R. J., & Maddrey, A. M. (2004). The biopsychosocial perspective of pain. In J. M. Raczynski & L. C. Leviton (Eds.), *Handbook of clinical health psychology* (Vol. 2, pp. 357–378). Washington, DC: American Psychological Association.

Gatchel, R. J., & Mayer, T. G. (2000). Occupational musculoskeletal disorders: Introduction and overview of the problem. In T. G. Mayer, R. J. Gatchel, & P. B. Polatin (Eds.), *Occupational musculoskeletal disorders: Function, outcomes, and evidence* (pp. 3–8). Philadelphia: Lippincott, Williams & Wilkins.

Green, J. A., & Shellenberger, R. (1999). Biofeedback therapy. In W. B. Jones & J. S. Levin (Eds.), *Essentials of complementary and alternative medicine* (pp. 410–425). Philadelphia: Lippincott, Williams and Wilkins.

International Association for the Study of Pain. (1979). Pain terms: A list with definitions and notes on usage. *Pain, 6,* 249.

Joint Commission on Accreditation of Healthcare Organizations. (2008). Nutritional, Functional, and Pain Assessments and Screens. Retrieved March 16, 2008 from http://www.jointcommission.org/AccreditationPrograms/Hospitals/Standards

Katz, J. (1999). Phantom limb pain. In A. R. Block, E. F. Kremer, & E. Fernandez (Eds.), *Handbook of pain syndromes: Biopsychosocial perspectives* (pp. 403–434). Mahwah, NJ: Lawrence Erlbaum.

Mayer, T. G., & Polatin, P. B. (2000). Tertiary nonoperative interdisciplinary programs: The functional restoration variant of the outpatient chronic pain management program. In T. G. Mayer, R. J. Gatchel, & P. B. Polatin (Eds.), *Occupational and musculoskeletal disorders: Function, outcomes, and evidence* (pp. 639–650). Philadelphia: Lippincott, Williams & Wilkins.

Melzack, P., & Wall, P. D. (1965). Pain mechanism: A new theory. *Science, 150,* 971–979.

Melzack, R. (1975). The McGill pain questionnaire: Major properties and scoring methods. *Pain, 1,* 277–299.

Melzack, R. (1999). Pain and stress: A new perspective. In R. J. Gatchel & C. Turk (Eds.), *Psychosocial factors in pain: Critical perspectives* (pp. 89–106). New York: Guilford.

Miaskowski, C. (1999). The role of sex and gender in pain perception and responses to treatment. In R. J. Gatchel & D. C. Turk (Eds.), *Psychosocial factors in pain: Critical perspectives* (pp. 401–411). New York: Guilford.

Milgrom, P., Mand, L., King, B., & Weinstein, P. (1995). Origins of childhood dental fear. *Behavior Research and Therapy, 33,* 313–319.

Mitchell, S. W. (1871). Phantom limbs. *Lippincott's Magazine of Popular Literature and Science, 8,* 563–569.

National Institutes of Health. (2007). The National Institutes of Health Consensus Development Program: Acupuncture. Retrieved May 31, 2007 from http://consensus.nih.gov/1997/1997Acupuncture107html.htm

National Institutes of Health. (1997, November). *Acupuncture: Consensus statement, 15*(5), 1–34.

Osterweiss, M. (1987). *Pain and disability: Clinical, behavioral, and public policy perspectives.* Washington, DC: National Academies Press.

Quadrel, M. J., & Lau, R. R. (1990). A multivariate analysis of adolescents' orientations towards physician use. *Health Psychology, 9,* 750–773.

Ratcliff, K. S. (2002). *Women and health in a gendered world.* Boston: Allyn & Bacon.

Rosenfeld, J. A. (2001). *Handbook of women's health: An evidence-based approach.* Cambridge, UK: University Press.

Rothenberg, M. A., & Chapman, C. F. (1989). *Dictionary of medical terms for the nonmedical person* (2nd ed.). New York: Barron's Educational Series.

Skevington, S. M. (2004). Pain and symptom perception. In A. Kaptein & J. Weinman (Eds.), *Health psychology* (pp. 182–206). Malden, MS: Blackwell Publishing.

Skevington, S. M., & Mason, V. L. (2004). Social influences on individual differences. In T. Hadjistavropoulos & K. D. Craig (Eds.), *Pain: Psychological perspectives* (pp. 179–208). Mahwah, NJ: Lawrence Erlbaum.

Turk, D. C., & Monarch, E. S. (2002). Biopsychosocial perspective on chronic pain. In D. C. Turk & R. J. Gatchel (Eds.), *Psychological approaches to pain management* (2nd ed., pp. 3–29). New York: Guilford.

Turk, D. C., & Okifuji, A. (2001). Matching treatment to assessment of patients with chronic pain. In D. C. Turk & R. Melzack (Eds.), *Handbook of pain assessment* (2nd ed.), pp. 400–416). New York: Guilford.

Vlaeyen, J. W. S., & Linton, S. J. (2000). Fear avoidance and its consequences in chronic musculoskeletal pain: A state of the art. *Pain, 85,* 317–332.

Von Korff, M. (1999). Pain management in primary care: An individualized stepped-care approach. In R. J. Gatchel & D. C. Turk (Eds.), *Psychosocial factors in pain: Critical perspectives* (pp. 360–373). New York: Guilford.

Wall, P. D. (1996). Comments after 30 years of the gate control theory of pain. *Pain Forum, 5*(1), 12–22.

Wright, A. R., & Gatchel, R. J. (2002). Occupational musculoskeletal pain and disability. In D. C. Turk & R. J. Gatchel (Eds.), *Psychological approaches to pain management* (2nd ed., pp. 349–364). New York: Guilford.

Zborowski, M. (1969). *People in pain.* San Francisco: Jossey-Bass.

# Chapter 11

# Applications of Health Psychology to Cardiovascular Disease

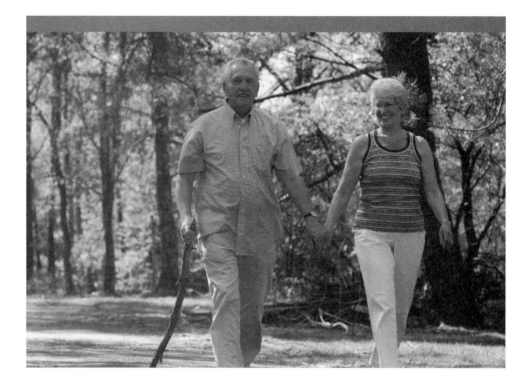

## Learning Objectives

After studying this chapter students will have the knowledge and skills to be able to:

1. Define the most important purposes and structures of the cardiovascular system.

2. Describe the types of health problems typically experienced within the cardiovascular system.

3. Explain biological, psychological, and sociocultural factors contributing to cardiovascular disease (CVD). Identify which are controllable and which are not controllable.

4. Summarize the major psychosocial explanations influencing the development of CVD.

5. Explain and evaluate forms of primary prevention for CVD, including prevention of both biological and psychosocial risks.

6. Describe screenings for biological and psychosocial risk factors.

7. Discuss biological and psychosocial factors involved in recovery from CVD.

8. Summarize types of rehabilitation programs available for CVD patients.

## Introduction

You survived childhood, adolescence, and early childhood by avoiding accidents and violence. As you age, your next major health hurdle will probably be **cardiovascular disease (CVD)**. Three important outcomes of CVD are heart attacks, cardiac arrest, and strokes. Perhaps you already know someone who had a heart attack or you have family members who are trying to keep their blood pressure under control to avoid strokes. Both are results of CVD, which is the leading cause of death and a major cause of disability in the United States (Centers for Disease Control [CDC], 2008).

CVD does not happen in one day or even in one year. It develops over several decades of life. The disease is a cumulative process reflecting lifestyle choices, personality, age, and genetic background. After completing this chapter, you will have new knowledge about preventing CVD in your life. This analysis uses the perspective of health psychology, because biological, psychological, and sociocultural factors contribute to this disease. For example, age (biological factor), hostility (psychological factor), and low income (sociocultural factor) can all contribute to diseases of the cardiovascular system. Prevention and treatment also require a biopsychosocial approach.

Students will recall that physicians of behavioral medicine and health psychology researchers apply behavioral science methods to understand health problems such as CVD. Consequently, much of the research is accomplished and authored by physicians and health psychologists working together. Some even refer to this field as cardiovascular behavioral medicine in order to emphasize the importance of human behavior and psychological and sociocultural factors. CVD may also be viewed as a response of our bodies or biological systems to challenges in the sociocultural environment, such as the widespread availability of inexpensive high-fat food. How much high-fat food is available on your campus?

We will first consider important biological concepts and then identify biopsychosocial risk factors leading to the development of CVD. Interestingly, most risk factors are under the control of every individual. Understanding risk factors or causes of disease aids us in discovering ways to prevent those diseases. When epidemiologists and other scientists talk

---

**cardiovascular disease (CVD)** Diseases of the cardiovascular system, which includes the heart and blood vessels. The system pushes blood, nutrients, oxygen, and waste products throughout the body.

about reducing risks to health and safety problems, they focus on three stages of prevention: primary, secondary, and tertiary. Primary prevention includes all efforts to avoid health and safety problems. For example, to prevent CVD it is beneficial to exercise aerobically on a regular basis. Secondary prevention refers to health screenings that make it more likely to know about diseases in early stages when treatment is more likely to be effective. You may have experienced common screenings for CVD, such as measurement of your blood pressure, heart rate, and blood cholesterol levels. Following the diagnosis of CVD, tertiary prevention efforts are used to prevent death and improve patients' quality of life. Biology, psychology, and social relationships play an important part in prevention, treatment, and recovery from CVD.

## Biological and Psychosocial Aspects of CVD

### Biological Aspects of CVD

We begin with biology because it is the aspect of CVD with which students are most familiar. What follows is a brief overview of important biological concepts.

Structures and Purposes of the Circulatory System
The cardiovascular system is essential to good health; *cardio* refers to the heart, while *vascular* refers to arteries and veins. Outcomes of CVD include **angina pectoris** or recurrent chest pain, heart attacks, deaths from cardiac arrest, and strokes. One purpose of the cardiovascular system is to move oxygenated, nutrient-rich blood to every cell in the body, enabling those cells to perform their diverse functions. Blood moves from the heart through the arteries. If you cut yourself and see bright red blood, it may be flowing from your arteries. Arteries can become so blocked that the billions of cells beyond the blockage do not receive necessary oxygen or nutrients. Without oxygen and nutrients, cells die. If cardiac arteries are blocked, then blood cannot nourish the cells of the heart muscle, and people begin to experience symptoms leading to cardiac arrest. If the blood flowing through arteries to the brain is blocked, then a stroke may result (see **Figure 11.1**).

Coronary arteries carry blood to the heart muscle cells, and arteries on the sides and backs of our necks carry blood from the heart to the brain. You can count your heart rate or the number of beats per minute by gently putting two fingers against the side of your neck just below your jaw. Feel for the pulse made by your heartbeat in a carotid artery. Find your radial pulse by pressing two fingers on the thumb side of your wrist. An infant's pulse is usually checked on the inside of the upper arm at the brachial artery.

---

**angina pectoris**  Recurrent chest pain caused by disease of the cardiovascular system.

**Figure 11.1**
Our cardiovascular system
includes the heart, lungs,
blood, arteries, and veins.

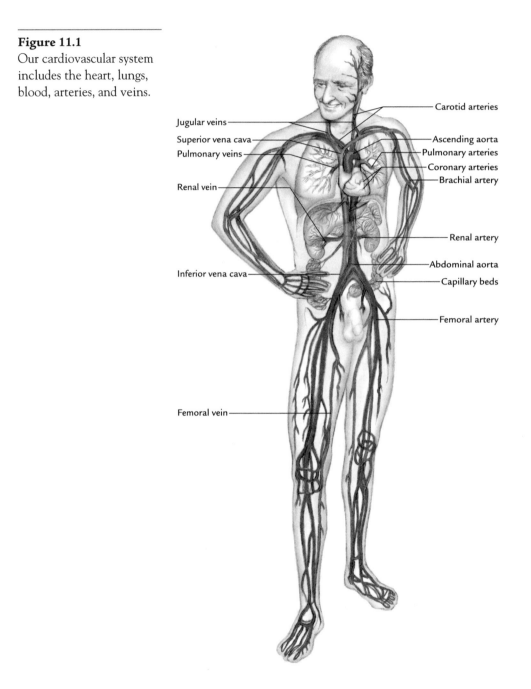

Problems Within the Cardiovascular System

Most deaths in the United States are the result of coronary heart disease (CDC, 2008a). As we grow older, two kinds of deterioration occur in our vascular systems, **arteriosclerosis** and **atherosclerosis**. Both have a negative impact on blood flow to the heart and brain and on the pressure exerted on the inside of artery walls. Mainly due to age and lifestyle choices, artery walls lose their flexibility or elasticity and become stiff. This is arteriosclerosis, which you may know as hardening of the arteries. When the heart beats, blood is pushed through stiff-walled arteries, causing blood pressure to rise to dangerous levels. Atherosclerosis refers to a second problem in the arteries that occurs when the inside walls of arteries are becoming lined with plaque or debris, including a waxy substance called **cholesterol** (Suchday, Tucker, & Krantz, 2002, p. 204). Plaque builds up inside arteries, restricting the amount of space available for blood to flow. Stiffness of artery walls (arteriosclerosis) plus plaque buildup (atherosclerosis) can be so extensive that blood flow to the heart or brain becomes blocked. Perhaps you heard someone say his or her coronary or carotid artery was 95% blocked. This means there is very little space through which oxygenated blood can flow. When blood flow to heart muscle cells is restricted, the heart is damaged, causing chest pain and myocardial infarctions, or heart attacks. The heart could also completely stop beating, which is cardiac arrest. Strokes occur when blood flow to the brain is restricted, and there is no oxygen to feed the brain cells. The cells die, and we may lose some capacity in our brains.

One of the first things that happens at a physical examination is that someone takes your blood pressure. Blood pressure is the force of blood on artery walls, and physicians rely on blood pressure readings to tell them about the health of arteries. There are two numbers to the measurement. The upper number, **systolic** pressure, reflects the force of blood on interior walls of arteries when the heart contracts. The lower number, **diastolic** pressure, is blood pressure measured when the heart relaxes. **Essential hypertension (EH)** occurs when

**arteriosclerosis**  Disorder of the arteries including the hardening of the artery walls and loss of elasticity, resulting in decreased blood flow to the heart and brain.

**atherosclerosis**  Disorder of the arteries in which plaque consisting of cholesterol and other fats lines the inner arterial wall and narrows the space through which blood can flow to the heart and brain.

**cholesterol**  A waxy fat or sterol existing in animal fats and the human body that forms deposits in blood vessels, clogging arteries and contributing to heart attacks and strokes.

**systolic**  The systole is the contraction of the heart that drives blood into the aorta and pulmonary artery; it is the top number reported in blood pressure readings.

**diastolic**  The diastole is the period between two contractions of the heart; it is the second or lower number given in blood pressure readings.

**essential hypertension (EH)**  Blood pressure considered too high for good health but with no known cause.

blood pressure is too high for good health. Scientists do not know all the causes of hypertension, but believe it reflects biology, such as age and genetic background; psychology, such as emotional or affective tendencies; and sociocultural lifestyle choices, including smoking and overeating. **Hypertension**, or high blood pressure, increases risks for strokes, heart attacks, and kidney disease. The renal system, including kidneys, plays a role in hypertension, because it is involved in controlling fluid volume. Hypertension may be asymptomatic and may go undiagnosed and untreated for long periods of time (American National Red Cross, 2005). Our blood pressure usually rises as we grow older.

### Serious Cardiovascular Conditions and Events

**Ischemia and Angina Pectoris Ischemia** is decreased blood supply to a body part, and myocardial ischemia is insufficient blood flow to meet the heart's metabolic demands (Suchday et al., 2002, p. 204). (See **Figure 11.2**.)

When plaque occludes coronary arteries, the heart muscle cells do not receive enough oxygenated blood and people usually experience chest pain. This pain may indicate an early stage of CVD known as angina pectoris. Different situations trigger or cause chest pain in people with angina. One biological situation is strenuous exercise, especially in cold weather. Other situations are psychosocial, such as elevated stress occurring while watching a favorite team lose the ball. Both situations cause blood pressure to rise and the heart muscle to work harder. When heart cells do not get enough oxygen, the muscle hurts. People with diagnosed angina recognize the pain and can stop it by slowing down their exercise rate or turning off the television. Some take nitroglycerin as a tiny pill under their tongue or through a skin patch. As the medicine moves into the bloodstream, it opens, or dilates, the coronary arteries and pain is relieved. If there is no relief from medication, a person may be having a heart attack and someone should call an ambulance.

**Heart Attacks or Myocardial Infarctions** A heart attack, or **myocardial infarction,** is an event indicating severe CVD. Coronary arteries are so blocked that not enough oxygenated

**hypertension** A disorder of the cardiovascular system in which the blood pressure is persistently above 140/90 mg HG.

**ischemia** Decreased blood supply to a body part; myocardial ischemia refers to insufficient blood flow to meet the heart's metabolic demands.

**myocardial infarction** A heart attack that destroys that part of the heart muscle that has lost its blood supply.

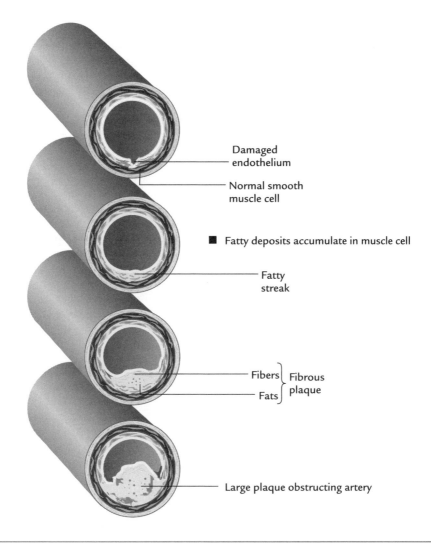

Damaged endothelium

Normal smooth muscle cell

■ Fatty deposits accumulate in muscle cell

Fatty streak

Fibers ⎱ Fibrous
Fats ⎰ plaque

Large plaque obstructing artery

**Figure 11.2** Due to lifestyle choices and age, the walls of the coronary and carotid arteries stiffen and become blocked with plaque.

blood is getting to the heart muscle, and muscle cells deprived of oxygen will die. Emergency medical service (EMS) should be called immediately. Angina pains and heart attacks warn people of CVD, so they can seek medical care to prevent death. Angina is an ongoing or chronic condition, while a heart attack is an event. Chest pain is considered the classic sign of a heart attack, but there are other signs and signals.

## Think About It!

### What to Do in an Emergency

IF YOU THINK YOU ARE HAVING A HEART ATTACK, CALL YOUR EMERGENCY MEDICAL SYSTEM IMMEDIATELY.

**Common or "classic" signs of heart attack**

- Uncomfortable pressure, fullness, squeezing, or pain in the center of the chest that lasts more than a few minutes, or goes away and comes back
- Pain that spreads to the shoulders, neck, or arms
- Chest discomfort with light-headedness, fainting, sweating, nausea, or shortness of breath

**Less common warning signs of heart attack**

- Atypical chest, stomach, or abdominal pain
- Nausea or dizziness (without chest pain)
- Shortness of breath and difficulty breathing (without chest pain)
- Unexplained anxiety, weakness, or fatigue
- Palpitations, cold sweat, or paleness

Not all of these signs occur in every heart attack. Sometimes they go away and return. If some occur, get help fast. IF YOU NOTICE ONE OR MORE OF THESE SIGNS IN ANOTHER PERSON (OR YOU HAVE THEM YOURSELF). DON'T WAIT. CALL 911 OR YOUR EMERGENCY MEDICAL SERVICES AND GET TO A HOSPITAL RIGHT AWAY!

**Be prepared**

- Keep a list of emergency rescue service numbers next to the telephone and in your pocket, wallet, or purse.
- Find out which area hospitals have 24-hour emergency cardiovascular care.
- Know (in advance) which hospital or medical facility is nearest your home or office.

**Take action**

- If you have heart attack symptoms that last more than a few minutes, don't delay! Immediately call 911 or the EMS numbers so an ambulance (ideally with advanced life support) can be sent for you quickly.
- If ambulance service isn't available in your area, immediately have someone drive you to the nearest hospital emergency room (or another facility offering 24-hour life support).

- If you're with someone who may be having heart attack symptoms, immediately call 911 or the EMS. Expect the person to protest—denial is common. Don't take "no" for an answer. Insist on taking prompt action.

- Give CPR (mouth-to-mouth breathing and chest compression) if it's needed and you're properly trained.

*Source:* Alters, S., & Schiff, W. (2009). *Essential concepts for healthy living* (5th ed.). Sudbury, MA: Jones and Bartlett Publications, LLC.

**Cardiac Arrest Cardiac arrest** is the most serious cardiac event. Heart muscles are so damaged that the cardiac rhythm is interrupted and the heart stops beating. Persons who are unconscious, not breathing, and have no pulse are experiencing cardiac arrest. Victims can sometimes be resuscitated through **cardiopulmonary resuscitation (CPR)** while waiting for EMS to arrive. CPR includes pressing down and then releasing the center of the victim's chest in a pumping motion, alternated with breathing into the victim's lungs. The American Red Cross and the American Heart Association train people in CPR. This training is often offered in first aid classes on campus. If bystanders know CPR, they may keep a person's blood circulating until an ambulance comes. An alternative in some locations is a battery-operated device known as an **automated external defibrillator (AED)** that can be used to start an arrested heart beating again. Most include exact instructions.

**Stroke Stroke**, another event associated with CVD, is due to blockage of blood flow to the brain. Strokes are the third leading cause of death in the United States, and every 45 seconds someone experiences a stroke (CDC, 2008b). Strokes increase after age 55 and are more likely to occur in men than in women. African Americans experience more strokes than white Americans. Major strokes may result in disability that requires rehabilitation. A carotid

**cardiac arrest** A stoppage of the heart leading to oxygen deprivation in important organs such as the lungs, brain, and kidneys.

**cardiopulmonary resuscitation (CPR)** The provision of external massage of the heart and oxygen by another person on someone who is experiencing cardiac arrest.

**automated external defibrillator (AED)** A device that analyzes heart rhythms and can tell when to administer a shock to a victim of cardiac arrest. The shock, defibrillation, may re-establish an effective heart rhythm.

**stroke** A cerebrovascular event in which oxygen is blocked in the blood vessels of the brain. The person may experience paralysis, weakness, an inability to speak, or death.

TABLE 11.1 Signs of Stroke

**Some or all of these signs accompany a stroke:**

Weakness, numbness, or paralysis on one side of the body

Loss or dimming of vision, particularly in one eye

Loss of speech, or difficulty speaking or understanding speech

Sudden, severe headache

Sudden dizziness, unsteadiness, or episodes of falling

*Source:* Alters, S., & Schiff, W. (2009). *Essential concepts for healthy living* (5th ed). Sudbury, MA: Jones and Bartlett Publishers.

artery could be 100% blocked, so immediate medical attention is required for stroke victims to prevent further brain damage. There are several warning signs of strokes. One is facial numbness similar to being anesthetized for dental work. People may feel dizzy, lose their balance, appear confused, or have difficulty speaking. Persons having strokes sometimes lose consciousness and are injured from the fall. When they regain consciousness, they may not be able to talk, see, or move one side of their body. About 75% of stroke patients experience muscle weakness or partial paralysis on one side of the body (Suchday et al., 2002, p. 225). **Table 11.1** lists the signs of stroke.

**Transient ischemic attacks (TIAs)** are mild strokes that come and go. In TIAs, symptoms may be difficult to identify. People experiencing mild strokes sense something is wrong, but are not sure what is happening. One signal of a TIA is not remembering what just happened or missing time. TIAs are useful because they warn us that blood flow to our brain was interrupted, and we need medical diagnosis and treatment.

## Psychosocial Aspects of CVD

Psychosocial aspects of CVD include some concepts already familiar to students from earlier chapters. These include stress, negative emotions or affect, personality traits, lifestyle choices, social isolation, and a variety of sociocultural factors including poverty, discrimination, and residing in neighborhoods with high rates of crime. Ischemia merged with stressful situations, in combination with individual ways of reacting to stress, may result in CVD, heart attacks, cardiac arrest, strokes, and death. Reactions to stressful situations may begin a chain of biological processes including increases in heart rate and breathing. These phys-

**transient ischemic attacks (TIAs)** A brief episode of insufficient blood supply to the brain.

iological changes enable us to defend ourselves or escape from danger. Powerful and damaging psychological responses to stressful social situations are often followed by potent reactions in the neurological, hormonal, endocrine, and immune systems. Some individuals appear to be particularly responsive to stressors and their reactions contribute to the development of CVD (Suchday et al., 2002, p. 205).

## Identifying Causes of CVD Using the Health Psychology Perspective

Most health psychologists and other scientists believe the causes of CVD are multifactorial and include biological, psychological, and sociocultural factors. It is unclear precisely which factors are more important, in part because researchers must work within ethical limitations when doing experimental studies. For example, it would be unethical to try to trigger heart attacks, cardiac arrest, or strokes in people to test hypotheses about stress, even though scientists believe stress contributes to cumulative artery wall damage, plaque buildup, and hypertension. Experiments with cynomolgus monkeys do demonstrate that stress causes injury to the endothelium of the coronary arteries (Manuck, Kaplan, Clarkson, Adams, & Shively, 1991).

What can be demonstrated in laboratories is that when human subjects are placed in stressful situations, such as hearing loud noises, recalling an incident that triggered intense anger, or doing difficult math tasks, then biological and psychosocial changes such as a rise in blood pressure and in expressions of frustration may occur (Gottdiener et al., 1994). If people already have plaque buildup in their arteries, then blood thickening due to stress could result in blockage of the coronary or carotid arteries. This is one reason why daily doses of blood thinners, such as aspirin, are sometimes advised for older people.

## Biopsychosocial Risk Factors for CVD

### Biological Risk Factors

Scientists trying to prevent CVD study **risk factors**. Some risks are biological, while others are psychological or sociocultural. Knowing about their risks makes it possible for people to eliminate or minimize some of those factors. For purposes of prevention, all three types of risk factors should be examined and understood. Biological risk factors can be non-modifiable, such as age; partially modifiable, such as blood pressure; or totally modifiable,

**risk factors**  Behaviors and conditions that put people at risk of certain illnesses such as heart disease.

such as smoking. The Framingham heart study produced a sample score sheet for estimating coronary heart disease risk that focuses mainly on biological risks. It includes age, total cholesterol, HDL cholesterol, blood pressure, diabetes, and smoking (CDC, 2008a).

Uncontrollable Risk Factors: Age and Genetic Background

From a biological viewpoint the greatest risk for CVD is age. The older we get, the more likely we are to develop vascular disease. Age is a non-modifiable risk factor, because there is nothing we can do to stop growing older. A second uncontrollable risk factor is genetic background. This risk refers to having a blood relative who died prematurely of heart disease or stroke. There is a greater likelihood of developing CVD if we descend from people who succumbed to CVD. The strongest connection will be with parents, but if grandparents, sisters, brothers, or even aunts or uncles have CVD, then you, as a genetic relative, are at greater risk than someone with a different genetic background. It has to be a direct blood connection, so an aunt or uncle related only by marriage has no genetic connection to you, and the relationship does not increase your risk. There is also evidence that there are genetically based risks for high cholesterol levels, high blood pressure, and a tendency toward excessive body fat, although it is generally believed those factors are mainly due to lifestyle choices.

Partially Controllable Risk Factors: Cholesterol, Hypertension, and Diabetes

High cholesterol levels can be prevented and treated. The lifestyle behavior most associated with high cholesterol levels is eating food containing saturated fat. This is discussed in the chapter on nutrition and weight control. Regular aerobic exercise and avoiding obesity are additional approaches to keeping blood cholesterol levels low. Medications are available to treat high cholesterol levels, but may have unpleasant side effects.

Arteriosclerosis and atherosclerosis contribute to CVD by causing blood pressure to rise, which damages artery walls. Hypertension may be partially genetic, but it reflects lifestyle choices, including smoking, alcohol use, and salt intake. Blood pressure can be improved by regular aerobic exercise, maintaining a healthy body weight, and taking medications.

Even young college students may have high blood pressure and should learn about their blood pressure numbers. To get a baseline measurement, go to the college health center and have your blood pressure taken at different times of day and different days of the week over the semester. Keep a record by writing the numbers down and briefly describing recent stressors in your life to see if stress might cause the numbers to rise.

Most cases of diabetes are due to lifestyle choices but may have genetic bases too. There are two general types of diabetes and both are risks for CVD. Type I diabetes is not well understood, but lifestyle choices are probably not a causal factor. This type of diabetes usually appears first during youth. Type II diabetes is associated with lifestyle choices that result in obesity. People with diabetes spend a great deal of time and thought maintaining the balance between their food intake and activity levels. Many use insulin to help maintain that balance. In addition to CVD, uncontrolled diabetes contributes to kidney disease, blindness, and amputations due to poor blood circulation. Diabetes is discussed more thoroughly in the chapter on chronic diseases.

## Psychosocial Factors Contributing to CVD

Health psychologists confirm that stressors trigger biological changes, including increases in heart rate, breathing patterns, blood pressure, and blood clotting mechanisms. No studies find that stressors directly contribute to CVD, although associations are found between stress and personality traits such as **hostility** (Martin & Brantley, 2004, p. 238–240). Some researchers suggest that long-term minor stressors are more likely to contribute to CVD than major events (Twisk, Snel, Kemper, & van Mechelen, 1999). Sudden cardiac arrest and strokes do occur in people with CVD when there is a sudden shocking event.

Stress and Lifestyle Risk Factors

Self-report research links psychosocial factors such as stress to lifestyle choices. People say they smoke, overeat, and abuse substances including alcohol to help them cope with stress. There is research evidence that stress interferes with positive health behaviors such as exercise (Martin & Brantley, 2004). Lifestyle choices such as smoking, abusing alcohol, overeating, and never exercising are independent risk factors for CVD. Studies show that chronic stress influences weight gain in caregivers of Alzheimer patients, paramedics, and fire fighters (Vitaliano, Russo, Scanlan, & Greeno, 1996; Gerace & George, 1996). Stressful events are also associated with changes in glucose and insulin response in obese patients (Seematter et al., 2000). Excessive body fat contributes to diabetes and hypertension, which are both additional risks for CVD. People are at greater risk for CVD when they choose inactive leisure-time activities. Watching television or videos and sitting to play video games are sedentary leisure-time activities typical of our culture. It is possible to run in place or peddle a stationary exercise bicycle while watching television, but few people choose to do so. All risk factors have an additive effect on total CVD risk. For example, if people smoke and have high cholesterol levels, they have a higher risk than they would have if they just had one or the other.

The CVD risk factors of smoking, alcohol use, eating patterns, and being sedentary are under the control of most people. Exceptions are infants, children, and adolescents being raised by adults who make poor lifestyle choices for themselves. For example, smoking is a completely controllable risk factor for CVD, except for children and teens who cannot escape the smoke exhaled by their caregivers. Alcohol use is common in many families, and children grow up and repeat family patterns. Nutritional choices are also controlled by parents and

---

**hostility** An attitude of antagonism toward others. It is believed to be a risk factor for CVD. Part of the Type A personality.

other caregivers until children are allowed to select their own food at school or when eating away from home. Exercise habits are similarly established by parents unless children take physical education classes in school or participate in after-school sports.

### Smoking and CVD

There is a clear statistical connection between smoking and CVD. Smoking tobacco products is the greatest lifestyle risk factor for CVD, and the most preventable (CDC, 2008a). Most people know that smoking causes cancer, but do not know about the robust statistical relationship between smoking and CVD. Unlike age and genetic background, this risk factor is 100% preventable. Smokers reduce their risk of vascular diseases when they stop smoking. Nonsmokers reduce their risks by avoiding smoke exhaled by other people.

### Obesity and CVD

Choosing unhealthy eating patterns is another lifestyle choice and totally preventable risk factor for vascular disease. Obesity refers to the accumulation of excessive amounts of body fat. Fat accumulates when we take in more calories than we use. The prevention of obesity is discussed in greater detail in the chapters on exercise and eating behaviors. Excessive body fat also contributes to diabetes and hypertension, which are additional risk factors for heart disease.

### Absence of Regular Exercise and CVD

Choosing to be sedentary is a third controllable risk for CVD. Lifestyle risk factors reflect a nation's culture and economy, and many people have sedentary jobs. People can offset being sedentary at work by being physically active away from work. Physical activity or regular exercise improves the health of the cardiovascular system, lowers cholesterol levels and resting blood pressure, and reduces excess fat on the body. People may become obese and at risk for CVD when they choose only sedentary leisure-time activities.

## Other Psychosocial Risk Factors Contributing to CVD

### Psychosocial Risks and Research Issues

Research results about the relationship between psychosocial factors and CVD are difficult to evaluate. It is not easy to compare studies when concepts such as anger, aggression, and hostility are defined and measured in different ways. It is also difficult to demonstrate a direct connection between psychological factors such as negative affect and infirmities such as heart disease. A second problem in the study of psychosocial risk factors is that much of the research is retrospective rather than prospective. Longitudinal prospective studies are difficult and expensive. Furthermore, it is unethical to set up experiments to cause heart attacks, strokes, or a symptom of CVD in order to test hypotheses. The greater the distance in time between a psychosocial risk and the diagnoses of vascular disease, the more difficult it is to establish causal connections.

A third problem in social science research is that anger and other negative emotions can trigger chest pain, but chest pain may also cause negative emotions. There is such enormous variation in human behavior it is difficult to confirm statistical relationships. It should also be noted that most studies on heart disease were based on men. As a result, we know less about CVD in women than we do in men.

Another set of problems is involved in researching the effect of culture on heart disease. Culture refers to the way of life of a people residing within a geographic area. Culture is pervasive, and from a research perspective it is not easy to isolate all the characteristics of cultures that might put people at risk for CVD. In addition, when behavioral scientists are products of the culture they study, it is very difficult for them to be objective, because most people believe their way of life is right, good, and normal. Some social scientists suggest that living in a highly competitive culture that emphasizes material rather than spiritual success contributes to CVD, while others counter by pointing to the health advantages of living in industrially and technologically advanced countries.

An additional research issue is that not all residents within a geographic area such as the United States are experiencing the general culture in the same way. Education, income, and other factors vary greatly. Lower income usually means less access to medical care, groceries, and healthful environments where walking for exercise is safe and the air is clear and clean. Low-income people are more likely to live in stressful social environments, and they tend to be more socially isolated. All of these factors contribute to poorer health and greater health risks. For example, heart disease risk is greatest among African American men living in high-stress poor neighborhoods (Polednak, 1998). Rates of essential hypertension are very high for African Americans and highest among those who live in lower socioeconomic circumstances. This points to both biological and psychosocial origins of the disease (Ng-Mak, 1999; Young, Waller, & Kahana, 1991).

Negative Emotional States

In prose and poetry, the heart is viewed as the body part most affected by emotions. People say their hearts feel differently when they are in love or when they are grieving. Personal traumas such as the death of a spouse or child, and community disasters such as floods and fires, are associated with sudden cardiac death. For example, residents of Tel Aviv had an increased incidence of sudden cardiac death following Iraqi missile strikes, and a significant increase in cardiac death occurred on the day of a California earthquake (Suchday et al., 2002, p. 206). People who display anger, aggression, and hostility are at high psychosocial risk for CVD. Anger is an emotional reaction, aggression is a behavior, and hostility is an ongoing tendency (Chesney, 1985).

Personality Traits and Stress

Our personality includes our characteristic ways of feeling and reacting. Personality reflects everything that happens, including living in a family, a neighborhood, going to school, and interacting with peers. Attitudes and reactions also reflect what we see on television, hear on the radio, and read about in newspapers or on the Internet. Personality traits influence reactions to stress and health behavior choices that put us at risk of CVD (Suchday et al., 2002, p. 208). Through retrospective research, health psychologists have identified personality characteristics common in patients with CVD, including hostility, anger, **cynicism**, and a feeling of being constantly pressed for time. Negative affect or emotions can become characteristic patterns of thinking and reacting in the face of adversity. Intense negative reactions such as anger and fear may also reflect stress from the social context in which people live, such as living in poverty, or being abused by caregivers.

Physicians have long noted links between personality characteristics and heart disease. In 1868, a German physician, T. von Deusch, described speaking loudly and excessive work habits as predictors of CVD. A few years later, Dr. William Osler wrote that mental worry and sudden shock could lead to chest pain (Williams, 1989). In the early part of the 20th century, physicians theorized that men with hypertension were people who had difficulty expressing their angry feelings. The Type A behavior pattern was linked to heart disease in the 1950s. Nevertheless, it is still difficult to specify the precise causality between CVD disease and personality.

The Type A Behavior Pattern

Has anyone ever said you had a Type A personality? In health psychology, a cardiac-disease-prone personality is known as the Type A personality. Two cardiologists, Friedman and Rosenman (1959), observed certain common personality traits and behaviors among their patients who had experienced heart attacks. They identified distinctive traits such as impatience, exasperation, and feeling constantly pressed for time. Time urgency was also related to competitiveness, irritability, and hostility. Patients' hostility often arose in response to events the observing physicians thought were trivial or unimportant.

In 1981, the National Heart, Lung and Blood Institute (NHLBI) recognized the Type A behavior pattern as a psychosocial risk factor for coronary heart disease (2008b). This area of biobehavioral research continues to develop. Friedman and Rosenman studied men already diagnosed with heart disease; it is difficult to know precisely which came first, heart disease or the Type A behavior pattern, or even if there was a connection. Later studies were prospective rather than retrospective, giving greater credibility to the research. In the 8-year Western Collaborative Group Study, a structured interview was used to distinguish between Type A and Type B men, none of whom had evidence of CVD before the study began (Rosenman et al., 1975). More men identified as Type A developed CVD than those identified as Type B. Researchers concluded that a Type A behavior pattern predicts an increased risk of CVD (Jenkins, 1976). Other research does not confirm the effect of Type A

---

**cynicism** Belief, attitude, or viewpoint that other people cannot be trusted. It is believed to be a risk factor for cardiovascular disease. Part of the Type A personality.

behavior pattern on CVD. Today scientists are trying to determine if the pattern is present prior to adulthood among high school students or even in children in elementary school. The earlier a personality pattern is identified, the more likely a person could change attitudes and behavior.

### Cynicism and Hostility

Inconsistent research findings on the Type A personality led researchers to examine specific personality characteristics (Suchday et al., 2002, p. 208). Not all components of the Type A personality are equally harmful. Hostility and cynicism are viewed as two factors most likely to damage the circulatory system. Both hositility and cynicism are complex concepts, and different studies define and measure them in different ways.

A physician, Redford Williams (1989), found premature death due to CVD, cancer, and other causes was more characteristic of people who scored higher on hostility measures. Cynicism, hostility, or a negative worldview may affect the likelihood of having supportive social relationships (Suchday et al., 2002, p. 209). Williams argued that people should believe in the goodness of others, be slow to anger, and avoid resentment and irritability. Williams thought that hostility was learned through childrearing practices and facial expressions, but genetic factors might also be involved.

Hostility, anger, and cynicism may also contribute to lifestyle behaviors inherently harmful to health. Overeating and use of tobacco, alcohol, and other substances can be reactions to social situations or the result of efforts to suppress hostility and anger (Rozanski, Blumenthal, & Kaplan, 1999). Being hostile, angry, and cynical is probably a learned response and hostile parents may set this example for their children.

## Primary Prevention of CVD

### Reducing Biological Risks of CVD

Many of the approaches listed below are familiar to you from earlier chapters. The first line of defense against CVD is avoiding tobacco smoke, alcohol, and other heart-damaging substances (CDC, 2008b). The first line of offense is regular exercise that requires sustained movement and elevates the heart rate and breathing, for 30 or more minutes, at least 5 days each week. This does *not* mean people must run or jog. The Centers for Disease Control (2008) suggests 30 minutes of brisk walking every day for everyone. Healthful eating patterns also help prevent CVD and are discussed in detail in an earlier chapter. Body fat is extra calories stored on the body. Maintaining the balance between calories consumed and calories used prevents the accumulation of excess body fat. Exercise and good nutrition help prevent obesity and diabetes. Exercise also helps to control hypertension and to manage high cholesterol levels.

### Reducing Psychosocial Risks of CVD

Stress damages our circulatory and immune systems, making us more susceptible to CVD. Several psychosocial risk factors are open to modification. We can avoid known stressors and change our damaging emotional reactions such as anger, hostility, and cynicism. By removing stress from our lives and changing habitual reactions, we reduce risks of CVD. Students may want to refer back to the chapters on stress and stress management. Techniques for changing Type A behavior patterns also exist (Friedman, 1996).

Work situations and personal relationships may be daily sources of stress. The kinds of jobs we hold may jeopardize our health and safety. This is particularly true when jobs make demands on us over which we have little control. Sedentary jobs also contribute to CVD.

High job turnover is an indicator of stress at worksites. Role conflict, role ambiguity, industrial mental hygiene, and healthy workplace design have all been factored into studies in occupational health psychology (Quick et al., 2004, pp. 234–235). Occupational stress research indicates that distinctive attributes of certain types of jobs may contribute to the development of cardiovascular disease in some people. For example, jobs with low control by workers and high demands from management predicted CVD in men, while women were more affected by high demands from their families and non-supportive bosses as well as by jobs over which they had little control (Suchday, Tucker, & Krantz, 2004, pp. 206–207). In addition to the demand/control aspects of work, an imbalance between effort and compensation adds stress (Steptoe & Ayers, 2004, p. 180). Both the type of work being accomplished and characteristics of the job environment may result in stress. These factors include noise, shift work, and working to a machine-based tempo. In a prospective study of 25 years, Kivimaki and colleagues (2002) concluded that the risk of dying from CVD was more than double for those with high job strain and an effort/reward imbalance.

## Secondary Prevention of CVD: Screening for Risk Factors

### Screening for Biological Risk Factors

You will recall that longitudinal research is *better* than retrospective studies at identifying health risks, but it is also more difficult and more expensive. The Framingham heart study is an important investigation of CVD and has gone on for more than 50 years (Voelker, 1998). This pioneering effort has enabled researchers to identify many of the risk factors, prevention strategies, and treatments for CVD. Every 2 years participants fill out forms and go through medical tests. The study helped identify high cholesterol, hypertension, smoking, and obesity as risk factors and found that aerobic exercise could reduce risk factors. About 5,000 people began the study, which now includes two generations of families. At this time 17,500 pieces of information exist on each subject or participant.

### Heart Rate, Blood Pressure, and Cholesterol Levels

Secondary prevention refers to identification of threatening factors before serious damage to health occurs. Many screenings for biological risk of CVD occur during routine checkups in clinical settings, including annual medical exams for adults at middle age or earlier if there is family history of CVD. Listening to hearts beat, measuring blood pressure, and taking body temperatures are noninvasive screenings because they do not require entering the bloodstream. At some point physicians may add glucose tolerance tests for diabetes and more invasive tests that might indicate heart disease. As a result of screenings, physicians may suggest blood pressure-lowering medication to prevent strokes or recommend specialists in CVD. The results of personal screenings often motivate people to change their risky behaviors to prevent heart attacks or strokes.

You will recall cholesterol is a substance in the blood that can accumulate in artery walls, restricting blood flow and contributing to CVD. National health agencies recommend certain cholesterol level limits for optimal health. When cholesterol levels exceed these levels, a person may be at greater risk for CVD. Recommendations change over the years. Cholesterol measurements include levels of total cholesterol, high-density lipoproteins (HDLs), and low-density lipoproteins (LDLs), and the ratio of total cholesterol to HDLs. Limiting saturated fat intake by careful selection of food and exercising regularly will improve blood lipid levels. In addition cholesterol-lowering medications are available. Medications do not cure high blood pressure or cholesterol levels and usually must be taken for the rest of one's life. Taking medications is more difficult if there are unpleasant side effects such as fatigue, weakness, dizziness, drowsiness, depression or affective distress, headaches, and sexual dysfunction. One perplexing result of several cholesterol-reduction studies is that while medications resulted in fewer CVD deaths, the number of deaths from accidents, suicides, and violence increased (Kaplan, Manuck, & Shumaker, 1992).

### Angiocardiograms, EKGs, and Treadmill Stress Tests

**Angiocardiograms,** EKGs, and treadmill stress tests are more complicated biological screenings. **ECGs** or **EKGs** screen electrical impulses made by the heart so doctors can locate abnormalities. A type of EKG stress test can be carried out while exercising on a treadmill to see how the heart performs under the stress of moving uphill at a fast pace. Sometimes chemicals are injected into the bloodstream to monitor blood flow to the heart before, during, and after the exercise stress test. If major blockage of coronary arteries is indicated, the patient may be immediately sent to the hospital for more diagnostic work and possible surgery.

### Gender Differences in Screenings

Most tests were developed using male patients. New research shows variations when women are tested. Angiocardiograms show plaque buildup inside the arteries. A recent finding is that women's coronary arteries may appear to be free of blockage even when arteries are clogged. The result is that women are not being diagnosed with CVD when, in fact, they have CVD and are at risk of heart attacks (Neighmond, 2006). One theory is that plaque in women is smooth rather than lumpy. There are other gender differences in screening.

---

**angiocardiogram** A series of x-rays of the heart while a contrasting medium is being passed through it; used to diagnose disorders of the heart.

**ECGs or EKGs** Electrocardiogram; a diagnostic procedure that graphically records the electrical activity of the heart.

For many years, physicians and scientists believed women were less likely to have heart disease than men. Now we know the gender difference is really an age difference. CVD appears at earlier ages in men than in women. One adverse consequence of this error is that many college textbooks list gender, or being male, as a risk factor for heart disease, implying that women are protected against the disease (American National Red Cross, 2005). Consequently, screening and treatment may be delayed.

Another gender difference in diagnoses of heart disease lies in CVD research. Most early studies included only men and scientists and physicians assumed that what was true of men was also true of women. They were mistaken. For example, the calculations for women doing treadmill stress tests must take into account the fact that women have more tissue on their chest walls. (See **Figure 11.3** to compare leading causes of death for males and females.)

Health Risk Analysis (HRA)

The **health risk analysis (HRA)** is a general screening tool for risks of CVD; it includes physiological conditions, health-related behaviors, and psychosocial factors. HRAs usually include questions about genetic background and health-related practices such as exercise and eating patterns. There may also be questions about one's ability to laugh, to make decisions without stress, to express angry feelings, to discuss personal problems with friends or professional counselors, and about general satisfaction with life.

Screening for Psychosocial Risk Factors

Screenings for psychosocial risk factors include questionnaires, face-to-face interviews, and possibly laboratory experiments. Students are already aware of the problems of validity and reliability associated with standardized surveys. Inconsistent results may be due to respondents' varying educational levels, perspectives, and current contextual factors. For example, answers to questions about hostility and cynicism may vary depending on what is going on in a person's life at the time the questions are answered. Over the years dozens of personality characteristics have been included among items but most focus on Type A behavior patterns: hostility, stress, negative affectivity, and pessimism (Smith & Ruiz, 2004, pp. 162–175).

**The Type A Behavior Pattern** Specific screening tools assess the Type A behavior pattern. Questionnaires and interviews include items about Type A characteristics such as competitiveness, time urgency, and hostility. If screening shows a tendency toward Type A behavior, then people can take steps to reduce this style of responding to stressors. One early example is the Jenkins Activity Survey, which focuses on impatience, striving, and competitiveness (Jenkins, Rosenman, & Zyzanski, 1974). Rosenman developed the Type A Structured Interview, which includes questions and problems focusing more on a respondent's

---

**health risk analysis (HRA)** A series of questions on topics that may indicate a high risk of some diseases, such as heart disease.

**Figure 11.3**
CVD is the number one
cause of death of both men
and women of all races and
all ages.

*Source:* National Center for
Heath Statistics. (2004).
Health, United States 2004.
Washington DC: U.S. Gov-
ernment Printing Office,
and Alters, S., & Schiff, W.
(2009). *Essential concepts for
healthy living* (5th ed.). Sudbury, MA: Jones and
Bartlett Publishers.

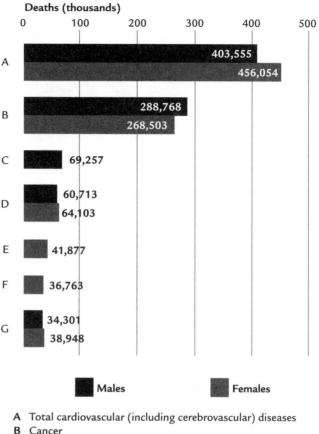

Deaths (thousands)

A  Total cardiovascular (including cerebrovascular) diseases
B  Cancer
C  Accidents
D  Chronic lower respiratory diseases
E  Alzheimer's disease
F  Pneumonia/influenza
G  Diabetes mellitus

style of responding rather than on the answers (Rosenman, 1978). The Framingham Heart study also produced a Type A scale, mainly assessing impatience and competitiveness (Haynes, Feinleib, & Kannel, 1980).

Friedman (1996) has written about both the diagnosis and treatment of Type A behavior patterns. He notes that people rarely describe themselves as being hostile, and consequently self-report questionnaires are less reliable for screening than face-to-face interviews. According to Friedman, diagnosis of Type A behavior must be done by trained professionals. His screening training program includes videotaped clinical examinations. Friedman emphasizes time urgency and free-floating hostility as central components of the behavior pattern.

In the appendices of his book are exercises to help reduce both time urgency and free-floating hostility. There are also techniques for enhancing one's sense of security and self-esteem.

**Screening for Hostility and Cynicism** These screening tools usually include statements about the extent to which a respondent believes others are untrustworthy or are a threat to safety and well-being. In early studies, a hostility scale was correlated with both vascular diseases and biological lifestyle choices such as smoking (Cook & Medley, 1954). During interviews, noteworthy factors included antagonistic behaviors by respondents toward interviewers such as challenging, confronting, and contradicting them. Some respondents exhibit hostility by withholding answers to questions. The Coronary Artery Risk Development in Young Adults Study (CARDIA) was a prospective study investigating CVD risk factors, including hostility, in 5,000 individuals. This study continued for 16 months and was completed in 1986 (Sherwitz & Rugulies, 1992). One important finding was that educational levels, gender, age, and race affect hostility, and hostility affects risks to arteries.

Screening for Cardiovascular Reactivity to Stressors
Health psychologists also screen for **cardiovascular reactivity**. It is defined as a consistent pattern of physiological change when a person is exposed to stressors (Matthews et al., 1986). Reactivity occurs in specific social contexts or settings. It may arise from such diverse origins as personality, race, hormones, early childhood experiences, and traumas during adolescence. Triggers of reactivity are varied. These may include environmental stressors such as barking dogs, psychological reactions such as intense anger, and physical stressors such as pain. Recent research indicates that exercising after exposure to a stressor can limit the duration of cardiovascular arousal and has the potential of improving health (Chafin, Christenfeld, & Gerin, 2008). In some experimental settings aerobically fit individuals showed less cardiovascular reactivity to psychological stress compared to non-exercisers (Fillingim & Blumenthal, 1992). Recent research indicates that heart rate response to stressors in laboratory situations does relate to the stress reaction in real life (Johnston, Tuomisto, & Patching, 2008). Interventions that may lessen cardiovascular reactivity are stress management, cessation of smoking, more healthful eating patterns, and regular aerobic exercise.

Screening for Job-Related Risk for CVD
One way to screen for job-related risk factors is to evaluate the social and physical aspects of worksites. For example, people can evaluate how much exercise their job requires during typical work days. Another issue is the nutritional content of food available for employee meals and snacks. A third worksite risk is exposure to smoke or other pollu-

cardiovascular reactivity A tendency of one's heart to act in response to some factors such as fright or some other stressor.

tants. Many worksites provide no opportunity for exercise and only high-fat food is available. Some employers offer health promotion programs at the worksite and employees are encouraged to make suggestions for improving everyone's health. Many worksites have medical personnel on staff. It is also worthwhile to inquire if automated external defibrillators (AEDs) are available at the worksite.

The social and relational aspects of work life can be screened for risk factors. The worksite is a social setting as well as a physical setting, because most work requires interaction among employees. Social support is important in preventing disease. Coworkers can be sources of friendship and social support, but they can also be sources of stress. Being sexually harassed at one's worksite is clearly damaging to both mental and physical health (Alexander, LaRosa, Bader, & Garfield, 2004). The chapters on stress emphasized that jobs with high demands but little control are often sources of stress for male employees. This is also true for women with the added frustration of having unsupportive bosses and high family demands (Suchday et al., 2002, p. 207). It is also possible to screen for conflict-prone and conflict-resistant organizations in relation to CVD (Stokols, 1992). In conflict-prone organizations, interpersonal conflict and poor health are more likely. Conflict-prone organizations lack common goals, are intolerant of others' opinions, and provide no means for resolving conflicts. Worksite factors combined with individual tendencies can act together to create unhealthy work situations.

**Screening for Social Support for Lifestyle Changes** The concept of social support refers to having close and beneficial relationships with family and friends. Social support buffers us from stress, provides access to resources, and increases compliance with health recommendations (Suchday et al., 2002, p. 207). Physicians advise people identified as being at risk for CVD due to smoking, obesity, and genetic background to change their lifestyles. This may include taking medications to reduce hypertension and cholesterol levels, stopping smoking, exercising regularly, and eating more nutritionally. As you know from other chapters, it is difficult to make lifestyle changes. The likelihood of following medical recommendations depends on people's knowledge and skills, their willingness to change, and the extent of their social support for making changes. Before making lifestyle changes, it is worthwhile for people to visit with family members, friends, and coworkers about their CVD risks and to ask for help in sustaining lifestyle changes. Partners, family members, and friends can encourage and even facilitate lifestyle changes by joining in healthful behaviors themselves. Emotional support, including boosting a person's self-confidence, will also be helpful (Amick & Ockene, 1994).

Tobacco use and cessation are related to social support. Tobacco is highly addictive and stopping its use is difficult. Most people must be highly motivated to stop smoking. If one's partner, good friends, or children smoke and do not intend to stop, then making a change will be more difficult. This is one reason why joining group programs for smoking cessation, weight loss, and regular exercise may be beneficial in behavior change. Group members can supply social support lacking at home.

## Tertiary Prevention: Treatment for CVD

Treatment follows screening and diagnosis. The goal of tertiary prevention is to avoid further deterioration in health, improve the quality of the patient's life, and prevent death. This may be accomplished through medications, surgery, lifestyle changes, and decreasing stress. Some procedures, such as surgery are highly invasive, while noninvasive treatment includes lifestyle changes, cognitive-behavioral therapy, and support groups. Rehabilitation, or regaining previous capacities, is also part of tertiary prevention and includes restoration of the physical, mental, and social health of the patient.

Being treated for a heart attack or stroke is a life-changing experience. People recover and then resume their lives realizing they have a serious chronic illness. The disease and its treatment become dominant components of patients' lives and the lives of their family members, friends, and even coworkers. For many there are constant physical reminders such as chest pain and shortness of breath. In the case of strokes, people may have lost the ability to walk, care for themselves, or speak clearly. A prevailing psychological factor is fear of having another heart attack or stroke. Family members and friends are also fearful they will do something that brings on another heart attack or stroke.

Patients have the right to know about their condition so they can make decisions about their own care. It is important for them to receive social support from their medical and rehabilitation teams, as well as family and friends. Many people are reluctant to question medical personnel or ask them to repeat or explain something that is difficult to understand. In other cases medical personnel talk to the family members rather than directly to patients. This makes patients feel their opinions are not valued or needed.

Clinical health psychologists are often involved in cardiac and stroke rehabilitation. Their role may include helping patients make psychological adjustments to the changes of living with a chronic condition. Medical doctors and health psychologists agree that managing stressors is important for those recovering from CVD. Most rehabilitation programs suggest ways for patients to maintain good emotional and social health along with good physical health. Therapists often focus on the important relationships patients have with their family, friends, and medical personnel. There is evidence that support groups made up of other patients are also beneficial for extending life expectancy (Maes & Boersma, 2004, pp. 11).

### Biological Tertiary Prevention

**Recognition of Symptoms of CVD Events**  Even after screening and treatment, many people still do not change behaviors putting them at risk. When people first experience symptoms they often deny or explain away their symptoms. For example, chest pain is attributed to indigestion after a big meal or a pulled chest muscle from mowing the lawn. Denial reflects an optimistic bias and results in delays in calling EMS. On the average, people wait 3 hours, but some wait as long as 24 hours before seeking medical care (Surwit, Williams, & Shapiro, 1982). Denial, optimistic bias, and delay increase the likelihood of greater damage to heart muscles or the brain in cases of stroke.

Stroke symptoms are different from symptoms of heart disease. While risk factors for all types of CVD are similar, symptoms are different. You will recall that in the case of TIAs, a person may not even be aware a stroke has occurred, because symptoms disappear in a short period of time. Possible stroke symptoms are confusion, unusual behaviors including difficulty speaking or moving, blurred vision, severe headaches, ringing in the ears, and loss of bowel or bladder control. To determine if a stroke has occurred, some physicians recommend asking the person to do three things based on the first three letters of the word *stroke*, such as asking the person to *s*mile, to *t*alk, and to *r*aise both arms over his or her head. If these are difficult for the person to do, then someone should call EMS immediately. Medication can prevent further brain damage and another stroke.

**Medical Treatments Including Surgery Angioplasty** is a medical procedure that improves blood flow to the heart. The procedure involves pressing accumulated plaque against the walls of the coronary arteries with a small balloon. The procedure increases the space through which blood can flow to heart muscle cells. Open-heart surgery is more invasive. The chest wall is opened to allow access to the coronary arteries that may be replaced with arteries taken from places in the patient's body or elsewhere. Arteries can also be held open with artificial devices. Cardiac surgery may involve other complicated medical procedures such as replacement of heart valves and/or complete heart replacements or transplants. Pharmacological treatment includes anti-ischemic drugs such as beta blockers and nitrates, and lipid-lowering drugs.

Biopsychosocial Tertiary Prevention: Cognitive-Behavioral Therapy
Multimodal rehabilitation programs increase survival rates by helping to prevent another heart attack or stroke, but one significant problem is patients' low adherence rates following their release from hospital settings. Rehabilitation research emphasizes optimizing patient functioning in all areas of life (Suchday et al., 2002, pp. 211–217). Surgical medical treatments are stressful for patients, family, and friends, so people recovering from cardiovascular surgery are encouraged to learn stress management techniques, to eat in healthier ways, to exercise regularly, and to stop smoking. Social support from family and friends is important in recovery from heart attacks, cardiac arrest, and strokes.

Post-treatment life may include adjustment to emotional changes in both heart and stroke patients. Patients do better when they get professional help with psychological difficulties, economic problems including work issues, and adjustments within the family. Patients often report trouble sleeping and being depressed. About 20% of heart attack patients experience

---

**angioplasty** A medical procedure that improves blood flow to the heart by pressing accumulated plaque against the walls of the coronary arteries with a small balloon. The procedure increases the space through which blood can flow to heart muscle cells and may relieve angina.

symptoms of depression including fatigue, irritability, hopelessness, helplessness, and suicidal ideation (Suchday et al., 2002, p. 209). Depression is associated with a three-fold risk of CVD mortality and morbidity. An NHLBI working group (2008c) is examining the role of antidepressants combined with cognitive therapy for this problem. Chronic stress and sleep deprivation may be responsible for some physical and emotional symptoms (Nicolson & van Diest, 2000).

Gender combined with age affects outcomes of rehabilitation, including coping mechanisms. For example, women may face more complex convalescent challenges because they are often older than men when CVD occurs. Women are more likely to be alone as a result of partner death, so they lack spousal support. Women are as likely to benefit from rehabilitation as men, but only about 20% of those in cardiac rehab programs are female. Personality is another factor in recovery. Research indicates Type A men are less likely to seek social support and Type A women can be even more resistant to lifestyle changes than men (Sotile, 1996).

Many patients face significant lifestyle changes, because all of the things known about primary prevention are also recommended during rehabilitation. Doctors tell patients to stop smoking, to stop eating high-fat food, to start exercising, and to lose weight. These recommendations may be perceived by patients as depressing restrictions on their lives. Sometimes previous recreational activities are prohibited so opportunities for fun are gone. Age, gender, ethnicity, income, educational level, and other social factors affect recovery from cardiovascular events.

Regardless of treatment, most patients have less energy and stamina. If jobs have unhealthy aspects or cause a great deal of stress, employees may request transfers or look for other jobs. If a patient's job requires lifting or other types of heavy physical labor, physicians may recommend changing jobs or retiring. Stress results from loss of income, as well as job changes. In the United States, a person's job is a source of self-identification and self-esteem. One of the first things we ask upon meeting someone is "What do you do?" Many people believe what they do for a living is the most important thing about them. Heart and stroke patients may feel useless when their occupational roles end.

Scientists are exploring whether or not social support improves outcomes following a heart attack. The Enhancing Recovery in Coronary Heart Disease Social Support Instrument (ESSI) assesses types of social support that have shown up in previous studies as being related to heart disease outcomes. The ESSI is a seven-item Likert-type self-report measuring such items as feelings of closeness and being loved, tangible support such as doing daily chores, giving good advice, and marital status support (Lett et al., 2007).

Generally, family members and friends are sources of social support and have a positive effect on rehabilitation. A recent study suggests that social relationships can improve morbidity and mortality by affecting recovery behaviors including medication adherence, attendance at rehabilitation programs, and general improvement in the quality of life (Malloy, Perkins-Porras, Strike, & Steptoe, 2008). Rehabilitation support groups consist of other patients in similar situations and their family members. Experienced professional counselors lead support groups. Common problems and solutions are shared among people in similar situations. Support groups can decrease the sense of isolation common to CVD patients. The Recurrent Coronary Prevention Project demonstrated that changes in hostility and Type A behavior patterns resulted in fewer reappearances of heart attacks compared to typical cardiac care programs during that same time frame (Friedman et al., 1996), but there continue to be inconsistent findings among programs (Suchday et al., 2002, pp. 215-217).

Programs Designed for Recovery from CVD

**The Opening Your Heart Program** Dr. Dean Ornish developed the Opening Your Heart Program, a non-invasive treatment following heart attacks (Ornish et al., 1990; Ornish, 1990). The program uses biological, psychological, and sociocultural strategies to reverse heart disease. The Lifestyle Heart Trial tested the effectiveness of a specific lifestyle change program on an experimental group of patients. The control group followed standard physician instructions. The experimental program required involvement of patients and their partners for 1 year. It included support group meetings twice a week, 1 hour of daily aerobic exercise, a low-fat vegetarian diet, smoking cessation, and stress management training.

Ornish's program is about healing the heart physically, emotionally, and spiritually, using lifestyle change rather than surgery or medications. When patients followed the program, their coronary arteries were less blocked and blood flow to their hearts increased. Ninety-one percent experienced a reduction in chest pain frequency, 42% reported shorter periods of chest pain, and 28% said their pain was less severe. Angiograms demonstrated reduction in blockage of coronary arteries. Ornish teaches patients ways to increase intimacy in their lives, and patients experienced positive changes in their psychosocial condition. They reported their lives were more meaningful and more under their control. Anger was reduced, there was less anxiety, depression, and Type A behavior. More recently, Ornish developed a video series encouraging good communication between heart disease patients and their family members. He confirms that social support helps with anxiety, depression, and morale.

**Hospital-Based Cardiac Rehabilitation Programs** These programs began in the 1970s and usually consist of a series of meetings that include exercise training to improve aerobic capacity along with the added benefit of improvement in mood. Rehabilitation incorporates education about cardiac risks and counseling on nutrition, psychological health, and returning to work. Health professionals in cardiac rehab programs can be sources of emotional support. Social support improves self-esteem and buffers the effects of stressful events including serious medical problems. Fellow patients support each other by talking about recovery experiences. In rehabilitation, social support improves the likelihood patients will stick with recommended medical and behavioral changes. Sometimes social support from fellow patients offsets the negative impact of family members who may become overly attentive, helpful, and sympathetic thus making patients feel even more helpless (Dracup, 1994). Group support is a powerful antidepressant and reduces feelings of isolation (Anderson, 1987).

**The Family Systems Approach** This is another program designed for rehabilitation and re-covery. Family members provide transportation for medical followup, encourage and partic-ipate in exercise and dietary changes, and are important to patients' psychosocial recovery. Sotile (1996) suggests a circular relationship between how patients act, how family and friends react, and how patients respond. He believes recovery for patients depends upon the entire family working together as a team. Sotile also recommends family stress management training and proactively addressing sexual aspects of rehabilitation. Patients fear resuming sexual relationships because they or their partners suspect sexual activity will trigger an-other heart attack or stroke. At least 70% of patients resume sexual activity within a year (Surwit et al., 1982).

**Developing a Trusting Heart** Psychological factors associated with heart disease include hostility, anger, stress, depression, social isolation, and lifestyle behavioral habits. An appro-priate intervention increases positive mental health (Johnson, 2004, pp. 13–14). Hostility corrodes social support of family and friends. A recent meta-analysis suggested that inter-ventions aimed at altering psychosocial patterns—for example Type A behavior patterns and hostility—lowered the rate of myocardial infarction among some patients (Suchday et al., 2002 pp. 209–216).

Redford B. Williams (1989) devised this program to help people reduce hostility through changes in attitude, feelings, and behaviors. He found that friendships and other forms of social support reduced risks of CVD. His research shows that if people learn to trust oth-ers and to limit their hostile and angry reactions, they will improve their heart health. Williams suggests a behavioral modification pathway to develop a more trusting heart, in-cluding keeping records of cynical thoughts, confessing hostility to others, stopping cyni-cal thoughts, reasoning with oneself, putting oneself in other people's shoes, laughing at oneself, practicing trust, learning, pretending each day is the last, and practicing forgiveness.

**Changing Ways of Expressing Anger** New ways of expressing anger is another part of reha-bilitation efforts. Gender differences occur in the way people express anger. Both women and men experience anger but express it differently (Siegman & Smith, 1994). Women tend to use words to convey anger, while men are more likely to communicate through physical actions. Interventions such as anger management help some women and men change habit-ual forms of rage or expression of anger. There is an important ethical issue involved in anger-management interventions, because anger may be an appropriate response to a social setting or relationship. One must weigh health risks against the benefits of recognizing and changing situations that result in anger (Chesney, 1985).

## Summary

The leading cause of death for people living in industrialized countries is cardiovascular dis-ease. This chapter applies the biopsychosocial approach of health psychology to CVD. Bi-ological aspects include structures, purposes, and problems of the circulatory system. Important health problems include angina, heart attacks, cardiac arrest, and strokes. Psychosocial aspects of CVD include stress, negative emotional states, personality traits such as cynicism and hostility, and the Type A behavior pattern, which reflects personality traits and common ways of responding to stressors.

Uncontrollable biological risk factors for CVDs include age and genetic background. Partially controllable risk factors are cholesterol levels, hypertension, and diabetes. Risk factors that are clearly controllable include smoking tobacco, poor nutritional practices, obesity, and a sedentary lifestyle. While biological factors contribute to damage of the cardiovascular system, psychological and social factors also play an important role. Stressful social and cultural conditions are implicated in the development of CVD. Psychosocial risk factors are more difficult to study than the biological because of ethical limitations on research and the difficulties of longitudinal studies.

Primary prevention includes choosing behaviors to prevent the deterioration of the body that put us at risk of CVD. Heart disease and strokes can be prevented through means discussed in detail in other chapters, including regular aerobic exercise, good nutritional practices, stopping smoking, and stress management. Secondary prevention includes screenings for heart rate, blood pressure, and cholesterol levels. Angiograms and treadmill stress tests are available in medical settings for further screening. There are many instruments for screening for psychosocial risk factors including assessments of the Type A behavior pattern, hostility, stress, cardiovascular reactivity, and expression of anger.

The goal of tertiary prevention is rehabilitation following cardiovascular events such as heart attacks, cardiac arrest, and strokes. An additional goal is to prevent further damage and death. In this chapter we examined treatments for CVD including invasive and noninvasive approaches. Many rehabilitation programs are available in hospital settings and usually include family members along with other patients in support groups.

Programs specifically designed for recovery from CVD include the Ornish Opening Your Heart Program, the family systems approach, changing ways of expressing anger, and writing about traumatic experiences.

## Review Questions

1. Explain the most important components of the cardiovascular system, including structures and their purposes.

2. Describe health problems typical of the cardiovascular system and their biological causes.

3. List and briefly explain psychosocial aspects of CVD.

4. Distinguish among the three types of prevention and give one example of each type related to CVD.

5. List risk factors for CVD that are biologically based, partially under individual control, and totally avoidable.

6. Explain primary prevention or the best ways to avoid CVD, including biological risks and psychosocial risks.

7. Briefly describe three common biological screenings for CVD. Based on your own experience with these screenings, state how accurate you believe each one is, and justify your answer.

8. Explain the content and purpose of a health risk analysis.

9. What are some gender-based problems when screening for biological risk factors?

10. Describe two types of psychosocial screenings for recognition of risks for CVD, one for personality traits and another for job characteristics.

11. Explain why you think people deny that their pain is a signal of CVD disease.

12. List and briefly explain two invasive options for tertiary prevention or treatment of CVD.

13. Describe two noninvasive options for tertiary prevention of CVD.

## Student Activity

Choose one of the following activities.

1. *Write a report about your own risks for CVD disease.*

   a. Find out your blood pressure numbers by going to the campus health center and having someone take your blood pressure. Student enrollment fees usually pay for this service. Ask the technician what your blood pressure is, what the ratio means, and whether or not your blood pressure is appropriate or is too high for a person your age. Write the number down for your report along with a description of your experience. (Have your blood pressure retaken on your birthday each year for comparison.)

   b. Evaluate your risks for CVD. Look back at the pages of this chapter on risk factors and evaluate your risks for heart disease and strokes.

   Age:

   Family's History:

   Risky Behaviors or Lifestyle Choices:

   Preventive Behaviors or Lifestyle Choices:

2. *In small groups or alone, interview a willing respondent who has experienced some form of CVD and has received treatment.*

   1. Write a summary of the interview and then present the information to the class or professor. Be sure to keep the name of your respondent anonymous, because this an important ethical issue in research.

   Suggested interview questions:

   1. When did you first learn you had (angina pectoris, a heart attack, cardiac arrest, TIA, or stroke)?

   2. How did you know something was wrong?

   3. Tell me what you did next.

   4. Describe any medical treatment you received.

   5. Describe any rehabilitation you completed.

   6. Tell me about suggestions made by your medical team to prevent another problem.

   7. Please describe how the illness changed your life.

   8. Add here any other questions you may have.

# References

Alexander, L. L., LaRosa, J. H., Bader, H., & Garfield, S. (2006). *New dimensions in women's health* (4th ed.). Sudbury, MA: Jones and Bartlett Publishers.

American National Red Cross. (2005). *First aid, responding to emergencies.* Yardley, PA: StayWell.

Amick, T. L., & Ockene, J. K. (1994). The role of social support in the modification of risk factors for CVD. In S. A. Shumaker & S. M. Czajkowski (Eds.), *Social support and CVD* (pp. 259–278). New York: Plenum Press.

Anderson, M. P. (1987). Psychological issues in cardiovascular rehabilitation. In J. W. Elias & P. H. Marshall (Eds.), *CVD and behavior* (pp. 151–178). Washington, DC: Hemisphere Publishing Corporation.

Carver, C., Scheier, M., & Pozo, C. (1992). Conceptualizing the process of coping with health problems. In H. S. Friedman (Ed.) *Hostility, coping and health* (pp. 167–188). Washington, DC: American Psychological Association.

Centers for Disease Control. (2008a). Heart Disease Facts and Statistics. Retrieved August 26, 2008 from http://www.cdc.gov/heartdisease/facts.htm

Centers for Disease Control. (2008b). About Stroke. Retrieved August 26, 2008 from http://www.cdc.gov/stroke/about_stroke.htm

Chafin, S., Christenfeld, N., & Gerin, W. (2008). Improving cardiovascular recovery from stress with brief post stress exercise. *Health Psychology, 27* (1, Suppl), S64–S72.

Chesney, M.A. (1985). Anger and hostility: Future implications for behavioral medicine. In M. A. Chesney & R. H. Rosenman (Eds), *Anger and hostility in cardiovascular and behavioral disorders* (pp. 277–290). Washington, DC: Hemisphere Publishing Corporation.

Cook, W. W., & Medley, D. M. (1954). Proposed hostility, pharisaic-virtue scales for MMPI. *Journal of Applied Psychology, 38,* 414–418.

Dracup, K. (1994). Cardiac rehabilitation, the role of social support in recovery compliance. In S. A. Shumaker & S. M. Czajkowski (Eds.), *Social support and CVD* (pp. 333–353). New York: Plenum Press.

Fillingim, R. B., & Blumenthal, J. A. (1992). Does aerobic exercise reduce stress responses? In J. R. Turner, A. Sherwood, & C. Light (Eds.), *Individual differences in cardiovascular response to stress* (pp. 203–215). New York: Plenum Press.

Friedman, M., & Rosenman, R. H. (1959). Association of specific overt behavior pattern with blood and cardiovascular findings. *Journal of the American Medical Association, 169,* 1286–1296.

Friedman, M. (1996). *Type A behavior: Its diagnosis and treatment.* New York: Plenum Press.

Friedman, M., Breall, W. S., Goodwin, M. L., Sparagon, B. J., Ghandour, G., & Fleischmann, N. (1996). Effect of type A behavioral counseling on frequency of episodes of silent myocardial ischemia in coronary patients. *American Heart Journal, 132,* 933–937.

Gerace, T. A., & George, V. A. (1996). Predictors of weight increases over 7 years in firefighters and paramedics. *Preventive Medicine, 25,* 593–600.

Gottdiener, J. S., Krantz, D. S., Howell, R. H., Hecht, G. M., Klein, J., Falconer, J. J., et al. (1994). Induction of silent myocardial ischemia with mental stress testing: Relationship to the triggers of ischemia during daily life activities and to ischemic functional severity. *Journal of the American College of Cardiology, 24,* 1645–1651.

Jenkins, C. D., Rosenman, R. H., & Zyzanski, S. J. (1974). Prediction of clinical coronary heart disease by a test for the coronary-prone behavior pattern. *New England Journal of Medicine, 23,* 1271–1275.

Jenkins, C. D., (1976). Recent evidence supporting psychological and social risk factors for coronary disease. *New England Journal of Medicine, 294,* 987–994, 1033–1038.

Johnson, N. G. (2004). Introduction: Psychology and health—taking the initiative to bring it together. In R. H. Rozensky, N. G. Johnson, C. D. Goodheart, & W. R. Hammond (Eds.), *Psychology builds a healthy world.* Washington, DC: American Psychological Association.

Johnston, D. W., Tuomisto, M. T., & Patching, G. R. (2008). The relationship between cardiac reactivity in the laboratory and in real life. *Health Psychology, 27*(1), 34–42.

Kaplan, R., Manuck, S., & Shumaker, S. (1992). Commentary to part two: Does lowering cholesterol cause increases in depression, suicide, and accidents? In H. S. Friedman (Ed.), *Hostility, coping, and health* (pp. 117–126). Washington, DC: American Psychological Association.

Kivimaki, M., Leino-Arjas, P., Luukkonen, R., Riihamaki, H., Vahera, J., & Kirjonen, J. (2002). Work stress and risk of cardiovascular mortality: Prospective cohort study of industrial employees. *British Medical Journal, 325,* 857.

Lett, H. S., Blumenthal, J. A., Babyak, M. L., Catellier, D. J., Carney, R. M., Berkman, L. F., et al. (2007). Social support and prognosis in patients at increased psychosocial risk recovering from myocardial infarction. *Health Psychology, 26,* 418–427.

Maes, S., & Boersma, S. N. (2004). Applications in health psychology: How effective are Interventions? In S. Sutton, A. Baum, & M. Johnston (Eds.), *The Sage handbook of health psychology* (pp. 299–325). Sage: Thousand Oaks, CA.

Malloy, G. J., Perkins-Porras, L., Strike, P. C., & Steptoe, A. (2008). Social networks and partner stress as predictors of adherence to medication, rehabilitation attendance, and quality of life following acute coronary syndrome. *Health Psychology, 27* (1), 52–58.

Manuck, S. B., Kaplan, J. R., Clarkson, T. B., Adams, M. R., & Shively, C. A. (1991). Behavioral influences on coronary artery disease: A nonhuman primate model. In H. S. Friedman (Ed.), *Hostility, coping and health* (pp. 99–108). Washington, DC: American Psychological Association.

Martin, P. D., & Brantley, P. J. (2004). Stress, coping, and social support in health behavior. In J. M. Raczynski & L. C. Leviton, *Handbook of clinical health psychology* (Vol. 2, 233–267). Washington, DC: American Psychological Association.

Matthews, K. A., Weiss, S. M., Detre, T., Dembroski, T. M., Falkner, B., Manuck, S. B., & Williams, R. B. (Eds.). (1986). *Handbook of stress, reactivity, and cardiovascular disease.* New York: John Wiley and Sons.

National Heart, Lung and Blood Institute, Department of Health and Human Services, National Institutes of Health (2008a). Risk Assessment Tool for Estimating Your 10-Year Risk of Having a Heart Attack. Retrieved August 26, 2008 from http://hp2010.nhlbihin.net/atpiii/calculator.asp?usertype=pub

National Heart, Lung and Blood Institute, Department of Health and Human Services, National Institutes of Health (2008b). NHLBI Study Finds Hostility, Impatience Increase Hypertension Risk. Retrieved August 26, 2008 from http://www.nhlbi.nih.gov/news/press/03-10-21.htm

National Heart, Lung and Blood Institute, Department of Health and Human Services, National Institutes of Health (2008c). Study of Heart Disease Patients Treated for Depression and Low Social Support Finds No Survival Benefit but Significant Improvement in Depression and Social Functioning. Retrieved August 26, 2008 from http://www.nhlbi.nih.gov/new/press/03-06-17.htm

Neighmond, P. (2006, July). *Detection changing for women's heart disease.* Retrieved November 15, 2006 from www.npr.org, National Public Radio Broadcast.

Ng-Mak, D. S. (1999). A further analysis of race differences in the National Longitudinal Mortality Study. *American Journal of Public Health, 89,* 1748–1751.

Nicolson, N. A., & van Diest, R. (2000). Salivary cortisol patterns in vital exhaustion. *Journal of Psychosomatic Research, 49* (5), 335–342.

Ornish, D., Brown, S. E., Scherwitz, L. W., Billings, J. H., Armstrong, W. T., Ports, T., et al. (1990). Can lifestyle changes reverse coronary heart disease?: Lifestyle heart trial. *Lancet, 336,* 129–133.

Ornish, D. (1990). *Dr. Dean Ornish's program for reversing heart disease.* New York: Ballantine Books.

Pennebaker, J. W. (1992). Inhibition as the linchpin of health. In H. S. Friedman (Ed.), *Hostility, coping, and health* (pp. 127–139). Washington, DC: American Psychological Association.

Polednak, A. P. (1998). Mortality among Blacks living in census tracts with public housing projects in Hartford, Connecticut. *Ethnicity and Disease, 8,* 36–42.

Quick, J. C., Piotrkowski, C., Jenkins, L., & Brooks, Y. B. (2003). Four dimensions of healthy work: Stress, work-family relations, violence prevention, and relationships at work. In R. H. Rozensky, N. G. Johnson, C. D. Goodheart, & W. R. Hammond (Eds.), *Psychology builds a healthy world* (pp. 223–273). Washington, DC: American Psychological Association.

Rosenman, R. H., Brand, R. J., Jenkins, D., Friedman, M., Struas, R., & Wurm, M. (1975). Coronary heart disease in Western Collaborative Group Study. Final follow-up experience of 8½ years. *Journal of the American Medical Association, 233,* 872–877.

Rosenman, R. H. (1978). The interview method of assessment of the coronary-prone behavior pattern. In T. M. Dembroski, S. M. Weiss, J. L. Chields, S. G. Hayes, & M. Feinleig (Eds.), *Coronary-prone behavior* (pp. 55–70). NY: Springer-Verlag.

Rozanski, A., Blumenthal, J. A., & Kaplan, J. R. (1999). Impact of psychological factors on the pathogenesis of CVD and implications for therapy. *Circulation, 99,* 2192–2217.

Seematter, G., Guenat, E., Schneiter, P., Cayeux, C., Jequier, E., & Trappy, L. (2000). Effects of mental stress on insulin-mediated glucose metabolism and energy expenditure in lean and obese women. *American Journal of Physiology, Endocrinology and Metabolism, 279,* 799–805.

Sherwitz, L., & Rugulies, R. (1992). Lifestyle and hostility. In H. S. Friedman (Ed.), *Hostility, coping and health* (pp. 77–98). Washington, DC: American Psychological Association.

Siegman, A. W., & Smith, T. W. (Eds.). (1994). *Anger, hostility, and the heart.* Hillsdale, NJ: Erlbaum.

Smith, T. W., & Ruiz, J. M. (2004). Personality theory and health behavior. In R. G. Frank, A. Baum, & J. L. Wallander (Eds.), *Handbook of clinical health psychology* (Vol. 3, pp. 143–199). Washington, DC: American Psychological Association.

Sotile, W. M. (1996). Psychosocial interventions for cardiopulmonary patients: A guide for health professionals. Champaign, IL: Human Kinetics.

Steptoe, A. & Ayers, S. (2004). Stress, health, and illness. In S. Sutton, A. Baum, & M. Johnston (Eds.), *The sage handbook of health psychology* (pp. 169–196). Thousand Oaks, CA: Sage.

Stokols, D. (1992). Conflict-prone and conflict-resistant organizations. In H. S. Friedman (Ed.), *Hostility, coping and health* (pp. 65–76). Washington, DC: American Psychological Association.

Suchday, S., Tucker, D. L., & Krantz, D. S. (2002). In S. B. Johnson, N. W. Perry, Jr., & R. H. Rozensky (Eds.) *Handbook of clinical health psychology* (Vol. 1, pp. 203–238). Washington, DC: American Psychological Association.

Surwit, R. S., Williams, R. B., & Shapiro, D. (Eds.). (1982). *Behavioral approaches to CVD.* New York: Academic Press.

Twisk, J., Snel, J., Kemper, H., & van Mechelen, W. (1999). Changes in daily hassles and life events and the relationship with coronary heart disease risk factors: A 2-year longitudinal study in 27–29 year old males and females. *Journal of Psychosomatic Research, 46,* 229–240.

Vitaliano, P. P., Russo, J., Scanlan, J. M., & Greeno, C. G. (1996). Weight changes in caregivers of Alzheimer's care recipients: Psychobehavioral predictors. *Psychology and Aging, 11,* 155–163.

Voelker, R. (1998). A "family heirloom" turns 50. *Journal of the American Medical Association, 279,* 1241–1245.

Williams, R. (1989). *The trusting heart: Great news about type A behavior.* New York: Times Books.

Young, R. F., Waller, J. B., Jr., & Kahana, E. (1991). Racial and socioeconomic aspects of myocardial infarction recovery: Studying confounds. *American Journal of Preventive Medicine, 7,* 438–444.

# Chapter 12

# Applications of Health Psychology to Cancer

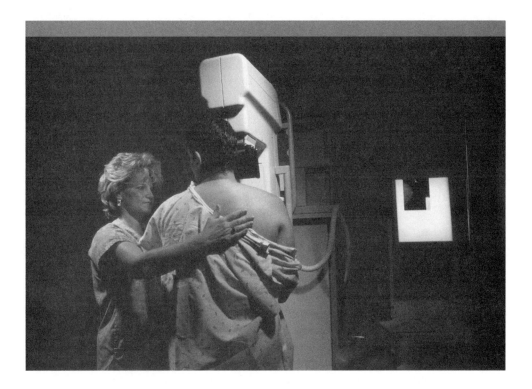

## Learning Objectives

After studying this chapter students will have the knowledge and skills to be able to:

1. Understand, define, and explain terminology associated with cancer.

2. Relate in detail the biological and psychosocial factors that contribute to the development of cancer.

3. Describe primary, secondary, and tertiary approaches to cancer prevention.

4. Write or talk about the many biopsychosocial factors associated with recovery from cancer.

5. Compare the most common cancers causing death in the United States at this time including precipitating factors.

6. Explain ways to reduce risks of all cancers.

## Introduction

**Cancer** is probably the most dreaded of all diseases. The word brings to mind a painful wasting disease. This is an outdated perception. There have been enormous advances in the diagnosis and treatment of cancer since the 1950s. Currently more than 10.5 million people in the United States have survived cancer and its treatments (American Cancer Society [ACS], 2007). Millions of cancer survivors are living long, happy, and successful lives. However, cancer is the second most likely cause of death in the United States, surpassed only by cardiovascular disease. About 1.4 million new cancer cases are diagnosed each year in the United States, plus more than 1 million skin cancers. In 2002, cancer killed 6.7 million people around the world, including 560,000 in the United States (ACS, 2007).

Health psychologists and health promotion specialists study ways to prevent cancer through the promotion of positive health practices and avoidance of known cancer-causing agents or carcinogens. Clinical health psychologists working in patient support make substantial contributions to improvement of patients' lives, especially in the areas of pain control and in the enhancement of mood and immune systems. Others focus on the psychology of stress management as an aid to recovery from cancer. The diagnosis of cancer is emotional and distressing. Clinical health psychologists develop methods that help in dealing with the fear, anger, guilt, and depression of cancer patients and their families. Relationships of cancer patients with family members, friends, and medical personnel are important to recovery and for responsible followup on testing and treatment regimens. Some people still believe that cancer is contagious and avoid visiting or touching people diagnosed with cancer. At one time, having cancer was shameful and hospitals did not put patients' names on hospital room doors in order to protect their privacy.

Loss of jobs and insurance coverage issues are other important sociocultural components of cancer treatment. The National Health Interview Survey (2006) revealed that 43.6 million Americans, or 14.8% of the population, had no health insurance (Centers for Disease Control [CDC], 2006a). Consequently about 16 million citizens are unable to obtain medical care due to cost. In addition, many health insurance policies limit coverage by a lifetime dollar amount and some people cannot get policies if they were ever diagnosed with any cancer, including skin cancer. About 40% of businesses do not offer health insurance to their employees.

One impediment to cancer research is the diversity of the disease itself. There are hundreds of variations of diseases sharing the name cancer. What all have in common is an abnormal growth of cells that interferes with nearby normal cell tissue and may eventually spread throughout the body. There is different terminology for each tumor type and different cancers have different risk factors. For example, overexposure to ultraviolet light, in-

---

**cancer** An abnormal malignant growth of cells that can invade nearby tissue and may spread throughout the body.

cluding tanning practices, is a risk factor for skin cancer, but smoking is a risk factor for a wide variety of cancers in the lungs, pharynx, esophagus, cervix, mouth, stomach, pancreas, liver, kidney, and bladder (see **Figure 12.1**). The risk factors remain unknown for some types of cancer. Cancer, with its variety of sites, causes, and management, continues to be a very complex disease to understand and treat.

The causes of many cancer types are linked to human behavior and in many cases are preventable. These behaviors include the use of tobacco, alcohol, dietary and exercise practices resulting in obesity, and sexual activity. Known causes of cancer are still widely promoted and available in this country. These include tobacco products, alcohol, high-fat foods, charred meat, and tanning beds. The mass media, including television, films, and music, continue to encourage irresponsible sexual activity even when it is known that some cancers are associated with having unprotected sexual intercourse. Some cancers are even a consequence of jobs.

## A Biopsychosocial Analysis of Cancer Risk Factors

### The Biology of Cancer

Cellular Biology

Cells have a limited life expectancy; we slough off and produce new cells constantly. The biology of cancer begins at the cellular level and utilizes a specialized vocabulary. A **neoplasm** is new cell tissue and may be benign or malignant. A **tumor** is a growth of tissue and can be localized or invasive. A **malignant tumor** grows and spreads. Usually **benign tumors** do not cause problems, but malignant neoplasms or cancerous cells increase if no natural or synthetic suppressants are available. Many cancers proliferate rapidly, invade adjoining healthy cells, and spread throughout the body. This process is called **metastasis**. Malignant cells can metastasize from the original site to distant areas in the body. Cancerous cells migrate through the bloodstream, the lymph system, and even across body cavities. There are hundreds of cancer types, but most are discussed in terms of their original site, even though there are variations in cancer types even within specific sites. Prevention and treatment are usually discussed in terms of the site of the original cancerous neoplasm.

**neoplasm** Any abnormal development of a cell; it may be benign or malignant.

**tumor** A growth of tissue characterized by cell increases; it may be benign or malignant.

**malignant tumor** A growth of tissue that is damaging to the body, such as a cancer that is invasive and spreads throughout the body.

**benign tumor** A growth of tissue that is noncancerous or nonspreading.

**metastasis** The spread of cancerous tissue from its original site through the lymphatic system, bloodstream, or across a body cavity.

**Figure 12.1**
Lung cancer is largely due to smoking and continues to be the major cancer killer for both women and men. The significant rise in lung cancer in women probably reflects the power of advertising aimed at young women by the tobacco industry.

*Source:* American Cancer Society, Inc., 2006.

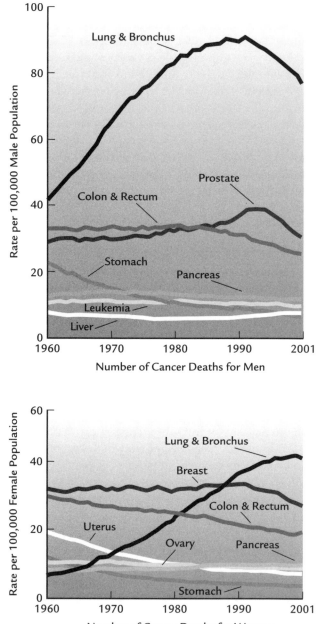

Changes in Cells

The causes of cancer are diverse and include the interplay of biological, behavioral, and environmental factors. From a biological standpoint, irritants or precipitating factors alter cells and promote the growth of a cancer. Radiation, viral infections, excessive sunlight exposure, and carcinogens such as tobacco, alcohol, and other chemical agents cause cellular changes, resulting in malignancy. **Carcinogens** change the **deoxyribonucleic acid (DNA)** of cell genes. In addition to human behavior, heredity or family history puts us at risk of some types of cancer. Some are associated with racial or ethnic categories. Environmental pollutants such as smoke also alter genetic material. The likelihood of many cancers increases with age. This indicates that exposure to carcinogens may take years to cause mutations. Some nutritionists suggest we consume phytochemicals from plant foods to neutralize the effects of free radicals that have detrimental effects on cell membranes and sometimes lead to cancer (Insel, Turner, & Ross, 2006).

Cancer Terminology

Terms such as **diagnosis** and **prognosis** are common to all medical fields. A medical diagnosis is the identification of a disease or an injury. A prognosis is the predicted outcome of treatment for disease or injury. A diagnosis of cancer is based on symptoms, medical history, physical examinations, laboratory tests, x-rays, CT scans, and other diagnostic tests. It is very difficult to make an accurate prognosis in cancer cases because so many variables affect outcomes. Biological, psychological, and sociocultural factors affect the outcomes of cancer diagnoses and treatments.

The three major approaches to cancer are surgery, or cutting away diseased tissue; **chemotherapy**, which destroys cancerous cells with chemicals; and **radiation**, which destroys diseased tissue with high-energy rays. Sometimes all modes are used in treatment.

---

**carcinogens** Substances capable of making body cells malignant or cancerous; a cancer-forming agent or a risk factor for cancer.

**deoxyribonucleic acid (DNA)** A large molecule found in the chromosomes of the cell nucleus that contains genetic information.

**diagnosis** Identification of a disease or injury following an evaluation of symptoms and health history.

**prognosis** Prediction of a probable outcome of a disease or injury.

**chemotherapy** Disease treatment using chemicals, including drugs such as antibiotics. The most common usage refers to drugs used to treat cancer.

**radiation** Electromagnetic energy emitted as rays used for both diagnostic work and in the treatment of some cancers. Radiation may cause severe burns and even trigger cancer development.

Other treatments include hormone therapy, biological therapy, and targeted therapy. Oncologists are physicians who specialize in cancer treatment. There are surgical oncologists and oncologists who specialize in chemotherapy and radiation. Cancer is a uniquely troublesome disease, because it can metastasize through the body and may require many different treatments or combinations of treatments that must be carefully timed.

## Biological Risk Factors for Cancer

Uncontrollable biological risks for cancer include age, gender, and family history. These are risks about which we can do very little except to practice healthy lifestyles. Aging is inevitable, and being older than 50 years means we are at greater risk for some cancers. This is why many recommended checkups for cancer begin at age 50.

Gender also puts us at risk of specific cancers. Females and males have different reproductive organs, so cancers associated with those areas of the body are different. For example, women are at risk for cancers of the breast, ovaries, and cervix. Men can have breast cancer, but it is rare. Men, especially young men, should be aware of risks for testicular cancer, because this is the most common cancer in men between the ages of 20 and 34. Most males are uncomfortable talking about their genitals and prostate, but 1 in 300 will develop testicular cancer and 1 in 6 will be diagnosed with cancer of the prostate. White men are more likely to develop testicular cancer than men of any other race. Men with a family history of testicular cancer have a higher risk. Abnormal or undescended testicles, even if corrected by surgery, are more likely to develop cancer.

The prostate is a gland about the size of a chestnut found at the neck of the urethra. It produces the fluid part of semen and forms part of the structure of the urethra. Cancer of the prostate is the second leading cause of cancer-related death among men in the United States, but if found early most survive this cancer. African American men have a higher risk of developing the disease. Cancer of the penis is very rare (1 in 100,000) but risk factors include the **human papillomavirus (HPV)**, poor genital hygiene, having many sexual partners, and using tobacco products (M.D. Anderson, 2008a, p. 3).

Family history puts us at risk of cancer. If a blood relative has had cancer, then we are at greater risk of that type of cancer too. Family history reflects ethnic and racial backgrounds as well as familial genetic factors. For example, people of northern European backgrounds who have light skin, light-colored eyes, red hair, and freckles are at greater risk of skin cancer. The frequency of nevus or congenital moles and birthmarks runs in families, and these can become cancerous.

---

**human papillomavirus (HPV)** A virus that may cause genital warts and/or the development of abnormal cells in the anus, cervix, penis, and vaginal tissue.

## Psychosocial Risk Factors for Cancer

More than 60% of all cancers can be attributed to lifestyle choices. These include risk factors with psychological, social, or cultural origins. Examples include tobacco and alcohol use, dietary practices, sexual behavior, occupational risks, and practice of other risky behaviors such as tanning by exposure to sunlight and tanning beds. There is also evidence that the viability of our immune function is compromised by both poor health habits and by stress. The stress of being diagnosed with cancer may result in depression and a reduction in natural killer cell activity, further endangering the body (Martin & Brantley, 2004, p. 239). Immune function is important in warding off acute infections acquired during treatments for cancer.

### Tobacco Use

Lung cancer is the leading cause of cancer death among women and men, and the most common cause of lung cancer is tobacco use (CDC, 2007). Tobacco and its smoke contain many known cancer-causing substances. Exposure to tobacco smoke, even if we are not smoking the cigarette, pipe, or cigar, puts us at risk of cancer. Deaths from lung cancer are decreasing, but among high school students, 25% of females and 32% of males continue to use some form of tobacco (CDC, 2006b). Prospective studies of tobacco-related mortality among men show there is no health benefit to switching from smoking cigarettes to using snuff or chewing tobacco (Henley, Thun, Connell, & Calle, 2005). Any culture in which the use of tobacco products is encouraged by example and through heavy advertising will be characterized by cancer deaths.

### Alcohol Use

Alcohol use contributes to cancers of the mouth, esophagus, head and neck, liver, colon, rectum, breast, pancreas, and bladder (West, Harvey-Berino, & Raczynski, 2004, p. 12). There is also a synergistic effect between smoking and alcohol use. This means people who combine smoking with alcohol are at even greater risk than if they used only one or the other. Chronic liver disease and liver cancer are associated with hepatitis infections (Clark, Rhodes, Rogers, & Lidden, 2004, p. 123).

### Sexual Practices

Sexual intercourse transmits several diseases associated with cancers. Both women and men are at risk of the human immunodeficiency virus (HIV) and acquired immunodeficiency syndrome (AIDS) from any unprotected penetrative sexual activity. AIDS is a progressive disease that destroys the immune system, making some cancers more likely, especially Kaposi's sarcoma.

Sexual behaviors are implicated in cancers of the cervix, penis, vagina, and vulva. Infection with HPV causes cervical dysplasia, which may lead to cervical cancer; nearly all cases of cervical cancer result from HPV. HPV is sexually transmitted and highly contagious. Regular Pap smears (examination of a sample of cervical cells) can detect precancerous or cancerous conditions at early stages. The accuracy can be affected by patient preparation, sampling techniques, variation in fixing and staining of the smear, and by interpretations of the pathologist. Chemotherapy and radiation may be used to treat cervical cancer.

### Dietary and Exercise Behaviors

Evidence suggests that about one third of cancer deaths are associated with obesity, physical inactivity, and poor nutrition (ACS, 2007). Obesity results from the combined effects of unhealthy nutritional and exercise behaviors. It is a known risk factor for endometrial, breast, and kidney cancers (West et al., 2004, p. 12). Obesity and high-fat content in foods, especially saturated fat, appear to increase our cancer risk.

Lower intake of high-fiber foods is characteristic of high-fat diets. The absence of sufficient fiber in our diets is another dietary choice associated with a higher incidence of cancer. International studies indicate that low fiber intake increases risks for colorectal and breast cancers. Unfortunately many residents of the United States consume well below the recommended 25 grams of fiber per day (West et al., 2004, p. 18). Fruits and vegetables contain fiber, so a high intake of fruits and vegetables is desirable for the fiber content as well as for the various vitamins they supply. Charred meat and large amounts of foods high in salt also increase cancer risks. The Food and Drug Administration (FDA) studies the ways foods and food additives add to cancer risk. Over the past several decades the agency has eliminated several additives from the marketplace. These include some nitrates and dyes added to foods to make them more appetizing.

### Overexposure to Ultraviolet Light

Skin cancer is the most common cancer in the United States. Exposure to ultraviolet radiation from sunlight and tanning beds is a risk factor for cancers of the skin. Being tanned is associated in some segments of society with appearing younger and healthy. More than 1 million skin cancers were diagnosed in 2006 (ACS, 2007).

### Occupational Risks

Some jobs and occupations put people at risk of cancer. For example, working in bars where smoking is allowed puts people at risk of lung cancer. Some jobs in the health care industry cause excessive exposure to radiation. Asbestos is carcinogenic. Workers unknowingly carried asbestos fibers home on their work clothes putting the health of their spouses and children at risk along with their own. Industrial workers are at risk of cancer by exposure to radiation and to toxic substances such as benzene, chromium, coal tar, creosote, and arsenic.

### Delay in Seeking Medical Advice: Stress, Income, and Immunity

This chapter began by noting that people dread cancer among all diseases. Fear of cancer and ignorance about treatment and survival rates are two psychosocial factors keeping people away from seeking medical care. This delay may prove fatal. People with lower levels of income and education are more likely to delay seeking medical care, because low income is associated with limited access to health care insurance, medical diagnosis, and treatment. A recent study using the National Cancer Database analyzed the records of 3.7 million patients diagnosed with cancer from 1998 to 2004 and found that early screening was less likely for uninsured patients (Sack, 2008). In another study, African American women were less likely to be diagnosed with breast cancer than European American women, and were more likely to die from the cancer. This racial disparity in survival is accounted for by reduced access to health care and because the quality of mammography tends to be lower in public hospitals and clinics where black women are more likely to be diagnosed (Ackerman, 2008). Further, people living in low-income housing areas may be at greater risk of cancer from air pollution and other carcinogens such as asbestos used in building material.

## Primary Prevention: Reducing the Risks of Cancer

### Avoiding Known Risk Factors

It is not accurate to say that all cancers can be prevented. Any book title suggesting that is misleading. It is true that many cancers are the result of human behaviors that can be avoided. Many components of tobacco smoke are known carcinogens; therefore, the cancers associated with tobacco use can be avoided by not using tobacco products and avoiding secondhand smoke. It is difficult for children to avoid smoke exhaled by caregivers, so they cannot do much about their risks until they leave home. Drinking alcohol is another avoidable behavior that contributes to cancers of the esophagus and pancreas. The combination of smoking and alcohol puts us at even greater risk for cancer.

### Improving Health to Avoid Some Cancers

#### Exercise

The higher your fitness level, the less likely you are to succumb to cancer. Several studies indicate that regular aerobic exercise has a protective effect with regard to the development of cancer (Sallis & Owen, 1999). There is a strong and consistent inverse relationship between cancer and physical activity on the job (Lee, 1994). Powell and Blair (1994) proposed that about a third of colon cancer deaths can be attributed to inactive lifestyles. Moderate exercise is beneficial to the immune system, which provides protection against some cancers and helps during recovery from cancer (Woods & Davis, 1994). Exercise decreases risks of breast cancer and cancer of the prostate by regulating hormone levels. Physical activity helps manage the stress and depression associated with cancer treatment (Bogart & Delahanty, 2004, p. 214).

#### Healthy Diets

Good nutritional practices reduce the risks of some cancers. Nutritionists recommend eating five to nine servings of fruits and vegetables, and whole grains every day. High-fiber diets give bulk to waste in the gastrointestinal tract and move body waste more quickly, so fragile cells are less likely to be exposed to carcinogenic substances. Exercise also shortens transit time. Cruciferous vegetables such as cabbage and broccoli have been associated with lower levels of cancer. Vegetables contain antioxidants that help destroy free radicals believed to contribute to cancer. Foods containing vitamins A and C are particularly protective against cancer. Avoiding a high-fat intake and avoiding obesity are believed to be protective. High-fat eating patterns, or taking in more than 30% of daily calories from fat, is associated with prostate, breast, and colorectal cancers. Breast cancer rates were 9% lower in the women who made healthful dietary changes when participating in the Women's Health Initiative (2006).

Avoiding Excessive Amounts of Sunlight and Tanning Beds
Skin cancer is very common in the United States, with more than a million people diagnosed each year (CDC, 2007). Malignant melanomas have increased more than 100% since 1973. The lighter your skin color, the higher your risk of skin cancer, but people of all skin colors can develop skin cancer (**Figure 12.2**). Tanning beds produce the same UV-A radiation as the sun. There are defenses against skin cancer. Wearing hats and sunscreen with sun protective factor when outdoors and avoiding the sun between 11 AM and 4 PM help with prevention. The sunscreen must protect against both UV-A and UV-B rays to be effective. Babies should never be exposed to direct sunlight, and sunscreens should not be applied to infants under 6 months of age.

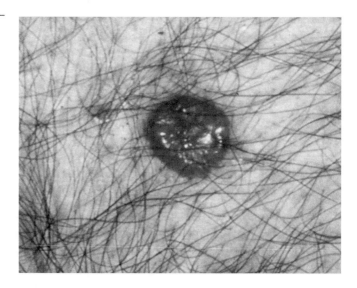

**Figure 12.2**
Tanning beds produce the same UV-A radiation as the sun.

# Secondary Prevention: Screening for Early Detection and Followup

## Self-Screening for Cancer

Keeping current about causes and signs of cancer helps avoid advanced malignancies. At our annual physical examinations we should call the attention of medical personnel to any signs of cancer. For example, consistent hoarseness or coughing can be signals of lung cancer. Unusual bleeding from the rectum is a sign of colorectal cancer. A lump or thickening in a breast or testicle may indicate cancer in those areas of the body. Breasts and testicles should be self-checked on a monthly basis (see "Think About It!" Early Detection May Save Your Life!). Breast self-exam (BSE) should be completed during the days between menstrual periods.

Young men, ages 20–34, are most susceptible to testicular cancer (M.D. Anderson, 2008a, p. 7). The monthly self-exam includes checking for changes such as lumps or enlargement in the testicles. Other symptoms include a heavy sensation in the groin or a dull ache in the groin or abdomen. Prostate cancer is more likely to occur in older men. Symptoms vary but may include frequent urination or difficulty with urination.

Every person should monitor the skin on the backs and fronts of their bodies for changes in warts or moles and any sores that do not heal. Moles that are bigger than a pencil eraser, or develop irregular borders, or change colors or shapes may indicate skin cancer (ACS, 2007). Changes in bowel or bladder habits may be a sign of any number of different problems including cancer. Persistent indigestion or difficulty swallowing are symptoms for a variety of cancers. Those who smoke, chew, or dip tobacco, or drink alcohol are at risk of oral cancers. Any changes in the interior of the mouth or nose may be indicative of precancerous conditions. White or velvety red patches and lumps or hardening of the tissue should be checked by medical personnel. Cancers always grow, but some grow so slowly they are more difficult to detect. Write down the date symptoms first appeared, as well as detailed descriptions of symptoms. This is valuable information for medical personnel. From a psychosocial aspect, self-awareness and self-screenings require vigilance and calendar-based organizational skills.

## Medical Screening

Early detection is one of the most important defenses against cancer death. Some screening for cancer is done at regular medical checkups, but people, including college students, must be willing to take the time to schedule those appointments. Females having regular gynecological exams should have their breasts checked for lumps and thickenings. Cervical cancer is diagnosed through pelvic exams and Pap smears. If there is any question about lumps or thickenings in the breast then the physician may suggest a further diagnostic procedure called a mammogram.

Medical personnel can check males for testicular and prostate cancer. Cancer of the prostate is checked first by digital rectal exams. The blood test for prostate cancer is for the

## Think About It!

## Early Detection May Save Your Life!

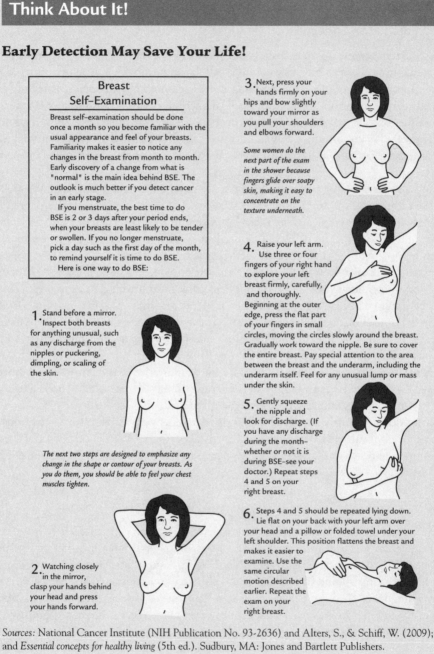

### Breast Self-Examination

Breast self-examination should be done once a month so you become familiar with the usual appearance and feel of your breasts. Familiarity makes it easier to notice any changes in the breast from month to month. Early discovery of a change from what is "normal" is the main idea behind BSE. The outlook is much better if you detect cancer in an early stage.

If you menstruate, the best time to do BSE is 2 or 3 days after your period ends, when your breasts are least likely to be tender or swollen. If you no longer menstruate, pick a day such as the first day of the month, to remind yourself it is time to do BSE.

Here is one way to do BSE:

1. Stand before a mirror. Inspect both breasts for anything unusual, such as any discharge from the nipples or puckering, dimpling, or scaling of the skin.

*The next two steps are designed to emphasize any change in the shape or contour of your breasts. As you do them, you should be able to feel your chest muscles tighten.*

2. Watching closely in the mirror, clasp your hands behind your head and press your hands forward.

3. Next, press your hands firmly on your hips and bow slightly toward your mirror as you pull your shoulders and elbows forward.

*Some women do the next part of the exam in the shower because fingers glide over soapy skin, making it easy to concentrate on the texture underneath.*

4. Raise your left arm. Use three or four fingers of your right hand to explore your left breast firmly, carefully, and thoroughly. Beginning at the outer edge, press the flat part of your fingers in small circles, moving the circles slowly around the breast. Gradually work toward the nipple. Be sure to cover the entire breast. Pay special attention to the area between the breast and the underarm, including the underarm itself. Feel for any unusual lump or mass under the skin.

5. Gently squeeze the nipple and look for discharge. (If you have any discharge during the month–whether or not it is during BSE–see your doctor.) Repeat steps 4 and 5 on your right breast.

6. Steps 4 and 5 should be repeated lying down. Lie flat on your back with your left arm over your head and a pillow or folded towel under your left shoulder. This position flattens the breast and makes it easier to examine. Use the same circular motion described earlier. Repeat the exam on your right breast.

*Sources:* National Cancer Institute (NIH Publication No. 93-2636) and Alters, S., & Schiff, W. (2009); and *Essential concepts for healthy living* (5th ed.). Sudbury, MA: Jones and Bartlett Publishers.

## Think About It!

### Early Detection Can Save Your Life!

#### Testicular Self-Examination

A simple procedure called testicular self-exam (TSE) can increase the chances of finding a tumor early. Men should perform TSE once a month—after a warm bath or shower. The heat causes the scrotal skin to relax, making it easier to find anything unusual. TSE is simple and only takes a few minutes.

- Examine each testicle gently with both hands. The index and middle fingers should be placed underneath the testicle while the thumbs are placed on the top. Roll the testicle gently between the thumbs and fingers. One testicle may be larger than the other. This is normal.

- The epididymis is a cordlike structure on the top and back of the testicle that stores and transports the sperm. Do not confuse the epididymis with an abnormal lump.

- Feel for any abnormal lumps—about the size of a pea—on the front or the side of the testicle. These lumps are usually painless.

If you do find a lump, contact your doctor right away. The lump may be due to an infection, and a doctor can decide the proper treatment. If the lump is not an infection, it is likely to be cancer. Remember that testicular cancer is highly curable, especially when detected and treated early. Testicular cancer almost always occurs in only one testicle, and the other testicle is all that is needed for full sexual function.

Routine testicular self-exams are important, but they cannot substitute for a doctor's examination. Your doctor should examine your testicles when you have a physical exam. You also can ask your doctor to check the way you do TSE.

*Source:* National Cancer Institute (NIH Publication No. 93-2636).

prostate-specific antigen or PSA. African American men should have their PSA tested regularly beginning at age 40. Other racial and ethnic categories should begin testing at age 50 unless there is a family history of prostate cancer.

Colorectal cancer may be detected by blood in a stool sample called a fecal occult blood test. This is usually done in conjunction with annual medical visits for adults beginning at age 50. The next diagnostic step would be a flexible sigmoidoscopy. A **colonoscopy** examines the colon and also allows precancerous polyps to be removed. Lung cancer can be detected

**colonoscopy** A medical procedure to examine the interior of the colon.

with a CT scan, but an early symptom is a persistent cough that is noticed by individuals or their companions.

# Tertiary Prevention: Coping with Cancer and Its Treatments

It is not yet possible to prevent all types of cancer, and we know it is helpful if people go into cancer treatment with overall good health and a lifelong history of good health practices. Research shows it is useful to recovery to have a positive mental outlook or optimistic attitude, and social support from family, friends, and coworkers (Ben-Zur, Gilbar, & Lev, 2001; Carver & Antoni, 2004; Helgeson, Snyder, & Seltman, 2004). Being informed and knowledgeable about all aspects of one's treatment is also very important (Bloom, 2002).

## Biological Aspects of Cancer Treatments

Choices of treatments depend upon the type of cancer, its location in the body, and stage of development. In general, treatment choices include surgery, radiation, chemotherapy, hormone or gene therapy, or some combination of these methods. All treatment modalities have side effects and usually create anxiety. For example sexual dysfunction is sometimes an outcome of cancer treatment, so the support of spouses and partners is essential (Yurek, Farrar, & Anderson, 2000). Pain is rarely a symptom of cancer in its early stages, but may be a side effect of treatments such as surgery. When cancer is advanced, medications can control the pain. Psychological interventions may be helpful with cancer-related fatigue (Jacobsen, Donovan, Vadaparampil, & Small, 2008).

Surgery
Surgery refers to removal of cancerous tissue plus surrounding tissue margins, and sometimes lymph nodes for diagnostic purposes. At times surgeons are unsure of the extent of a cancer's growth and are unable to provide answers about treatments or prognosis until they examine the interior of a patient's body. Surgery has a number of different biological side effects. These may include aftercare from anesthesia, including breathing exercises; intravenous (IV) administration of fluids containing medication, nutrients, and blood; and followup tests. Surgery for shallow skin cancers can usually be accomplished under a local anesthesia in physicians' offices. In some cases surgical removal of parts of the body are necessary including sections of the colon, prostate, or breast.

Psychosocial preparation for surgery includes preoperative discussions with patients and family members about possible outcomes of surgery. Many hospitals provide videos for patients and their families to take home and watch prior to surgery. This is to help them better understand procedures. Videos also show how to accomplish aftercare for the patient. In some cases surgery will result in disfigurement, but there are options for reconstructive surgery following recovery. Hospitals also provide pamphlets and detailed written instructions about post-surgical care. It is important for patients and families to understand the time and place for followup appointments that are central to effective cancer treatment.

Radiation

Radiation therapy is another treatment for cancer. This refers to electromagnetic energy emitted in the form of rays or particles. Radiation is used for diagnosis as well as for cancer treatment. Radiation interferes with the growth of cancerous cells and can destroy tumors. Radiation also has side effects. Symptoms depend on the amount of radiation, the exposure time, and the part of the body affected. Radiation may temporarily cause nausea, vomiting, headaches, and diarrhea. There may be hair loss and bleeding. A main danger of radiation is the loss of healthy cells near the tumor. For this reason it helps to continue to follow healthy lifestyle practices when undergoing radiation, especially following good nutritional practices.

Chemotherapy

This term refers to treatment for cancer using chemicals. Cancer-fighting drugs are injected into a vein or taken by mouth so the chemical can travel through the body. Drugs can slow and even stop the proliferation of cancer cells, and new chemical treatments are being developed every year. Chemical agents used in cancer treatment have assorted side effects including nausea and vomiting. In many cases patients and physicians must also contend with suppression of bone marrow function. Food aversions may be directly associated with chemotherapy, although it is essential for recovery that patients continue to take nourishment. Anti-nausea treatments usually help control this side effect. Some kinds of chemotherapy may result in premature menopause with attendant discomforts. Other options for cancer treatment are hormone therapy, gene therapy, and immunotherapy.

## Psychosocial Aspects of Cancer Diagnosis and Treatment

It is wonderful to hear news that a cancerous growth has been treated effectively, but neither cancer patients nor their families are ever quite the same following the diagnosis of cancer. They continue to worry that the cancer will return or show up in some other part of the body. Psychosocial factors affect both quality of life and outcomes in cancer patients (Cruess, Schneiderman, Antoni, & Penedo, 2004, p. 55). Highly publicized cases such as Lance Armstrong's extraordinary victories in the Tour de France (see **Figure 12.3**) demonstrate that people can recover from cancer (Armstrong & Jenkins, 2000, 2003).

Emotional Distress

Distress is one psychological reaction to the diagnosis and treatment of cancer. A variety of negative emotions may be triggered in patients, including anger, worry, anxiety, fear, depression, helplessness, hopelessness, and even guilt and shame. There may be fears about death and pain, job loss, cutting back on social and recreational activities, and time lost to treatment modalities. Family members and friends of cancer patients go through a similar array of emotional reactions upon hearing the news of a cancer diagnosis. They often believe they must carefully control their facial expressions as well as what they say to patients in order not to add to their emotional burden.

**Figure 12.3**
Lance Armstrong's extraordinary victories in the
Tour de France demonstrate that people can recover
from cancer and continue to excel.

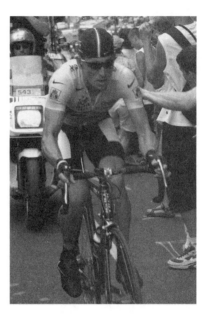

A recent study of surviving cancer patients suggests that psychosocial variables are more important than medical variables in adjusting to diagnosis, treatment, and survival of breast cancer (Carver et al., 2005). At 5 to 13 years following treatment, patients completed mailed questionnaires for the study. Patients who were initially well adjusted to the disease were more likely to remain so, regardless of medical differences. Marital status, the personality trait of optimism, and positive self-reports predicted psychosocial well-being among long-term survivors.

### Economic Change

Change in socioeconomic conditions may be a consequence of cancer diagnosis and treatment. Many patients cannot work while in treatment, and may be concerned about the loss of their jobs. It is an additional worry and economic burden if family members are solely dependent on the patient's income. Another economic concern is medical care costs. Cancer treatment can be very expensive, and without good medical coverage, the costs of treatment may be overwhelming.

### Relationships

Relationships are affected by cancer diagnosis and treatment (Alferi, Carver, Antoni, Weiss, & Duran, 2001). Family members and friends help by reminding their loved ones about dates for diagnostic work and regular medical checkups, and by providing transportation and other types of support. They may also be involved in encouraging individuals to follow up on any questionable results. Communication between the individual and family members is critical, because family members and close friends may be called upon to help with decisions about treatment. It is difficult to watch loved ones suffer through cancer treatment. Hair loss, weight change, nausea, and vomiting all affect one's self-esteem, as well as one's relationships with others, including children and parents. Sometimes patients must be isolated from others, including their children, because of the suppressed immune function some treatments cause. Fatigue, sleep problems, and loss of sexual interest have negative effects on family relationships. Family and friends may avoid physical touching, including hugging, for fear of hurting a patient. For the good of patients, all positive social relationships should continue throughout diagnosis and treatment.

### Support Groups

Groups of similar patients are very helpful in dealing with the stress and strain of cancer diagnosis and treatment. Every member of the group is going through or has already gone through similar situations. Patients may not feel obligated to maintain the pretense of cheerfulness that they keep up around family and friends. In support groups patients can talk about their emotional reactions and about the difficulties of treatment and aftercare. Sometimes there is practical advice, such as how to deal with nausea or hair loss. Problems in relationships with family members, friends, and coworkers can also be shared in confidential support group sessions.

### Stress

The connection between cancer and stress is of great interest in health psychology. It is well accepted that diagnosis and treatment of cancer will result in stress for patients, their families, and friends. Ways of coping with that stress is an important area of research. Many of the psychological interventions discussed in the earlier chapters on pain and stress management are helpful to cancer patients. Relaxation training may be particularly helpful with management of stress associated with cancer (Andersen, 2002). Other helpful approaches are biofeedback, guided imagery, and progressive muscle relaxation.

### Adherence to Treatment

Faithfully maintaining treatment protocols and consistency in receiving treatments are essential to recovery from cancer. This is especially an issue for patients in treatment for months or even years. A patient's quality of life may deteriorate during treatment. Adherence to medical regimens is less likely when treatments result in nausea, vomiting, hair loss, or fatigue. Fatigue and weight loss are among the most depressing and discouraging symptoms of cancer treatments.

### Exercise

Exercise is helpful for virtually all individuals diagnosed with cancer, but it should be individualized for patient limitations (Schwartz, 2003). Adjustments should be made for pain, fatigue, shortness of breath, and any disabilities following surgery and bed rest. There is also the possibility of nerve damage and loss of flexibility. Moderate, regular aerobic exercise is beneficial from biological and psychosocial perspectives. Strength training for muscle main-tenance and even bone redevelopment is possible. Stretching and other flexibility exercises can maintain joint range of motion following surgery. Exercise can even reduce feelings of fatigue in women with breast cancer who undergo chemotherapy (Schwartz, Mori, Gao, Nail, & King, 2001).

Complementary and Alternative Medicine

Complementary and alternative medicine may be used in addition to traditional Western medical approaches, but patients are advised to check with their oncologists before using these alternatives, because they may be harmful under some circumstances. Before relying on web sites for cancer advice, patients can check for bias, purpose, audience, and origin (master of domains) at the web site of the National Council Against Health Fraud (2002).

Complementary health care practices are not taught widely in medical school and usu-ally are not reimbursed by insurance companies. A variety of alternative medicine approaches are discussed in other chapters, including chiropractic; biofeedback; massage therapy; acupuncture for pain, nausea, and dry-mouth control; Chinese and Asian traditional prac-tices (including those from Tibet and India); guided imagery; herbal medicine; humor or clown therapy; hypnosis; Pilates, spirituality; and centering prayer.

**Reiki** uses universal life energy to relax, and reduce stress and pain by reconnecting the mind and the body along with other forms of exercise, meditation, massage, and relaxation (M.D. Anderson, 2008b). Additional complementary methods are nia dance play, tai chi, aromatherapy, holistic medicine, **osteopathic** and homeopathic medicine, naturopathic therapy, Feldenkrais awareness through movement, and pet therapy. Aromatherapy is an ancient approach that uses botanical oils such as lemon oil, eucalyptus oil, and sandalwood for relaxation. Osteopathic medicine or osteopathy attempts to restore the body structure by manipulating its parts. Practitioners of homeopathic medicine treat disease with sub-stances that produce effects different from those produced by cancer. Reflexology uses pres-sure points to massage the feet and restore the flow of energy in the body. Native American medicine men or shamans promote healing by altering levels of consciousness using sweat lodges, dancing, smoking, and inhaling or eating psychoactive plants.

---

**Reiki** An alternative or complementary medicine that uses universal life energy to relax, and reduce stress and pain by reconnecting the mind with the body.

**osteopathic medicine** A form of medical therapy that emphasizes the relationship of organs to the musculoskeletal system and restores body health by manipulating bones and muscles.

## Specific Types of Cancer: Their Causes and Treatments

### Lung Cancer

Lung cancer is the leading cause of cancer death among women and men (CDC, 2007). Even if the disease spreads to other parts of the body it is still called lung cancer. Smoking is responsible for 87% of all lung cancer cases in the United States (M.D. Anderson, 2007a). Other risks for lung cancer are family history; environmental exposure, especially to radon and asbestos, radiation, arsenic, air pollution (such as byproducts of combustion of fossil fuels), and environmental tobacco smoke; and lung diseases such as tuberculosis (TB). Symptoms specific to lung cancer vary but include a persistent cough; blood-streaked sputum; chest, arm, or shoulder pain; voice change; coughing up blood; shortness of breath; wheezing or hoarseness; repeated bouts of pneumonia or bronchitis; swelling of the neck and face; and clubbing of fingers. There are no effective screenings prior to the presentation of symptoms. X-rays, lab analysis of phlegm cells, fiber optic screenings, biopsies, CT scans, and blood tests are used for diagnosis. Treatment options include surgery, radiation, chemotherapy, and targeted biological therapies.

### Breast Cancer

Breast cancer is the leading cancer cause of death among Hispanic women and second only to lung cancer among other female population segments. About 178,500 new cases of invasive breast cancer are expected annually. Of those, about 2,000 will occur in men (ACS, 2007). Most cases occur in women age 50 and older. Risk is higher if the woman's first menstrual period occurred before the age of 12, if menopause began after age 55, or if a woman never had children or had her first child after age 30. Other risk factors are using hormone replacement therapy or oral contraceptives, obesity, high-fat diets, physical inactivity, and alcohol use. Symptoms include lumps or masses in the breast, enlarged lymph nodes in the armpit, and changes in the appearance of a breast, including nipple discharge and scaliness. All lumps are not cancerous. Many are due to a fibrocystic condition responding to hormonal changes associated with menstrual periods.

Self-screening includes monthly breast self-exams. Medical screening includes clinical breast examinations every 1 to 3 years after age 20, annually after age 40, and mammograms yearly after age 40. Following a suspicious mammogram, physicians may recommend further tests, including ultrasound, fine-needle aspiration to examine fluid in tumors, or a biopsy. Surgical options include removal of the lump or removal of the entire breast, which can be followed by reconstructive surgery (Miller, 2008). Chemotherapy, radiation therapy, and hormonal therapy are additional treatment options. Tamoxifen, an antiestrogen hormone, may be used as followup treatment for some types of breast cancers. It inhibits breast tumor growth. Other followup tests include chest x-rays, scans, blood tests, and medical examinations. Death rates from breast cancer are decreasing (ACS, 2007).

## Prostate Cancer

This is the second leading cause of death among men after lung cancer. About 200,000 men are diagnosed each year with prostate cancer and 30,000 die. Factors that put men at risk include age, race, and a high-fat diet. African American men and Jamaican men of African descent have the highest prostate cancer incidence rates in the world (ACS, 2007). Medical screening includes a digital exam of the prostate gland and blood analysis for PSA, beginning at ages 45 to 50. When the PSA in the blood rises to a certain level, a biopsy is recommended in order to search for cancerous cells, which are then graded and assigned to one of four stages. A radionuclide bone scan may be recommended to determine if the cancer has metastasized to the bones. Following a diagnosis of cancer a patient has options regarding treatment based on medical recommendations. There are at least three surgical options for removal of the prostate and adjacent tissue. Male hormones sometimes boost the growth of prostate cancer cells, so hormonal therapy may be used to block the supply of hormones to the cancer. Radiation is another option. **Brachytherapy** consists of tiny radioactive seeds placed inside or near tumors. A medical oncologist may also recommend followup chemotherapy.

## Colorectal Cancer

Cancers of the colon and rectum are the third leading cause of cancer death in the United States for women and most men (ACS, 2007). Cancer cells in the colon or rectum multiply uncontrollably, begin to damage surrounding tissue, and may spread to other parts of the body. The best chance for surviving colorectal cancer is early detection, but sometimes there are no symptoms in early stages. Primary screening is an annual fecal occult blood test. Symptoms include rectal bleeding, blood in the stool, prolonged diarrhea or constipation, a change in the size or shape of the stool, abdominal pain or cramping, and the urge to have a bowel movement when there is no need. Some cancers begin as polyps that become cancerous and bleed and may obstruct the intestine. This cancer is most common in people over the age of 50. Other risk factors are family history, inflammatory bowel disease, the lack of physical activity, obesity, high-fat diets, cigarette smoking, and alcohol. Physical screening should begin at age 50 with a flexible sigmoidoscopy every 5 years and a colonoscopy every 10 years. Risk reduction includes regular exercise, maintaining an ideal weight, quitting smoking, and limiting alcohol consumption. In 2005 there were 56,000 deaths, and about 145,000 new cases in the United States. Surgery is the most common treatment prior to metastasis. Chemotherapy and radiation are also used. Fewer than 40% of cases are diagnosed before the cancer

---

**brachytherapy** Medical approach to cancer using tiny radioactive seeds placed inside or near tumors to destroy them.

spreads (M.D. Anderson, 2007b). Chemotherapy, radiation, and immunotherapy are other treatment options.

## Lymphomas

About 20,000 deaths due to Hodgkin **lymphoma** and non-Hodgkin lymphoma occur annually (ACS, 2007). Symptoms include sores that bleed easily and do not heal, lumps or thickening, ear pain, coughing up blood, and persistent red or white patches. Known risk factors are smoking, smokeless tobacco, and excessive consumption of alcohol. Sometimes this cancer shows up in the oral cavity and is identified by dentists. Radiation therapy, surgery, and chemotherapy are used for treatment.

## Childhood Cancer

Childhood cancers are rare but about 10,000 new cases occur a year in the United States (ACS, 2007). About a third of cancer deaths of children are from **leukemia**. Symptoms include bone and joint pain, weakness, bleeding, and fever. Other childhood cancers occur in the brain, sympathetic nervous system, kidneys, eyes, and bone. There are pediatric oncologists, nurses, social workers, and psychologists available to assist children and their families. The goal in cancer treatment of children is to return them to their normal social environment as soon as possible. Teens are especially bothered by disfigurement due to cancer treatment. Children sometimes mistakenly view cancer as a punishment and blame themselves. Talk therapy may be necessary. Children's developmental levels are affected if treatments go on for long periods of time. Isolation to protect against infection is always difficult for children.

## Summary

This chapter explores biopsychosical aspects of cancer, its development, detection, and treatment. Cancer begins at the cellular level when the DNA of cells is altered. The causes of these changes can have biological or psychosocial origins. Important terminology of cancer diagnosis and treatment includes the words *neoplasm, malignancy, metastasis, carcinogenic, immune function, diagnosis, prognosis, radiation, surgery,* and *chemotherapy*. Non-modifiable risk factors about which we can do very little include age, gender, and family history. Psychosocial risk factors that we can influence include the use of tobacco and alcohol, dietary practices and exercise, sexual behavior, tanning practices, occupational choices, and delay in seeking medical advice due to fear and ignorance.

**lymphoma** Cancer in lymph tissues.

**leukemia** Cancer of the blood; a malignant neoplasm of blood-forming tissue.

Primary prevention to reduce the risks of cancer includes healthy lifestyles, including regular aerobic exercise, low-fat and high-fiber eating patterns, managing stress, and avoiding excessive amounts of ultraviolet radiation. Early detection is very helpful in recovering from cancer because it increases treatment options. People can self-screen for testicular, breast, and skin cancer. Medical personnel screen for these plus cervical, prostate, lung, and colorectal cancers. Treatments include surgery, radiation, and chemotherapy. Psychosocial aspects of treatment include allaying fears and emotional distress, making economic provisions for diagnosis and treatment, and maintaining high levels of social support from family and friends. Support groups made up of patients with similar cancers may also help in dealing with side effects of treatments and with emotional adjustment. Stress management, adherence to treatment protocols and timing, exercise, and various approaches of complementary medicine may be beneficial.

Lung cancer causes more deaths in the United States than any other cancer. The vast majority of lung cancer is due to exposure to tobacco smoke. Early diagnosis is difficult, but there are several signals of most lung cancers. Breast cancer is the second most likely type of cancer in women and prostate cancer is second in men. Women are encouraged to self-examine their breasts monthly and seek medical care if there are changes. Prostate cancer is found through digital rectal exams by medical personnel followed by a biopsy. Colorectal cancer is the third most common type of cancer death in the United States. It is first diagnosed through fecal occult blood tests and then by microscopic examinations of the colon. Lymphomas and childhood cancers are also major concerns.

## Review Questions

1. List several of the many complexities that still abound with regard to cancer and cancer treatment.

2. Using a biological viewpoint, explain the most important aspects of the disease called cancer. In your answer include unique terminology, including neoplasm, malignancy, metastasis, carcinogens, diagnosis, prognosis, diagnostic tools, and general treatments.

3. Discuss the three general biological risk factors for cancer and what can be done to offset the effects of those risks.

4. List and briefly explain psychosocial risk factors for cancer.

5. Explain the various ways that dietary choices put us at risk of cancer.

6. Briefly discuss the relationship between cancer and the immune system. State what can be done to reduce damage to our immune function.

7. Describe primary prevention for cancer.

8. Describe self-screening efforts people should utilize to avoid advanced cancers.

9. List the types of screenings by medical personnel that are recommended on a regular basis.

10. Briefly describe the three most common approaches to cancer treatment.

11. Explain five psychosocial aspects of cancer diagnosis and treatment.

12. Discuss the three most common causes of cancer deaths in the United States.

## Student Activity

Interview someone who has recovered from cancer. Using the issues discussed in this chapter, take the person through the whole process beginning with the self-screening, initial diagnosis, treatment, and followup. In your questions emphasize any psychosocial factors that helped in recovery. Write an essay based on the information from the interview and this chapter. Keep your interview subject's name confidential, although you may give gender and approximate age.

## References

Ackerman, T. (2008, February 5). Wider disparity here in breast cancer toll. *Houston Chronicle* (pp. A1, A9).

Alferi, S. M., Carver, C. S., Antoni, M. H., Weiss, S., & Duran, R. E. (2001). An exploratory study of social support, distress, and life disruption among low-income Hispanic women under treatment for early stage breast cancer. *Health Psychology, 20*, 41–46.

American Cancer Society. (2007). *Cancer facts and figures 2007*. Atlanta, GA: American Cancer Society.

Anderson, R. (2002). Biobehavioral outcomes following psychological interventions for cancer patients. *Journal of Consulting and Clinical Psychology, 70*, 590–610.

Armstrong, L., with Jenkins, S. (2003). *Every second counts*. New York: Broadway Books.

Armstrong, L., & Jenkins, S. (2000). *It's not about the bike: My journey back to life*. New York: Putnam.

Ben-Zur, H., Gilbar, O., & Lev, S. (2001). Coping with breast cancer: Patient, spouse, and dyad models. *Psychosomatic Medicine, 63*, 32–39.

Bloom, J. R. (2002). Surviving and thriving? *Psycho-Oncology, 11*, 89–92.

Bogart, L. M., & Delahanty, D. L. (2004). Psychosocial models. In R. G. Frank, A. Baum, & J. L. Wallander (Eds.), *Handbook of clinical health psychology* (Vol. 3, pp. 201–248). Washington, DC: American Psychological Association.

Carver, C. S., & Antoni, M. H. (2004). Finding benefit in breast cancer during the year after diagnosis predicts better adjustment 5 to 10 years after diagnosis. *Health Psychology, 23*, 595–598.

Carver, C. S., Smith, R. G., Antoni, M. H., Petronis, V. M, Weiss, S., & Derhagopian, R. P. (2005). Optimistic personality and psychosocial well-being during treatment predict psychosocial well-being among long-term survivors of breast cancer. *Health Psychology, 24*(5), 508–516.

Centers for Disease Control, National Center for Health Statistics (2006a). New CDC Report Documents Percentage of People Without Health Insurance. Retrieved November 1, 2007 from http://www.cdc.gov/nchs/press room/07 newsreleases/insurance.htm

Centers for Disease Control and Prevention. (2006b). Youth risk behavior surveillance—United States. *Morbidity and Mortality Weekly Report, 55 (SS-5)* 1–108.

Centers for Disease Control and Prevention. (2007). United States Cancer Statistics. Retrieved June 29, 2007 from http://www.cdc.gov/cancer/npcr/uscs/2003/facts_major.htm

Clark, L. F., Rhodes, S. D., Rogers, W., & Lidden, L. (2004). In J. M. Raczynski & L. C. Leviton (Eds.), *Handbook of clinical health psychology* (Vol. 2, pp. 121–146). Washington, DC: American Psychological Association.

Cruess, D. G., Schneiderman, N., Antoni, M. H., & Penedo, F. (2004). Biobehavioral bases of disease processes. In R. G. Frank, A. Baum, & J. L. Wallander (Eds.), *Handbook of clinical health psychology* (Vol. 3, pp. 31–79). Washington, DC: American Psychological Association.

Helgeson, V. S., Snyder, P., & Seltman, H. (2004). Psychological and physical adjustment to breast cancer over 4 years: Identifying distinct trajectories of change. *Health Psychology, 23,* 3-15.

Henley, S. J., Thun, M. J., Connell, C., & Calle, E. E. (2005). Two large prospective studies of mortality among men who use snuff or chewing tobacco. *Cancer Causes Control, 16*(4), 347-358.

Insel, P., Turner, R. E., & Ross, D. (2006). *Discovering nutrition* (2nd ed.). Sudbury, MA: Jones and Bartlett.

Jacobsen, P. B., Donovan, K. A., Vadaparampil, S. T., & Small, B. J. (2007). Systematic review and meta-analysis of psychological and activity-based interventions for cancer-related fatigue. *Health Psychology, 26*(6), 660-667.

Lee, I. M. (1994). Physical activity, fitness, and cancer. In C. Bouchard, R. J. Shephard, & T. Stephens (Eds.), *Physical activity, fitness, and health* (pp. 814-831). Champaign, IL: Human Kinetics.

Martin, P. D., & Brantley, P. J. (2004). Stress, coping, and social support in health and behavior. In J. M. Raczynski & L. C. Leviton (Eds.), *Handbook of Clinical Health Psychology* (Vol. 2, pp. 233-267). Washington, DC: American Psychological Association.

M.D. Anderson Cancer Center. (2007a). Lung Cancer Basics. Retrieved June 29, 2007 from http://mdanderson.edu/org/diseases/lung

M.D. Anderson Cancer Center (2007b). Colorectal Cancer Basics. Retrieved June 29, 2007 from http://mdanderson.edu/org/diseases/colorectal

M.D. Anderson Cancer Center (2008a). House call: What you should know about male cancers. *OncoLog, Report to Physicians, 53*(1), 3.

M.D. Anderson Cancer Center, Place of Wellness, Integrative Medicine Program. (2008b). This information came from a print copy for March/April 2008. It may be accessed at www.mdanderston.org/placeofwellness

Miller, K. D. (2008). *Choices in breast cancer treatment.* Baltimore, MD: The Johns Hopkins Press.

National Council Against Health Fraud. (2002). NCAHF Position Statement on White House Commission on Complementary and Alternative Medicine. Retrieved August 27, 2008 from http://www.ncahf.org

Powell, K. E., & Blair, S. N. (1994). The public health burdens of sedentary living habits: Theoretical but realistic estimates. *Medicine and Science in Sports and Exercise, 26,* 851-856.

Sack, K. (2008, February 18). Study: Late cancer diagnosis linked to lack of insurance. *Houston Chronicle,* p. A15.

Sallis, J. F., & Owen, N. (1999). *Physical activity and behavioral medicine.* Thousand Oaks, CA: Sage Publications.

Schwartz, A. L., Mori, M., Gao, R., Nail, L. M., & King, M. E. (2001). Exercise reduces daily fatigue in women with breast cancer receiving chemotherapy. *Medicine and Science in Sport and Exercise, 33*(5), 718-23.

Schwartz, A. L. (2003). Cancer. In J. L. Durstine & G. E. Moore (Eds.), *ACSM's exercise management for persons with chronic diseases and disabilities* (pp. 166-172). Champaign, IL: Human Kinetics.

West, D. S., Harvey-Berino, J., & Raczynski, J. M. (2004). Behavioral aspects of obesity, dietary intake, and chronic disease. In J. M. Raczynski & L. C. Leviton (Eds.), *Handbook of clinical health psychology* (Vol. 2, pp. 9-41). Washington, DC: American Psychological Association.

Women's Health Initiative. (2006). The diet/health connection: Results from the WHI dietary study. *WHI Matters, 11,* 2-3.

Woods, J. A., & Davis, J. M. (1994). Exercise, monocyte/macrophage function and cancer. *Medicine and Science in Sports and Exercise, 26,* 147-156.

Yurek, D., Farrar, W., & Anderson, B. L. (2000). Breast cancer surgery: Comparing surgical groups and determining individual differences in postoperative sexuality and body-change stress. *Journal of Consulting and Clinical Psychology, 68,* 697-709.

# Chapter 13

# Applications of Health Psychology to Chronic Illness

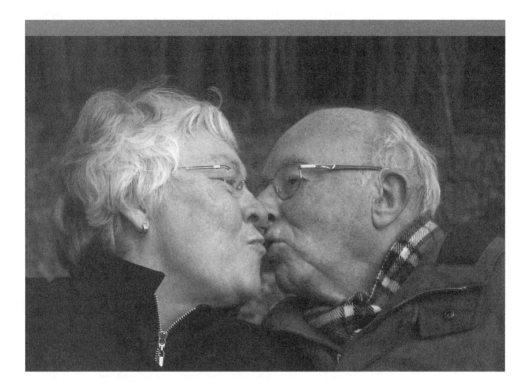

## Learning Objectives

After studying this chapter students will have the knowledge and skills to be able to:

1. Distinguish between chronic and acute illness and give examples of each type.

2. Recount important biological aspects of dealing with a chronic disease.

3. Discuss psychological aspects of living with a chronic disease, including emotional and cognitive responses.

4. Describe goal setting and other perspectives that may be helpful to individuals dealing with a chronic disease.

5. Sum up the concept of social support and give examples of sources for such support.

6. Discuss important biopsychosocial aspects of COPD, diabetes, HIV/AIDS, arthritis, asthma, and osteoporosis.

7. Explain the biopsychosocial aspects of life for patients with Alzheimer's disease and their caregivers.

## Introduction

Heart disease, stroke, and malignant neoplasms (cancers) are the three leading causes of death in the United States (National Vital Statistics System [NVSS], 2008). In rank order, the next primary causes of death are diseases of the lower respiratory system, unintended injuries or accidents, diabetes mellitus, and Alzheimer's disease. In many instances deaths are preceded by a period of illness. In addition to information on causes of death, several federal and state government agencies collect data on chronic illnesses. These reports reveal the extent of morbidity or restrictions on daily activities in a population.

For statistical purposes, the extent of chronic illness is determined through self-reports. Respondents or their proxies are asked about any chronic, unremitting conditions with which they have been diagnosed over the past 12 months (National Center for Health Statistics [NCHS], 2008). Medical advances have actually helped make chronic illness and disabilities more prevalent. More people are surviving serious illnesses and injuries. Chronic diseases affect more than 105 million Americans and account for more than 70% of all health care costs (Hoffman & Rice, 1996). Demographic factors such as low income, limited educational opportunities, and racism are associated with more behavioral risks and more chronic diseases (Orleans, Ullmer, & Gruman, 2004, p. 472).

### Types of Chronic Illness

This chapter focuses on seven categories of chronic illness, including **chronic obstructive pulmonary diseases (COPD)**, **diabetes mellitus**, HIV/AIDS, **arthritis**, **asthma**, **osteoporosis**, and **Alzheimer's disease**. Chronic obstructive pulmonary disease is a leading cause of death in the United States and a major cause of chronic illness. Diabetes is a chronic illness that contributes to deaths from cardiovascular and renal disease. HIV/AIDS is a contagious disease affecting the immune system. Arthritis is one of the most common chronic

**chronic obstructive pulmonary disease (COPD)**  Nonreversible lung disease, including emphysema and bronchitis; often caused by smoking.

**diabetes mellitus**  A complex chronic disorder of metabolism due to lack of insulin or having insulin that the body cannot use.

**arthritis**  A disorder that inflames joints resulting in swelling and pain.

**asthma**  A disorder that interferes with breathing and is characterized by wheezing. Mucus in the respiratory system results in inflammation of the bronchi.

**osteoporosis**  A disease resulting in fragile bones due to bone loss; outcomes include fractures, back pain, deformity, and loss of height.

**Alzheimer's disease**  A loss of cognitive ability especially memory. It usually occurs in old age and results in personality changes and confusion.

conditions contributing to lifelong suffering and disability. Asthma is a serious chronic respiratory disorder affecting millions of people, including children, teens, and adults. Alzheimer's disease and osteoporosis are two debilitating chronic illnesses that are more characteristic of older people. There are many other types of chronic illness characterized by physical, mental, and emotional conditions that limit the ability of adults to perform necessary activities such as working and doing household chores.

## Confronting Chronic Illness

Chronically ill people face major obstacles during their lifetime, including dealing with confusing health care systems, financial problems, changes in family functioning, unpredictable energy levels, and diminished self-esteem. Many behaviors and health issues already discussed are closely involved in chronic illness. These include dietary and exercise patterns, obesity, substance abuse, smoking, and risky sexual behaviors. Stress and pain, discussed earlier, are two crosscutting issues that are important in the management of chronic diseases. Healthy People 2010 sets forth national health objectives and identifies the burden of behaviors putting everyone's health at risk (U.S. Department of Health and Human Services [DHHS], 2000). **Table 13.1** provides information on noise levels that can lead to permanent hearing loss.

## Health Psychology and Chronic Illness

Chronic health problems cause biological, psychological, and sociocultural challenges. The fact that chronic diseases are usually the result of human behavior contributed to the development of the field of health psychology. Improvements in chronic disease management from a behavioral standpoint are vital to reducing health care costs and improving patient outcomes in diabetes, asthma, arthritis, hypertension, coronary heart disease, and other chronic diseases (Von Korff, Gruman, Schaefer, Curry, & Wagner, 1997). This is an opportune time for health psychologists to find more effective ways to change damaging behaviors and to reduce the burdens of chronic disease (Orleans et al., 2004, p. 465).

From a career standpoint there are several ways for health psychologists to approach chronic disease. Health psychologists join interdisciplinary medical teams to help patients deal with psychosocial aspects of chronic illness. Video-conferencing or other interactive electronic technology offers opportunities to participate in home care of people experiencing chronic illness (Johnston, Wheeler, Deuser, & Sousa, 2000). Health psychologists also work on research teams in universities and other organizations to find ways to prevent behaviors putting people at risk of chronic disease. They are developing new approaches or modifying existing theories of behavior change. Developmental psychologists often focus on chronic illnesses specific to life stages. Noncompliance with medical recommendations continues to be a major issue for study in health psychology. Health psychologists can apply the biopsychosocial model of health to improve our understanding of patients facing the difficult effects of chronic illness and disability. Being a clinical health psychologist is relatively new among the health professions, but professional opportunities include health care research in

TABLE 13.1    Noise Levels Produced by Daily Activities and Machines

A noise level above 85 dB can damage hearing and cause hearing loss over time.

| Source of noise | Sound level (dB) |
| --- | --- |
| Firearms | 140 to 170 |
| Jet engines | 140 |
| Rock concerts | 90 to 130 |
| Amplified car stereos | 140 (at full volume) |
| Portable stereos (e.g., iPods) | 115 (at full volume) |
| Power mowers | 105 |
| Jackhammers | 100 |
| Subway trains | 100 |
| Video arcades | 100 |
| Freeway driving in a convertible | 95 |
| Power saws | 95 |
| Electric razors | 85 |
| Crowded school buses | 85 |
| School recesses or assemblies | 85 |
| Hair dryer | 60 to 90 |
| Normal conversation | 40 |
| Quiet room | 10 |

Source: Edlin, G., & Golanty, E. (2007). Health and wellness (9th ed.). Sudbury, MA: Jones and Bartlett Publishers.

prevention and rehabilitation as well as primary, secondary, and tertiary patient care (Papas, Belar, & Rozensky, 2004, p. 298).

## Acute Health Problems Compared to Chronic Health Problems

Chronic diseases and disabilities are conditions that persist throughout one's life. A chronic illness is distinguished from an acute illness by duration. An acute illness or injury is short lived. It usually lasts no longer than a few months. Recovery is achieved through the immune system's natural response, by medical intervention, or both. The common cold is an example of an acute illness that lasts 10 to 14 days. A broken arm is another example of an acute or short-term injury. Infectious diseases were once the great killers in our society, but antibiotics and vaccines have reduced the incidence of disease or made treatment possible.

Confusion about distinguishing chronic illness from an acute illness can be seen in such health problems as headaches and asthma. Headaches affect most of us at one time or another and are usually acute or short lived. Migraines are severe and intermittent headaches that can last for hours or days, but there is no consistently identified neurological cause (Breier & Fletcher, 2002, p. 193). Migraines, unlike other headaches, recur and may be treated effectively with prescription medication. Most of us have headaches, but we do not view them as a chronic illness. We use over-the-counter medications such as aspirin to alleviate the pain. People with migraine headaches identify themselves as having a chronic health problem.

Some chronic illnesses or conditions feature acute episodes or outbreaks. An example of a chronic illness with acute episodes is asthma. An asthma attack is severe, but it can be treated with prescription medication. However, even after an attack the person is still said to have the illness of asthma, meaning he or she is likely to experience other episodes related to that condition. Asthma is a chronic illness.

Diseases of long duration have a powerful impact on the quality of life of patients and on the lives of their caregivers. Chronic health problems require extraordinary coping and stress management. Many impairments and restrictions must be dealt with every hour of every day.

## General Dimensions of Chronic Illness

### Biological Aspects of Chronic Illness

#### Physical and Mental Changes

Permanent alterations to the body and mind occur as a result of chronic illness and injuries. For example, each year nearly 11,000 people are hospitalized with an injury to the head or spine due to automobile accidents and falls (American National Red Cross, 2005). Many of these injuries become chronic health problems for patients and their families. Deterioration may be immediate or progressively worsen over a long period of time. Deterioration includes objective differences observable by others. Some examples are paralysis, limping, deformity, incontinence, breathing difficulty, ashen or bluish skin, flushing, vomiting, seizures, bleeding, sweating, loss of balance, lesions on the skin, speech difficulty, fainting, and the inability to use or move a limb.

There may be less-noticeable changes or subtle signs such as swelling of body parts and personality changes. Other symptoms are known only if the patient talks about them. Some examples are anxiety, restlessness, dizziness, weakness, insomnia, nausea, feeling bloated, thirst, loss of sensation or numbness, deafness, and pain. Pain categories include headaches, stomach aches, muscle aches, and joint tenderness. Psychosocial symptoms include frustration, depression, and a concern about being a burden to one's family and friends.

#### Medical Care

Medical efforts in emergency rooms, hospitals, and clinics cause emotional and physical changes in patients. Many medical treatments are invasive and disturbing, and treatments are complex. Patients may require special transportation vehicles, hours of waiting at treatment centers, and numerous visits with medical personnel. These issues usually continue for the rest of a patient's life. Treatments may be expensive and financially burdensome. Completing insurance forms is usually a tedious and complicated process. Many times patients turn to complementary health care to augment traditional medical treatments. For example, practitioners of homeopathy are often sought for help with arthritis, asthma, headaches, and depression (Gardea, Gatchel, & Robinson, 2004, p. 352). Chiropractic care may include spinal manipulation for asthma.

### Adherence to Medical Advice

Medical recommendations are always part of treating any chronic disease. Medications must be carefully scheduled and systematically tracked. Diabetes patients with kidney disease have frequent sessions at dialysis centers to clean their blood. Making medical appointments and remembering to keep them can be burdensome. Limitations and treatments at school or workplaces are bothersome and sometimes resented by fellow students or employees.

## Psychological Aspects of Chronic Illness

### Emotional Outcomes

There are almost always emotional consequences of being treated for chronic illness or disability. Patients struggle to maintain their individual identity in the face of their health problems. They experience the loss of the integrity of their body, their work life is interrupted, their future is threatened, and they may lose economic independence. Often cognitive changes are added to physical effects. Negative emotional states can be a direct result of facing a chronic illness or disability. Psychological responses may include depression, guilt, anxiety, anger, bitterness, and grief.

Patients with chronic illness typically experience both medical and psychological problems. Depression and anxiety are common. Primary care physicians may not have the time or background to recognize and treat these complications (Tucker, Phillips, Murphy, & Raczynski, 2004, pp. 456–457). Specific risk factors for depression being comorbid with chronic illnesses are being a young adult, a female, having a family history of depression, having a history of substance abuse, and low social support. Depressed patients have greater impairment than other patients who are not depressed particularly those with diabetes, arthritis, and lung disease (Tucker et al., 2004, p. 456).

There are indirect emotional outcomes of chronic illness. Patients' self-esteem is often damaged. For example, body image is the mental picture we hold about our physical appearance. When our body is disfigured, that image is affected, causing stress. Shame is another issue. Some chronic illnesses are viewed as dishonorable by many regardless of origin. This was true of leprosy in previous centuries. It is currently true of HIV/AIDS. Friends and family members often fear contagion from stigmatized diseases and this fear tends to further isolate patients adding to their loneliness and depression.

### Thoughts or Cognitions

Characteristic ways of thinking develop and revolve around having a chronic illness. Some people minimize or deny serious health problems. Distancing themselves from the problem is sometimes helpful, because many people do not want to be identified by their disease or disability. Teens and children especially want to avoid appearing different from their peers.

### Seeking Control

Being independent and in charge of one's life is important to most adults. Fear of dying and of losing control over oneself is worrisome. One way for people to gain control over their lives is to seek more information about their condition once it is diagnosed so they can make plans for their future. Setting goals and keeping records of progress are psychologically based ways to move towards a more normal existence. Looking forward to work and social events and resuming exercising are examples of goals to be set and achieved. Being able to take care of one's own medical needs often gives people a greater sense of achievement and independence. One example is people with diabetes deciding they can manage to give themselves insulin injections and prepare healthful foods. There are other accomplishments to record, such as improved pain control, improvement in body strength, and being less fearful, bitter, or angry. The sooner people resume a near-normal lifestyle the better it is for their emotional states. Patients are most encouraged by any improvement in their lives for which they are responsible.

### Optimism

Optimism is helpful in facing chronic disease or disability. An optimistic attitude promotes solution-focused changes. Optimistic patients are more likely to adhere to medical schedules and to receive social support from friends, family members, coworkers, and medical practitioners. In large hospitals, people often see others who appear to be worse off than they are, and this may lead to positive feelings such as gratitude about their own condition. The ability to sympathize with others and make downward comparisons often lifts patients' spirits. Optimism also improves immune function, persistence in treatment regimens, and enables patients to rebound from medical disappointments (Peterson & Bossio, 1991).

### Finding Meaning

Regaining a sense of coherence and meaning in one's life is beneficial. Many patients do not want to be viewed as sick or as victims deserving of pity. Most of the chronically ill and disabled are not clinically depressed and do not view themselves as helpless or hopeless victims. Some learn to find positive aspects about their illness or disability (Tomich & Helgeson, 2004). Others have religious or spiritual convictions that render meaning to all experiences whether good or bad.

## Social Aspects of Chronic Disease

As is true of almost all human situations, social support, including monetary support, is important for the well-being and continued progress of people with disabilities and chronic illnesses. Maintaining social support is an excellent goal for anyone, but especially for those with chronic health problems. There is sometimes a tendency to withdraw from others when we are ill or disabled. Other times chronically ill people simply lack the energy to carry on a conversation or even to smile. Some are reluctant to expose their altered physical appearance in public. Still others do not want their friends to see the extent of their deterioration. Some are ashamed of their condition. Studies show that having positive social relationships or social support is central to maintaining a positive outlook in the face of chronic illness or disability.

### Economic Issues

Recent research indicates that poverty is strongly associated with having three or more chronic illnesses. This circumstance is most characteristic of adults between the ages 45 and 64 who cannot maintain job responsibilities (NCHS, 2008). Illnesses include hypertension, heart disease, stroke, emphysema, diabetes, cancer, asthma, and arthritis. The relationship between poverty and chronic health problems reflects both the impact of low income on health and of poor health on income (Freidland, 2003).

### Family Relationships

Chronic illness affects the biological, psychological, and social well-being of patients and their family members in a variety of ways. Good relationships among family members are important components of maintaining social support and avoiding social isolation. Family roles adjust, authority figures change, and adjustments in sources and amounts of financial support often follow a diagnosis of chronic illness. Sometimes parents become too weak to be involved in the rights and duties of parenting and surrogates must step in to help. Important medical appointments disrupt family routines. Child and adolescent siblings sometimes resent the attention being given to an ailing sister or brother. Adhering to medical regimens must often be encouraged by those living with or near patients.

### Social Support Outside of the Family

It is often beneficial for patients and family members to seek social support from outside the family. Many organizations are available to provide assistance and support including information, transportation, medical care, medications, prostheses, wheelchairs, and crutches. A friend or an immediate member of the family may be willing to take responsibility for reaching out to the various groups for needed resources, although it is better if the patient does this. Many religious organizations and civic clubs are also involved in patient support. Fellow patients with similar problems and needs can be excellent sources of comfort and practical advice.

Support Groups and Professional Help
Many hospitals, clinics, and other health agencies sponsor support groups for patients with similar conditions. Patients learn that their problems and feelings of frustration and anger are common and that it is acceptable to express these aloud in a support group. No one understands the chronically ill and disabled as well as others who are similarly affected. Support groups provide useful information as well as emotional reassurance.

Many clinical psychologists, social workers, and other professionals working in health care prefer working with chronically ill or disabled people because it is a rewarding occupation. Patient education about biological, psychological, and social changes is an important issue. Giving control back to patients includes teaching them about wound care, pain control, rehabilitation techniques, relaxation routines, and medication use. Emotional support is given through conversations with patients. Patients may be helped by writing or journaling about their distress.

## Seven Specific Chronic Illnesses

### Chronic Obstructive Pulmonary Disease

The increasing prevalence of respiratory diseases is linked to two human factors, cigarette smoking and air pollution (Creer, Bender, & Lucas, 2002, p. 239). Chronic obstructive pulmonary disease (COPD) is the fourth leading cause of death in the United States and is increasing in our population especially among women (DHHS, 2000). It includes emphysema, chronic bronchitis, and other diseases that block airflow in the lungs. A person with COPD is chronically disabled, because the damage to the lungs is permanent. Currently between 10 and 24 million people are affected by COPD (Centers for Disease Control [CDC], 2003a). Each year COPD accounts for thousands of deaths, hospitalizations, emergency room visits, and outpatient visits with medical personnel.

The Biology of COPD
COPD is diagnosed as nonreversible pulmonary or lung function impairment (CDC, 2002). The lung air sacs overinflate, leading to a breakdown in their walls and a significant decrease in respiratory function. In the case of emphysema, this means patients lose the capacity to exhale all the air from their lungs, so they often feel they are dying. Other breathing-related symptoms are chronic coughing and **dyspnea**, or labored breathing and difficulty when trying to move about a room or outdoors. Tobacco use is the key risk factor in the development and progression of COPD, but asthma, air pollution, genetic factors, and respiratory

---

**dyspnea** Difficult or labored breathing upon movement; shortness of breath associated with lung disorders such as COPD.

infections also play a role (CDC, 2003a). COPD rates in women are rising faster than in men, probably reflecting increased smoking by women since the 1940s. Early detection is possible by measurement of pulmonary function. The most important aspect of treatment is to avoid tobacco smoke. Coughing is treated with medication.

Psychosocial Aspects of COPD

Patients with COPD find that every effort to breathe is blocked. Imagine expending enormous effort every time you exhale. Many patients take oxygen tanks on wheels wherever they go. Physical and emotional stress make breathing even more difficult. Other limitations include the inability to work, to do simple household chores, or to maintain independent living conditions. Patients must often rely on others for daily care and economic support.

Smoking is the major risk factor for COPD (NIH, 1997). Tobacco is highly addictive and patients face the fact that they must eliminate exposure to tobacco smoke for the rest of their lives. Two goals of rehabilitation are symptom reduction and increased participation by patients in everyday activities. These are achieved with exercise training that has a rehabilitative component and learning social skills and medical management (Creer et al., 2002, pp. 247–248).

## Diabetes

Diabetes is a group of diseases distinguished by the lack of sufficient or effective insulin. Dangerously high levels of blood glucose or sugar in the blood can lead to serious health complications, including heart disease and death. There are three general forms of diabetes. **Type I diabetes**, sometimes called juvenile-onset diabetes, requires insulin by pump or injection. Risks for this kind of diabetes are not well understood, but the disease is probably due to an autoimmune destruction of insulin-producing cells resulting in insulin deficiency. The prevalence of type I is 1 to 2 cases per 1,000 people in North America (Wysocki & Buckloh, 2002, p. 67). In addition to insulin, other requirements are dietary control, regular exercise, and frequent medical checkups. A second type of diabetes, **gestational diabetes**, is associated with pregnancy and may disappear after the woman gives birth. Women who develop gestational diabetes are at increased risk for **type II diabetes**.

**type I diabetes**  A complex and chronic disorder; a form of diabetes mellitus that tends to appear early in life.

**gestational diabetes**  A form of diabetes appearing during pregnancy; it usually disappears after delivery but is a risk factor for type II diabetes.

**type II diabetes**  A form of diabetes usually appearing in adulthood but now appearing in obese young people.

Type II diabetes, once known as adult-onset diabetes, is becoming more common in our society. This is largely due to increases in obesity in adults, teens, and children. About 66% of adults are overweight and of those 32% are obese. Furthermore, 19% of children, ages 6–11, are overweight, as are 17% of adolescents ages 12–19 (NCHS, 2008). Currently about 54 million adults have pre-diabetes (CDC, 2005). The best means of prevention is to follow good nutritional practices and exercise regularly to avoid obesity throughout one's life.

The Biology of Diabetes

Two dangerous diabetic emergencies are comas and shock (American National Red Cross, 2005). Both stress and physical exercise can lower levels of insulin, bringing on decreased consciousness, severe headaches, and comas. Patients on insulin who fail to take adequate nourishment may experience insulin shock. Diabetes is a complex illness to treat because it damages tiny blood vessels. All forms of diabetes increase risks for heart and kidney disease, blindness and other ocular problems, neuropathy or loss of sensation in the feet, and amputations due to the inability of the body to heal sores and injuries. About two thirds of all lower-limb amputations occur in people with diabetes (CDC, 2005). According to recent prospective studies, very tight glycemic control results in fewer complications. On diabetes management teams, health psychologists are very useful in helping patients to integrate demanding medical regimens into their daily lives (Wysocki & Buckloh, 2002, p. 67).

Cancer and diabetes often coexist, because the risk of diabetes is increased among cancer patients. People with diabetes and cancer may be unable to exercise and will experience muscle loss causing greater insulin resistance (M.D. Anderson, 2006). Steroids used in some cancer treatments may cause higher blood glucose levels. During chemotherapy some people have difficulty eating adequately and keeping food down.

Psychosocial Dimensions of Diabetes

Psychosocial dimensions of diabetes include the fact that diabetes must be carefully controlled to prevent further deterioration in health. Unfortunately adherence to medical regimens is often low among people with diabetes. Glucose levels must be carefully monitored and kept in balance, but only about one fourth of diabetics check their glucose levels the recommended three times a day. Half of the people with diabetes are unable to recognize the symptoms of the onset of comas or shock (CDC, 2005). Knowledge, skills, and self-efficacy are essential for self-management of this disease (Wysocki & Buckloh, 2002 pp. 68–73), but adherence to the demanding treatment regimens is difficult for most patients (Anderson, 1996).

Emotional reactions to a diagnosis of diabetes include disbelief, denial, anger, anxiety, and depression. Stress management is important, because stress causes changes in blood glucose levels in about half of all diabetics. Another source of distress is disruption in family life. Caring for a diabetic child requires constant vigilance. Both diabetic children and their parents often construct explanations for the presence of the disease. Parents may feel guilty, and children sometimes believe their parents failed to protect them. One consequence is that children resist required routines. Dietary restrictions are difficult for everyone, but especially for diabetic adolescents who want to be like their peers and not have adults constantly monitoring their behavior. Excitement and anticipation of positive events such as dates, proms, or football games can cause dangerous changes in glucose levels.

## HIV/AIDS

Health psychologists, especially those interested in psychoneuroimmunology, study psychological factors, human behavior, and stress in an effort to understand the consequences of infectious diseases including HIV/AIDS. Research conclusions are mixed, but the progression of infectious disease reflects environmental factors and host vulnerability, both of which comprise psychosocial factors (Ironson, Balin, & Schneiderman, 2002, pp. 6–25).

HIV stands for human immunodeficiency virus; acquired immune deficiency syndrome (AIDS) is the last stage of an HIV infection. HIV/AIDS is better understood than ever before, but there is no cure, so prevention efforts become paramount. About 1 million people in the United States are living with HIV/AIDS. Unfortunately one fourth of that million are unaware of their infection, making infection of others more likely. The Centers for Disease Control keep surveillance data on HIV infections to provide a more complete picture of the infectious disease (see **Figure 13.1**).

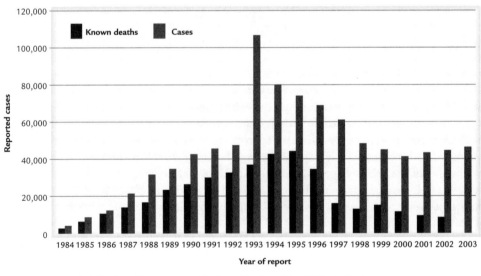

Notes: Includes Guam, Puerto Rico, the U.S. Pacific Islands, and the U.S. Virgin Islands.

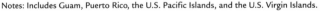

**Figure 13.1** HIV/AIDS is a chronic disease.

*Sources:* National Center for Health Statistics. National Vital Statistics System. U.S. Dept. of Health and Human Services. Centers for Disease Control and Prevention.

The Biology of HIV/AIDS

HIV is different from other viruses because it attacks the immune system, destroying white blood cells and making the body unable to defend itself against common infections. Symptoms include fever, weight loss, fatigue, and swollen lymph glands. The virus is a blood-borne pathogen and is present in semen, breast milk, blood, and vaginal secretions. It is most likely to be spread by having unprotected anal, vaginal, or oral intercourse with someone infected with HIV; by sharing contaminated needles; or by being exposed before or during birth or through breast feeding. At one time blood transfusions were also a source of infections, but blood in the United States has been tested for HIV antibodies since 1985.

## Think About It!

### Eliminating or Reducing Your Risk of HIV Infection and Other STIs

#### How to Eliminate Your Risk of Becoming Infected with HIV or Other STIs

Abstain from sex. If that is not an option:

- Do not have sex with HIV-infected individuals or those infected with any STI.
- Engage in sex only in a monogamous relationship in which it is certain that neither partner is infected.
- Abstain from using drugs.

*Note:* People in certain professions, such as health care workers and police officers, have additional risks of infection due to the nature of their work. Such risks are not eliminated by these practices. These people can become infected with hepatitis B virus or HIV if their blood mixes with the blood or bodily secretions of an infected person.

#### How to Reduce Your Risk of Becoming Infected with HIV or Other STIs

- Reduce your number of sexual partners.
- Avoid having sex with high-risk partners.
- Avoid having sex with people you do not know well.
- Avoid having sex while under the influence of drugs, including alcohol.
- Use a new latex condom during each act of sexual intercourse.
- Never share needles or syringes.

*Source:* Alters, S., & Schiff, W. (2009). *Essential concepts for healthy living* (5th ed.). Sudbury, MA: Jones and Bartlett Publishers.

In the early 1980s about 150,000 people in the United States were infected with HIV every year. Due to education and behavior change the rate has now decreased to approximately 40,000 people a year. About 75% of the HIV/AIDS patients are male adolescents and adults (CDC, 2007a). Since the late 1990s, treatment advances have led to a decrease in AIDS deaths. Drug regimens are complex and may cause serious side effects, making adherence difficult. Health psychologists work in the two areas of maintaining adherence to medications and adopting safer sex behaviors.

### Psychosocial Aspects of HIV/AIDS

Psychological and social responses to HIV/AIDS are important factors. Due to its sources and fear of contagion, HIV is a stigmatized disease. Patients are not likely to tell others for fear of prejudice and discrimination in social relationships, jobs, and recreational activities. As of 2007, 47 states, and the District of Columbia use confidential name-based reporting for HIV surveillance (CDC, 2007).

HIV is life threatening, so depression and anxiety are associated with both diagnosis and treatment (Carey & Vanable, 2004). There is evidence that high stress combined with greater depression predicts disease progression. Studies also show that active coping is beneficial to health, while denial, fatalism, and negative expectancies are not (Ironson et al., 2002, p. 12). HIV-infected women with chronic depression were twice as likely to die as those with no or few depressive symptoms (Ickovics et al., 2001).

Adherence to medical regimens is essential and stress management can improve both length and quality of life. Modifiable behaviors to prevent future infections are safer sex, not sharing needles, and selecting an AIDS-knowledgeable physician. Psychologists teach people ways to deal with any partner who resists using a condom by forcing a discussion of their reasoning and being assertive about avoiding the risks of HIV (Antoni et al., 1991). Cognitive-behavioral therapy can teach people ways to reduce stress, correctly evaluate stressful situations, improve coping skills, and modify endocrine and immune responses (Antoni & Schneiderman, 1999).

Psychologists have applied the transtheoretical model of behavior change to HIV/AIDS education (Ironson et al., 2002, p. 25). Pre-contemplators are given information about changing their risky behaviors, contemplators are motivated to set goals to change their behavior through increases in self-efficacy and social support, and in later stages individuals receive reinforcement to maintain the behavioral changes and deal with relapses.

## Arthritis

Arthritis, an inflammation of the joints, is the leading cause of disability in the United States (see **Figure 13.2**).

Arthritis and other musculoskeletal conditions are the most frequently mentioned cause of limitations among working-age adults (NCHS, 2008). Arthritis includes more than 100

**Figure 13.2**
Arthritis is the leading cause of disability in the United States.

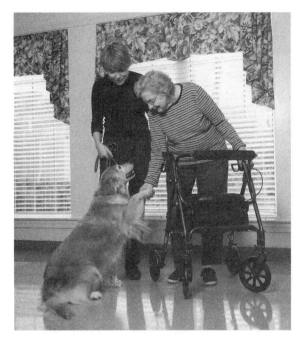

different diagnostic categories. Five examples are **osteoarthritis**, gout, rheumatoid arthritis, lupus, and fibromyalgia. About 45 million adults, or 1 in 5, have been diagnosed with some form of arthritis (CDC, 2007b; 2008a). Millions with diabetes, heart disease, and high blood pressure also have arthritis added to the burden of chronic illness. Arthritis accounts for about 750,000 hospitalizations each year and 36 million medical visits. About two thirds of the people with arthritis are under the age of 65 and include young children. Juvenile rheumatoid arthritis begins in childhood while lupus tends to appear in young women. If untreated, Lyme disease infections from ticks may result in arthritis. Young people should be aware that recreational and occupational joint injuries are also risk factors for later osteoarthritis. Being overweight or obese is a risk factor for osteoarthritis of the knees. Arthritis is not an inevitable outcome of aging. Behavior modification and early treatment can reduce symptoms and disability (CDC, 2008a). The Arthritis Foundation states that 4.6 million Americans have rheumatoid arthritis and 300,000 children have some form of juvenile arthritis (Arthritis Foundation, 2008).

**osteoarthritis** The most common form of arthritis; it occurs mainly in old age.

The Biology of Arthritis

Symptoms of arthritis and other rheumatic diseases include pain, swelling, redness, and stiffness in joints. Arthritis makes movement painful and awkward, because it usually affects joints in the hands, knees, hips, back, and feet. Osteoarthritis is associated with pain, bone spurs, and deformity. Women are three times more likely than men to be affected by rheumatoid arthritis, in which inflammation destroys both cartilage and bone. Other symptoms are fever, muscle aches, and fatigue. Some forms of arthritis, such as lupus and rheumatoid arthritis, may affect other organs, causing more complications for patients. Acute gouty arthritis, associated with excess uric acid crystals in a joint, often causes pain at the base of the largest toe.

Psychosocial Aspects of Arthritis

Psychosocial factors in arthritis include patient distress, lack of adequate social support, and decreases in coping skills (Bradley & Alberts, 1999). A common reaction to this disease is frustration and distress due to limitations of activities involving movement, including walking and lifting. Pain and fatigue also interfere with activities of daily life at both the workplace and home. Negative affect and mood disorders are common in people with rheumatic diseases (Huyser & Parker, 2002, pp. 410–411). Pain and lack of sleep affect stress, and stress, in turn, affects pain and lack of sleep.

Health psychologists find that learned helplessness and low self-efficacy are characteristic cognitive factors in patients, but are cautioned about suspecting patients of exaggerating pain to avoid work (Huyser & Parker, 2002). Helplessness refers to a global state by which people believe they lack ways to relieve sources of stress (DeVellis & Callahan, 1993). People who feel helpless are more likely to report higher levels of pain, depression, and impairment (Huyser & Parker, 2002, p. 414). Self-efficacy refers to confidence in one's ability to accomplish tasks, and low self-efficacy is associated with low adherence to arthritis treatment routines (Bandura, 1997).

Treatment with corticosteroids relieves inflammation, but may contribute to depression, interfere with sleep, increase susceptibility to infections, and cause peptic ulcers. Nonsteroidal anti-inflammatory drugs (NSAIDs) control symptoms, but may prove toxic to kidneys. Antirheumatic drugs include gold shots and methotrexate. Sleep improvement and pain reduction may be achieved by using antidepressants. It is preferable for treatment to focus on weight loss, exercise, and avoiding lifting.

Arthritis may result in embarrassing unsightly distortions in joints due to swelling, spinal deformation, and gait abnormalities. Some patients must rely on wheelchairs. Swollen joints in fingers are especially visible and make hand movements painful and difficult. Sexual activity may be awkward and even painful. Coping is improved through education and seeking information about the disease. Social support from friends and family members, particularly partners, positively affects patients' abilities to deal with the stressors of arthritis. People with arthritis are encouraged to exercise to improve their aerobic capacity, strength, and flexibility for purposes of both prevention and rehabilitation (Minor & Kay, 2003). Exercise recommendations include low-impact activities and avoidance of stair climbing and contact sports to ensure joint protection. The Arthritis Foundation web site includes information on pain control and has self-help programs including aquatics and tai chi (Arthritis Foundation, 2008).

## Asthma

Asthma refers to a chronic disease that causes narrowing in the airways and obstruction of lungs by mucus. Morbidity is a major problem, because asthma troubles millions of people and is one of the most common chronic diseases in children. Asthma has increased in the United States since the 1980s. It accounts for 1.8 million visits to emergency rooms, 10.4 million physician office visits, and 465,000 hospitalizations each year (CDC, 2003b).

### The Biology of Asthma

The main effects of asthma are breathing difficulties, tightness in the chest, wheezing sounds, and coughing. Risk factors for asthma attacks include infections, family history, and triggering factors in the environment such as air quality, climate, cockroach droppings, tobacco smoke, pet dander, dust mites, and some chemicals. Due to these risk factors, asthma attacks are more likely to occur in low-income urban areas. Asthma is also associated with allergies affecting nasal and sinus cavities. Medical treatments include the use of bronchodilators and corticosteroids. Beta agonists may also prevent asthma attacks.

Some medications have caffeine-like side effects, causing anxiety and hand tremors. Antihistamines can cause drowsiness. High doses of corticosteroids may cause depression and anxiety in both children and adults, and psychosis in adults (Creer et al., 2002, p. 261). Variation in severity of the disease affects exercise recommendations, because exercise sometimes triggers asthma attacks. General recommendations are sub-maximal intensity (75%), shorter duration, noncompetitive sports, and airflow measurement about 6 to 8 minutes following exercise (Clark, 2003).

### Psychosocial Aspects of Asthma

Both psychological and social factors are associated with asthma and other allergic disorders. Stress and negative emotions probably worsen the condition. Marital or family discord, depression, panic, anger, and hyperventilation can trigger attacks in both adults and children (Creer et al., 2002, pp. 252–253). Lower socioeconomic levels, family living conditions and practices, and environmental factors are also associated with the disease. Frequent absence from school may undermine cognitive development. It is difficult to assess existing research, because parents are relied upon to report the diagnosis, severity, medication use, and symptom control of their children (Creer et al., p. 254). Ethnic or racial minority status is a risk factor. For example, about 16% of African American boys are affected by asthma (CDC, 2006). Asthma attacks, sleeping difficulties, and emergency room visits interrupt patients' lives and the lives of other family members. Self-management training includes education about avoidance of triggers, keeping asthma diaries, the correct use of controller and reliever drugs, self-monitoring, and written management plans for parents of children with asthma (NIH, 1997). Biofeedback training and relaxation techniques may be helpful (Sarafino, 2004).

## Osteoporosis

Osteoporosis is the most common type of bone disease. An estimated 10 million Americans have it. An additional 18 million people have low bone mass or osteopenia, and without action on their part the disease becomes osteoporosis (NIH, 2008) (see **Figure 13.3**).

Osteoporosis is a chronic disease characterized by progressive loss of bone density, thinning of bone tissue, and vulnerability to fractures. It is most characteristic of women and men over 50. It occurs earlier in young women who limit calorie intake and exercise vigorously to the point that menstrual periods cease. In some cases this condition is called *anorexia athletica* (Fink, Burgoon, & Mikesky, 2006, pp. 345–348). The CDC recently put up an animated Internet site, "Powerful Bones, Powerful Girls," with a downloadable journal to encourage young women to take care of their bones by eating calcium-rich food and doing weightbearing exercises such as tai chi (CDC, 2008b).

Osteoporosis is a chronic condition consisting of reduced bone mass or density resulting in deformities. It is the most common cause of bone fracture injuries, which number about 1.5 million each year (Riggs & Melton, 1995). Fractures mainly occur in the hip, spine, wrist,

**Figure 13.3**
Osteoporosis is the most common type of bone disease and affects millions of Americans.

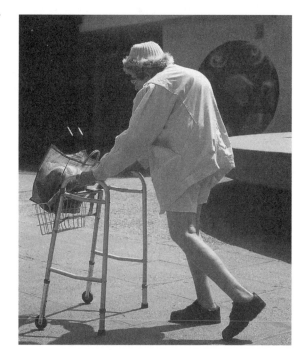

and forearm. The hip is a joint and the break actually occurs in the femur, which is a very large and important bone. About half of older patients with hip fractures never regain the same level of independence, and a fourth require institutional care (Maricic, 1996). Twenty percent of hip fracture victims die within a year of the fracture (Leibson, Tosteson, Gabriel, Ransom, & Melton, 2002).

The Biology of Osteoporosis
This disease is preventable. Once diagnosed it is treatable. It can be prevented through life-long healthy eating practices, including food rich in calcium such as cheese, milk, and fish, and through supplements of vitamin D. The body can manufacture sufficient vitamin D if exposed to 10 to 15 minutes of sunshine three times a week but supplements may be necessary. Osteoporosis is also prevented by doing weightbearing exercises regularly throughout life, because skeletal muscle pulling against bone cause bones to increase in density. Smoking and alcohol use put bone mass at greater risk (Office of the Surgeon General, 2007). Most risk factors are under the control of the individual, but estrogen deficiency and some medications also put people at risk. Heredity is a risk factor and may account for 40% to 60% of variance in bone mass (Huyser & Parker, 2002, p. 406).

There are no symptoms in the early stages of the disease and loss of height or fractures are often the first signs. Osteoporosis is diagnosed by bone densitometry using low-dose x-rays that assess bone for mineral loss and thinning. Treatment goals are to control pain, slow or stop bone loss, and prevent fractures by reducing the risk of falls. Bisphosphonates or calcitonin, plus calcium and vitamin D supplements may be recommended.

Psychosocial Aspects of Osteoporosis
Osteoporosis triggers major changes in the lives of patients and their families. Deformities and fractures negatively affect body image, self-esteem, and mood. Patients are anxious about falling. Fractures often prevent patients from regaining their ability to walk and maintain their independence. Many patients report deterioration in their quality of life, including significant financial expense. Injured patients live in fear of breaking another bone, pain and suffering, surgery, and losing contact with family and friends. Institutionalized patients debilitated by fractures often feel isolated, hopeless, and helpless. Rehabilitation is often painful, so many choose to remain in wheelchairs for the rest of their lives.

## Alzheimer's Disease

Alzheimer's disease is a chronic degenerative brain disorder associated with loss of cognitive capacity. It is believed to affect about 4.5 million people at this time in the United States (NIH, 2007). The greatest risk factor is old age. The disease is difficult to diagnose because loss of mental capacity can also be a result of mental deterioration due to aging and vascular diseases. Alzheimer's disease is often confused with the effects of depression, excessive alcohol use, and drug reactions. This disease is especially difficult for family members and other caregivers, because symptoms often include personality changes including suspiciousness, wandering behaviors, disorientation, and hallucinations. Spousal caregivers report high levels of stress, depression, and anxiety, and experience negative changes in their immune systems (Forlenza & Baum, 2004, p. 100).

Victims may become mute, incontinent, and completely dependent on the care of others. There is no known cure, but treatments slow the onset of some symptoms. Ginkgo biloba has demonstrated efficacy in treating patients with Alzheimer's disease and vascular dementia. After one year in a randomized controlled study, 309 patients suffering from Alzheimer's disease scored significantly higher on the geriatric evaluation by relative's rating instrument and the Alzheimer's disease assessment scale (Gardea et al., 2004, p. 355). It is often the patients' caregivers who need social support. In Florida the Alzheimer's Caregiver Support Online includes telephone-based education and support for caregivers of individuals with progressive dementia (Glueckauf, Nickelson, Whitton, & Loomis, 2004, p. 387).

The Biology of Alzheimer's Disease

The cause of Alzheimer's is not well understood although it is the most common form of dementia in older persons. It may coexist with other forms of dementia associated with loss of blood flow to brain cells. Alzheimer's usually begins with mild forgetfulness for recent events or the names of familiar people. During autopsies, pathologists find the brain tissue of people with Alzheimer's disease contains abnormal clumps of plaque and neurofibrillary tangles. Preliminary evidence suggests control of blood pressure, weight, and cholesterol may help reduce risks as well as staying physically, mentally, and socially active (Alzheimer's Association, 2007).

## Think About It!

### Steps You Can Take to Reduce the Risk of Dementia

Generally speaking, actions that promote good health also reduce the risk of Alzheimer's disease and other forms of dementia later in life. Some research supports the following risk-reduction strategies:

**Physical exercise:** Moderate exercise such as walking several times a week.

**Omega-3 fatty acids:** Consuming more of these fatty acids that are found in fish.

**Mental activity:** Staying mentally active, even doing crossword puzzles or playing challenging games such as chess.

**Healthy diet:** Eating healthfully; maintaining normal weight.

**B vitamins:** Supplementing B vitamins, especially folic acid.

**Ginkgo biloba:** Extracts of this herbal remedy may slow or stabilize the progression of dementia.

*Source:* Edlin, G., & Golanty, E. (2007). *Health and wellness* (9th ed.). Sudbury, MA: Jones and Bartlett Publishers.

Psychosocial Aspects of Alzheimer's Disease

Alzheimer's affects memory and reasoning. This chronic illness is particularly devastating to family members, friends, and other caregivers who come under an enormous amount of stress due to the behavior of patients with this disease. Seventy percent of Alzheimer's patients live at home, and the disease places physical, emotional, and financial stress on caregivers. The negative effects on caregivers are so significant that the Alzheimer's Disease and Related Disorders Association cites 10 warning signs of caregiver stress: denial of the permanence of the condition, anger at the victims for their lack of comprehension, withdrawal from their own friends, anxiety, depression, exhaustion, sleeplessness, moodiness, an inability to concentrate, and developing their own health problems.

## Summary

The focus of this chapter is the application of the biopsychosocial approach to chronic illness. Unlike acute disease and injury, chronic health problems endure for a lifetime, creating extensive problems for millions of patients, their families, and friends. Biological aspects of chronic illness include coping with pain and deterioration in body organs and structures. Medical treatment is often invasive, expensive, and burdensome. Adherence to medical recommendations is essential to maintaining life and preventing further deterioration. There are a variety of negative emotional reactions to chronic illness, but some measure of relief may be achieved through support groups and by keeping a journal about the experience. Benefits also accrue to patients who set goals, record their accomplishments, and find meaning in the experience. An optimistic attitude is of great benefit from a psychological viewpoint.

Chronic obstructive pulmonary disease (COPD) refers to permanent obstruction of breathing, resulting in severe limitations to any physical activity. Diabetes requires constant monitoring to maintain ideal blood glucose levels in the body. Heart and kidney disease, blindness, and amputations are possible outcomes of uncontrolled diabetes. Following nutritional dietary patterns and exercising regularly reduce the risks of adult-onset and gestational diabetes.

HIV/AIDS is a chronic disease affecting the immune system. It is most likely to be spread through unsafe sex with infected partners and intravenous drug use, so it is a highly stigmatized disease. Fears about public opinion often keep infected people from seeking medical testing and treatment. Arthritis is a chronic disease involving pain, swelling, and stiffness in the joints. It can severely limit day-to-day activities. Asthma is a chronic disease affecting the lungs of millions of children and adults. Attacks are triggered by exposure to pollutants such as cigarette smoke. Medication controls breathing problems following an attack. Osteoporosis and Alzheimer's disease are chronic diseases more characteristic of older people. Osteoporosis, a weakening of the bones, is the most common cause of fractures. It may also result in characteristic deformity of the upper end of the spine. Following fractures, many patients become dependent and never regain their previous quality of life. Alzheimer's disease refers to a progressive deterioration of the brain which may eventually result in the inability of patients to care for themselves. Caregivers suffer considerable distress from the emotional strain of caring for patients with Alzheimer's.

## Review Questions

1. Explain the differences between chronic and acute illness and give several examples of each type.

2. Summarize important biological aspects of dealing with a chronic disease.

3. Discuss psychosocial aspects of living with a chronic disease, including emotional and cognitive responses to the situation.

4. Describe approaches that may be helpful to individuals dealing with a chronic dis-

ease including changing attitudes or perspectives.

5. Define the concept of social support and give examples of sources of such support.

6. Summarize important biological and psychosocial aspects of COPD, diabetes, HIV/AIDS, arthritis, asthma, and osteoporosis.

7. Explain the psychosocial aspects faced by patients with Alzheimer's disease and their caregivers.

## Student Activity

Interview a person experiencing a chronic disease or someone caring for a person with a chronic illness. Assure the interviewee of confidentiality. Use the biopsychosocial approach of health psychology and the information in this chapter to develop questions for the interview, which must be approved by your professor. At the beginning of the interview ask general questions about the disease and about people's perceptions about maintaining health and independence. Consider biological, psychological, and sociocultural factors that may have contributed to the disease, including the lack of exercise, a healthy diet, and other health-related behaviors.

Next, explore what your subject currently does in response to the disease from biological, psychological, and sociocultural perspectives to maintain health. Ask about social support from friends and family members. Additional questions might include the difficulties of adhering to medical regimens. Take the information and meet in class with students who interviewed patients with the same disease. Categorize and bring together all the information from several subjects and present this information to the class and in a paper.

## References

Alzheimer's Association. (2007). The Year in Alzheimer Science. Retrieved April 18, 2007 from http://www.alz.org

American National Red Cross. (2005). *First aid: Responding to emergencies instructor's manual.* Yardley, PA: StayWell.

Anderson, B. J. (1996). Involving family members in diabetes treatment. In B. J. Anderson & R. R. Rubin (Eds.), *Practical psychology for diabetes clinicians* (pp. 43–52). Alexandria, VA: American Diabetes Association.

Antoni, M. H., Baggett, L., Ironson, G., LaPerriere, A., August, S., Klimas, N., et al. (1991). Cognitive-behavioral stress management intervention buffers distress responses and immunologic changes following notification of HIV-1 seropositivity. *Journal of Consulting and Clinical Psychology, 59,* 906–915.

Antoni, M. H., & Schneiderman, M. (1999). HIV and AIDS. In A. Bellack & M. Herson (Eds.), *Comprehensive clinical psychology* (pp. 238–275). NY: Elsevier Science.

Arthritis Foundation. (2008). Learn About Arthritis. Retrieved August 28, 2008 from http://www.arthritis.org/learn-about-arthritis.php

Bandura, A. (1997). *Self-efficacy, the exercise of control.* NY: Freeman and Company.

Bradley, L. A., & Alberts, K. R. (1999). Psychological and behavioral approaches to pain management for patients with rheumatic disease. *Rheumatic Disease Clinics of North America, 25* (1), 215–232.

Breier, J. I., & Fletcher, J. M. (2002). Diseases of the nervous system and sense organs. In S. B. Johnson, N. W. Perry, Jr., & R. H. Rozensky (Eds.), *Handbook of clinical health psychology: Vol. 1* (pp. 173–201). Washington, DC: American Psychological Association.

Carey, M. P., & Vanable, P. A. (2004). HIV/AIDS. In A. J. Christensen, R. Martin, & J. M. Smyth (Eds.), *Encyclopedia of health psychology* (pp. 135–140). New York: Kluwer Academic/Plenum.

Centers for Disease Control and Prevention. (2002). Chronic obstructive pulmonary disease surveillance—United States, 1971–2000. *Mortality and Morbidity Weekly Report* 51(SSO6), 1–16. Atlanta, GA: U.S. Department of Health and Human Services.

Centers for Disease Control and Prevention. (2003a). *Facts about chronic obstructive pulmonary disease.* Atlanta, GA: U.S. Department of Health and Human Services.

Centers for Disease Control and Prevention. (2003b). Self-reported asthma prevalence and control among adults. *Mortality and Morbidity Weekly Report. 52*(17): 381–384. Atlanta, GA: U.S. Department of Health and Human Services.

Centers for Disease Control and Prevention. (2005). *National diabetes fact sheet: General information and national estimates on diabetes in the United States, 2005.* Atlanta, GA: U.S. Department of Health and Human Services, Centers for Disease Control and Prevention.

Centers for Disease Control and Prevention. (2006). QuickStats: Percentage of children aged <18 years with current asthma, by race/ethnicity and sex—United States, 2001–2004. *Mortality and Morbidity Weekly Report 55*(07): 185. Atlanta, GA: U.S. Department of Health and Human Services.

Centers for Disease Control and Prevention. (2007a) *HIV infection reporting, basic information, and a glance at the HIV/AIDS epidemic.* Retrieved July 14, 2007 from http://www.cdc.gov/hiv/resources/factsheets.htm

Centers for Disease Control and Prevention. (2007b). *Targeting arthritis, reducing disability for nearly 19 million Americans.* Atlanta, GA: U.S. Department of Health and Human Services.

Centers for Disease Control and Prevention. (2008a). Arthritis, Osteoporosis, and Chronic Back Conditions. *Healthy People 2010.* Retrieved April 11, 2008 from http://www.hhs.gov

Centers for Disease Control and Prevention. (2008b). Powerful Girls have Powerful Bones. Retrieved April 11, 2008 from http://www.cdc.gov/powerful

Clark, C. J. (2003). Asthma. In J. L. Durstine & G. E. Moore (Eds.), *ACSM's exercise management for persons with chronic diseases and disabilities* (2nd ed. pp. 105–110). Champaign, IL: Human Kinetics.

Creer, T. L., Bender, B. G., & Lucas, D. O. (2002). Diseases of the respiratory system. In S. B. Johnson, N. W. Perry, Jr., & R. H. Rozensky (Eds.), *Handbook of clinical health psychology: Vol.*

*1* (pp. 239–282). Washington, DC: American Psychological Association.

DeVellis, R. F., & Callahan, L. F. (1993). A brief measure of helplessness in rheumatic disease: The helplessness subscale of the Rheumatology Attitudes Index. *Journal of Rheumatology, 20,* 866–869.

Fink, H. H., Burgoon, L. A., & Mikesky, A. E. (2006). *Practical applications in sports nutrition.* Sudbury, MA: Jones and Bartlett.

Forlenza, M. J., & Baum, A. (2004). Psychoneuroimmunology. In R. G. Frank, A. Baum, & J. L. Wallander (Eds.), *Handbook of clinical health psychology: Vol. 3* (pp. 81–114). Washington, DC: American Psychological Association.

Freidland, R. B. (2003). Multiple chronic conditions. *Data profiles, challenges for the 21st century: Chronic and disabling conditions: Number 12.* Georgetown University Center on an Aging Society. November.

Gardea, M. A., Gatchel, R. J., & Robinson, R. C. (2004). Complementary health care. In R. G. Frank, A. Baum, & J. L. Wallander (Eds.), *Handbook of clinical health psychology: Vol. 3* (pp. 341–375). Washington, DC: American Psychological Association.

Glueckauf, R. L., Nickelson, D. W., Whitton, J. D., & Loomis, J. S. (2004). In R. G. Frank, A. Baum, & J. L. Wallander (Eds.), *Handbook of clinical health psychology: Vol. 3* (pp. 377–411). Washington, DC: American Psychological Association.

Hoffman, C., & Rice, D. (1996). *Chronic care in America: A 21st century challenge.* Princeton, NJ: Robert Wood Johnson Foundation.

Huyser, B. A. & Parker, J. C. (2002). Rheumatic diseases. In S. B. Johnson, N. W. Perry, Jr., & R. H. Rozensky (Eds.), *Handbook of clinical health psychology: Vol. 1* (pp. 399–441). Washington, DC: American Psychological Association.

Ickovics, J. R., Hamburger, M. E., Valhov, D., Scheonbaum, E. E., Schuman, P., Boland, R. J., et al. (2001). Mortality, CD4 cell count decline, and depressive symptoms among HIV-seropositive women. *Journal of the American Medical Association, 285,* 1466–1474.

Ironson, G., Balin, E., & Schneiderman, N. (2002). In S. B. Johnson, N. W. Perry, Jr., & R. H. Rozensky (Eds.), *Handbook of clinical health psychology: Vol. 1* (pp. 5–36). Washington, DC: American Psychological Association.

Johnston, B., Wheeler, L., Deuser, J., & Sousa, K. H. (2000). Outcomes of the Kaiser Permanente Tele-Home Health Research Project. *Archives of Family Medicine, 9*(1), 40–45.

Leibson, C. L., Tosteson, A. N., Gabriel, S. E., Ransom, J. E., & Melton, L. J. (2002). Mortality, disability, and nursing home use for persons with and without hip fracture: A population-based study. *Journal of the American Geriatric Society, 50*(10);1644–1650.

Maricic, S. H. (1996). Rheumatic diseases of aging: Osteoporosis and polymyalgia rheumatica. In S. T. Wegener, B. L. Belza, & E. P. Gall (Eds.), *Clinical care in the rheumatic diseases* (pp. 191–195). Atlanta, GA: American College of Rheumatology.

M.D. Anderson Cancer Center. (2006). Survivorship issues: Keepig diabetes an issue, not a trouble. *Network: A Publication of the Anderson Network, Summer,* 5. Houston, TX: The M.D. Anderson Cancer Center.

Minor, M. S., & Kay, D. R. (2003). Arthritis. In J. L. Durstine & G. E. Moore (Eds.), *ACSM's exercise management for persons with chronic diseases and disabilities,* (2nd ed., pp. 210–216). Champaign, IL: Human Kinetics.

National Center for Health Statistics. (2008). *National Health and Nutrition Examination Survey Data for all Ages.* Retrieved April 10, 2008 from http://www.cdc.gov/nchs

National Institutes of Health. (2008). *Osteoporosis.* Retrieved April 11, 2008 from http://nih.gov

National Institutes of Health, National Institute on Aging. Alzheimer's General Information. Retrieved August 28, 2008 from http://www.nia.nih.gov/Alzheimers

National Institutes of Health, National Heart, Lung, and Blood Institute. (1997). Highlights of the Expert Panel Report 2: Guidelines for the Diagnosis and Management of Asthma. Retrieved August 28, 2008 from http://www.nhlbi.nigh.gov/guidelines/asthma

National Vital Statistics System. (2008). Deaths: Final Data for 2005. *National Vital Statistics Reports, 56*(10): April 24, 2008. Retrieved August 28, 2008 from http://www.cdc.gov/nchs/fastats/deaths.htm

Office of the Surgeon General. (2007). *Bone health and osteoporosis: A Surgeon general's report.* Retrieved April 11, 2008 from http://www.surgeongeneral.gov/library/bonehealth/

Orleans, C. T., Ulmer, C. C., & Gruman, J. C. (2004). The role of behavioral factors in achieving national health outcomes. In R. G. Frank, A. Baum, & J. L. Wallander (Eds.), *Handbook of clinical health psychology: Vol. 3* (pp. 465–499). Washington, DC: American Psychological Association.

Papas, R. K., Belar, C. D., & Rozensky, R. H. (2004). The practice of clinical health psychology: Professional issues. In R. G. Frank, A. Baum, & J. L. Wallander (Eds.), *Handbook of clinical health psychology: Vol. 3* (pp. 298–319). Washington, DC: American Psychological Association.

Peterson, C., & Bossio, L. M. (1991). *Health and optimism.* New York: Free Press.

Riggs, B. L., & Melton, L. J. III. (1995). The worldwide problem of osteoporosis: Insights afforded by epidemiology. *Bone* (Suppl. 5), 505S–511S.

Serafino, E. P. (2004). Asthma. In A. J. Christensen, R. Martin, & J. M. Smyth (Eds.), *Encyclopedia of health psychology* (pp. 19–21). New York: Kluwer Academic/Plenum.

Tomich, P. L., & Helgeson, V. S. (2004). Is finding something good in the bad always good? Benefit finding among women with breast cancer. *Health Psychology, 23*(1), pp. 16–23.

Tucker, J. A., Phillips, M. M., Murphy, J. G., & Raczynski, J. M. (2004). Behavioral epidemiology and health psychology. In R. G. Frank, A. Baum, & J. L. Wallander (Eds.), *Handbook of clinical health psychology: Vol. 3* (pp. 435–464). Washington, DC: American Psychological Association.

U.S. Department of Health and Human Services. (2000). *Healthy People 2010: Understanding and improving Health* (2nd ed.). Washington, DC: U.S. Government Printing Office.

Von Korff, M., Gruman, J., Schaefer, J., Curry, S. J., & Wagner, E. H. (1997). Collaborative management of chronic illness. *Annals of Internal Medicine, 127*(12), 1097–1102.

Wysocki, T., & Buckloh, L. M. (2002). Endocrine, metabolic, nutritional, and immune disorders. In S. B. Johnson, N. W. Perry, Jr., & R. H. Rozensky (Eds.), *Handbook of clinical health psychology: Vol. 1* (pp. 65–99). Washington, DC: American Psychological Association.

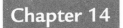

# Chapter 14

# Applications of Health Psychology to Diversity Issues

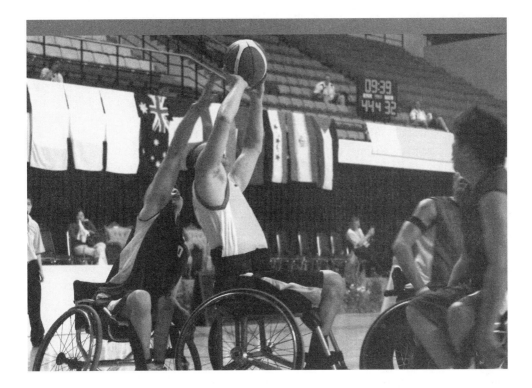

## Learning Objectives

After studying this chapter students will have the knowledge and skills to be able to:

1. Give an overall description of populations whose health problems are related to inequities in the U.S. culture.

2. Explain the ways poverty affects health, health care, and life expectancy.

3. Give examples of how biological, psychological, and social disparities related to race, ethnicity, and national origin affect health.

4. Discuss and give examples of ways biological, psychological, and social disparities in health are related to being female in the United States.

5. Discuss biological, psychological, and social disparities in health and health care related to physical, psychological, and social disabilities.

6. Discuss biological, psychological, and social disparities in health and health care
   related to age.

## Introduction

Many health problems are associated with biological factors such as age, gender, and ethnic
or racial origin. In other cases, illness and injury correlate with sociocultural factors, including economic conditions such as poverty. Third, unsafe behaviors are more prevalent
in certain populations, reflecting both biological and psychosocial origins. A few examples
are drunken driving, smoking, and substance abuse. Two psychologically based risk factors contributing to illness and injury are emotional problems and mental disabilities. This
chapter ties together some of these disparate facts by examining biopsychosocial factors
influencing health among diverse population groupings.

An effort was made throughout this textbook to be inclusive, so all chapters include references to the ways health issues specifically relate to gender, age, and ethnicity or race. Unfortunately many populations are underrepresented in studies in behavioral medicine and
health psychology so we know less about them. Exceptions are research projects specifically
aimed at members of populations delineated by age, gender, income, race, ethnicity, national
origin, or disability.

In this chapter the biopsychosocial approach of health psychology is used to understand
health issues for populations affected by poverty, discrimination, and disabilities. The chapter especially focuses on biology-based health problems linked to psychosocial risk factors.
Many health problems cluster within groupings in populations. An obvious gender example is that breast cancer is most often found in females, but only males experience prostate
cancer. Members of both genders develop heart disease, but their symptoms, diagnoses, treatments, and prognoses are often different. Young people are at risk for some diseases partly
as a result of the quality of care they receive while growing up. Adolescent health is affected
by socially driven tendencies to use tobacco, alcohol, weapons, and drive recklessly. The health
of older persons often reflects lifestyle choices they made earlier in their lives. Health risks
also mirror the value system of the culture in which they exist. Prejudice and discrimination
toward others are part of value systems and influence health. Health risks are influenced by
poverty, ethnicity, race, age, gender, and disabilities, regardless of individual lifestyle patterns.

For example, individuals living at lower socioeconomic levels experience both poorer
health and less safety from injuries. The United States prides itself on being tolerant of and
welcoming to people from diverse origins, but the reality for many is a disadvantaged health
status reflecting racial and ethnic background, immigration status, and national origin.
Many people with mental and physical disabilities are also subject to discrimination. Variations in sociocultural status result in disparities in health and health care. A different conceptual model is the socio-psycho-physiological framework of health and illness (Rugulie, Aust,
& Syme, 2004). This approach directs attention to the impact of social structure on physiological and psychological conditions and processes. The social and economic structure,

particularly the distribution of wealth, is the overarching factor at the top of this framework.

## Health and Sociocultural Characteristics

### Health and Income

Health problems are aggravated by lower levels of education, substandard housing, more dangerous occupations, and limited access to medical care. The most obvious health disparities reflect economic status. Epidemiologists have known for decades that health mirrors wealth. People with lower incomes are less likely to experience a long and healthy life compared to those with higher incomes. Earning power is an outcome of educational levels and hiring practices.

The government defines poverty for purposes of providing federal and state assistance, but the official poverty line underestimates the actual cost of living in the United States. Poverty statistics are based on definitions developed by the Social Security Administration. Poverty line thresholds vary by family size, number of children in the family, and, in some cases, ages of the adults in the family. Thresholds are updated annually by the United States Bureau of the Census to reflect changes in the Consumer Price Index for all urban consumers. In 2000, the average poverty threshold for a family of four was $17,603 (National Health Interview Survey, 2008). About 13% of all Americans live below this line, but millions more are economically disadvantaged. African Americans and Hispanic Americans have double the percentage of poverty of other racial and ethnic groups. Living on a lower income often means living in crowded, unsanitary housing in hazardous and polluted neighborhoods where stress levels are extremely high. Beliefs and behaviors also reflect socioeconomic status. Health beliefs and behaviors reflect social norms in neighborhoods and in the workplace (Kaplan, Everson, & Lynch, 2000). Low-income populations are less likely to eat healthily and exercise regularly, and are more likely to smoke (Emmons, 2000).

The most recent information from National Health Interview findings shows that the percentage of persons in excellent health increased with increased levels of education and family income (Adams, Lucas, & Barnes, 2008, pp. 5–6). Some highlights of the latest report are as follows:

- College graduates were more than twice as likely as persons who had not graduated from high school to be in excellent health.
- Persons with private health insurance were more likely than persons with other types of health insurance or uninsured persons to be in excellent health.
- Poor adults were three to four times more likely than those who were not poor to require help with activities of daily living and instrumental activities of daily living.
- Persons with the least education and the lowest incomes were the most likely to be unable to work due to health problems.

- Persons in the lowest income group were about four times more likely than persons in the highest income group to delay medical care due to cost and about eight times more likely to not get needed medical care. About 23 million persons delayed medical care in the last year due to cost.

Impoverished people are less likely to have health care insurance. They may not be able to afford to take time off from work to seek medical care. Both factors interfere with preventive health care services. People without resources often delay diagnoses and treatment for both illnesses and injuries. This postponement, based in socioeconomic conditions, increases the likelihood of chronic disease, disability, and premature death. Income influences the likelihood of stress including low job security, lack of control, and moods and emotions, including hostility and depression (Allgower, Wardle, & Steptoe, 2001). The distribution of wealth often reflects ethnic and racial minority status.

## Health and Race, Ethnicity, and National Origin

Over the last 100 years the United States has become more diverse. About 30% of the population belongs to a racial or ethnic minority group (Census Bureau, 2001). American Indian and Alaska Natives, black or African Americans, Hispanic or Latino Americans, Native Hawaiian and other Pacific Islanders, and Asian Americans are more likely to be poor and less likely to be as healthy as European Americans (Office of Minority Health and Health Disparities [OMHHD], 2008) (see **Figure 14.1**). Members of these groups experience a disproportionate burden of preventable disease, death, and disability (OMHD, 2008). For example, low-income populations, minorities, and children living in inner cities experience more emergency department visits, hospitalizations, and deaths due to asthma than the general population (OMHD, 2008). Recent immigrants, especially illegal immigrants, experience even lower socioeconomic status and levels of education, greater language difficulties, and discrimination. As a result they are more likely to experience inequities in health care. An important point made in the introduction was that poverty and minority status are often related.

It is difficult for social scientists to separate and evaluate the impact of dual or coexisting factors on health and safety. **Life expectancy** is one calculation commonly used to assess health differences by race, ethnicity, and national origin (U.S. Department of Health and Human Services [DHHS], 2006). For example, life expectancy at birth for blacks is 73 years and 78 years for whites.

---

**life expectancy** Actuarial tables provide estimated length of life based on gender, age, and other factors. It is a calculation commonly used to assess health differences by race, ethnicity, and national origin by the U.S. Department of Health and Human Services.

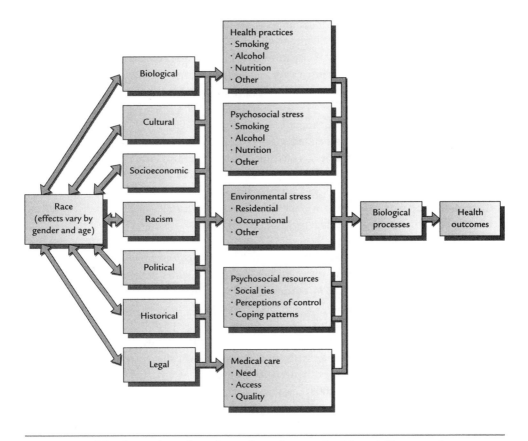

**Figure 14.1** This figure show the relationship of race to health and illustrates the biopsychosocial approach to health outcomes.

*Sources:* Williams, D.R. (1993). "Race in the Health of America: Problems, issues and Directions," MMWR, 42 (RR-10):9; and McKenzie, J., Pinger, R., & Kotecki, J. (2008). *An introduction to community health* (6th ed.). Sudbury, MA: Jones and Bartlett Publishers.

National statistics on causes of death are based on death certificates and make comparisons possible among groupings (National Center for Health Statistics, 2007). In the United States, the six major causes of death in descending order are heart disease, cancer, stroke, respiratory diseases, accidents or unintentional injuries, and diabetes, but these vary by ethnicity. Compared to other racial categories, Hispanic, American Indian/Alaska Native, and Asian/Pacific Islanders are more likely to die of accidents than other groupings. Death from diabetes is more common for blacks, Hispanics, American Indian/Native American, and Asian American/Pacific Islanders than for European Americans. Heart disease is the leading cause of death for all racial/ethnic groups except Asian or Pacific Islanders, who are more likely to die of cancer. In most instances death due to Alzheimer's disease is associated with being long-lived. Alzheimer's is the sixth leading cause of death for whites, but ranks 14th, 13th, and 12th for blacks, American Indian/Native American, and Asian American/Pacific Islanders, respectively. Scientists are still trying to sort out the influence on health risks of genetic susceptibility compared to suboptimal living conditions.

Biological Aspects of Race or Ethnicity

Some diseases are specifically associated with racial and ethnic groups. Three examples are osteoporosis, sickle-cell anemia, and type II diabetes. Osteoporosis is a greater risk for European and Asian American women than members of other racial and ethnic groups. First, members of these two populations are more likely to begin life with smaller bone size. Other factors implicated in osteoporosis are lack of calcium and vitamin D in the diet, limited exposure to sunlight, smoking, and lack of regular weightbearing exercise.

**Sickle-cell disease** is a group of genetic disorders characterized by the predominance of protein hemoglobin S (HbS) in red blood cells (Thompson & Gustafson, 1996). This blood disease occurs mostly in African Americans but also in some Mediterranean-origin populations. Red blood cells are especially important for carrying oxygen and storing iron. The term *sickle cell* refers to red blood cells being crescent-shaped, leading to anemia. Some symptoms of sickle-cell anemia are fatigue, weakness, headaches, joint pain, dizziness, and an enlarged spleen. When both parents carry the sickle-cell genetic trait, then a major concern becomes transmission to their children. Patients with sickle-cell disease may experience damage to bone marrow, heart, kidneys, spleen, and are at greater risk of stroke than others (Brown, Mulhern, & Simonian, 2002). Medical management is a lifelong issue.

Type II or adult-onset diabetes is associated with older age, obesity, history of gestational diabetes, inactivity, family history, and race or ethnicity. Complications of diabetes include heart disease and high blood pressure, blindness, kidney disease, and amputations (Wysocki & Buckloh, 2002). The prevalence rate for diabetes among American Indians in the southern United States and southern Arizona is about 27%, or nearly a third of that population. About 13% of blacks, 10% of Hispanic Americans, and 9% of whites are estimated to have diabetes (CDC, 2005a). Mexican Americans are 1.7 times as likely to have diabetes as non-Hispanic whites.

Psychosocial Aspects of Race, Ethnicity, and National Origin

Certain behaviors put people at risk regardless of genetic background, but some are also associated with income and minority status. For example, smoking puts people at risk of cancer, heart disease, and chronic obstructive lung disease (Fisher, Brownson, Heath, Luke, & Walton, 2004). Research on smoking among adults in the United States indicates that

**sickle-cell disease (SCD)**  A hereditary blood disease in which blood cells are abnormally shaped. It occurs mainly in people of African descent and causes a form of anemia.

about 32% of American Indian and Alaskan Natives smoke. Data on other groups show 22% of whites and blacks currently smoke, as do 15% of Hispanics, and 13% of Asians (CDC, 2006a). The ratio may change, because recent data about smoking among teens indicate that about 26% of whites, 12% of blacks, and 22% of Hispanics begin smoking in high school (CDC, 2006b). If these percentage differences prevail over time, then higher rates of smoking-related diseases in some groupings are expected in the future.

HIV/AIDS frequently reflects poverty, lifestyle choices, gender, and minority status. Behavioral risks include unprotected sexual intercourse and intravenous drug use (Ironson, Balbin, & Schneiderman, 2002). In 2005, the CDC estimated that about 40,000 people become infected each year in the United States, and of those diagnosed with HIV/AIDS during 2005, 49% were black, 31% were white, and 18% were Hispanic (2005b).

## Health and Gender

Gender, being female or male, is an important issue affecting health. **Sexism**, or prejudice and discrimination based on gender, continues to influence health and safety in addition to race, ethnicity, education, socioeconomic status, and age. Discrimination against people based on their gender is a pattern of behavior existing in most cultures and reflects enduring societal structures. **Social structure** refers to the existing order or the general social context within which people live out their lives. The term includes the organization of a society's historical, political, economic, family/kinship, religious, and educational systems. The social structure in the United States continues to be gender-biased, despite changes made in the 20th century including women being allowed to vote, to own property, and to seek certain types of jobs. In the United States women continue to be marginalized in many facets of life, including education, business, and sociopolitical processes. Pay inequities, inadequate child care arrangements, and restrictions on control of reproduction persist to plague women's physical and emotional health.

Gender discrimination adds to the impact of ethnic, racial, and economic inequalities. Women of African, Hispanic, Asian, Native, and European American background often experience lower levels of health and health care than males of the same ethnic and racial origins. About a third of women who head households live in poverty, which is a major contributor to illness and injury. The combined effects of poverty, discrimination, inability to provide for one's children, and fear of violence are sources of enormous stress for women (Ratcliff, 2002).

**sexism** Discriminatory actions, thoughts, and statements directed against people based on their biological status as a female or male.

**social structure** The organizational components within which people live. The term includes the political, economic, family/kinship, religious, and educational systems of a nation or country.

**Domestic violence** and sexual harassment continue to influence women's mental and physical health. Unrealistic beauty standards for women are common in our society. These expectations contribute to distorted body image, disordered eating practices, and excessive exposure to tanning, putting women at risk of skin cancer. Women are also exposed to hazards in their homes and workplaces. Up until very recently, no major longitudinal studies focused on women's health or health care. Variations in causes of illness and injury reflect biological, psychological, and sociocultural factors specific to gender.

Biological Aspects of Being Female

Women have a greater life expectancy than men: 81 years compared to 76 years (DHHS, 2006). Women have lower rates of injury, but higher rates of illness. Women are more likely than men to experience osteoporosis and some autoimmune disorders. Breast cancer in men is rare, but 1 in 8 women will develop the disease in their lives. Cardiovascular disease is the leading cause of death in women, but heart disease was considered a male disease up until about 1989. Heart attacks continue to be treated less aggressively in women and are more likely to be fatal for women than for men. Stress, mental health, and substance abuse are additional issues for women whose experiences with these health problems are different from men's. Due to the feminist movement in the 1960s and publications of the Boston Women's Health Collective in the 1970s and since, women's health is now being given more attention than ever before (Boston Women's Health Collective, 1973).

HIV/AIDS is a particular problem for poor minority women, who often contract it through heterosexual intercourse and needle sharing. Nevertheless, women were not included in HIV/AIDS clinical trials until 1993 (Ratcliff, 2002). Women are excluded from many health studies and are underrepresented in drug trials. Exclusion occurred partially due to fears about the side effects of the drugs if women were pregnant and also due to drug companies' concerns about the effects of menstrual cycles on research outcomes. In many cases it was assumed women were just like men, but with a smaller body size. During the previous century, the biology of women's health mainly included reproductive concerns. Hormones, menstruation, menopause, and maturation continue to be treated as medical problems requiring medical treatment. Two national women's health studies have brought women's health to the attention of both the general population and the medical community. The Nurse's Health Study is based on questionnaires completed by participating nurses who are women. The National Women's Health Initiative is an ongoing study that includes medical data, controlled experiments, and information about lifestyle and disease and accident occurrence. Women's health is gaining research recognition (Stanton & Gallant, 1995; Gallant, Keita, & Royak-Schaler, 1997; Etaugh & Bridges, 2004; Alexander, LaRosa, Bader, & Garfield, 2004).

---

**domestic violence**  Coercion of a family member or partner by physical, social, or psychological action. It includes child abuse and spousal abuse.

## Psychosocial Aspects of Being Female

On a worldwide basis, women still have less access than men to education, income, gainful employment, sports, and health care. For example, women were once limited to running only half the court in basketball games. It took legislative change for women to gain greater access to athletics, scholarships, and related rights (Tricard, 2008; Snooks, 2000).

### Sexual Violence

Sexual violence is a specific health risk that is greater for women than for men. It is an important and emerging area of concern in the United States and throughout the world. **Sexual violence** refers to nonconsensual sexual activity and includes threats, intimidation, peeping, taking nude photos, unwanted touching, and rape (CDC, 2008a). Global sexual violence problems include gang rapes in wartime and in prisons, sexual trafficking, and child marriages.

In the United States, 1 in 6 women, and 1 in 33 men report experiencing an attempted or completed rape at some time in their lives (Tjaden & Thoennes, 2000). Sexual violence includes **sexual harassment** in schools, neighborhoods, and at job sites. An estimated 20% to 25% of college women experience attempted or complete rape during their college career (Fisher, Cullen, & Turner, 2000). Among high school students 11% of females and 4% of males reported having been forced to have sex (CDC, 2008a). Sexual violence contributes to a number of health problems, including unwanted pregnancy, chronic pain, stomach problems, and sexually transmitted diseases. Emotional effects include fearfulness, anxiety, anger, and stress leading to eating disorders and depression. Globally, sexual violence is a common and serious health problem affecting millions of people.

## Health and Disabilities

One of every seven people in this country has a physical, intellectual, or emotional disability affecting quality of life. In many cases, disability is complicated by poverty. Health and health-related behaviors such as exercise and eating are affected by physical and mental limitations. Social isolation of people with disabilities further contributes to biopsychosocial difficulties. Public attitudes and environmental obstacles exacerbate quality of life. The Americans with Disabilities Act and recent court decisions have provided some relief, but many problems still exist in this country for persons with disabilities (see **Figure 14.2**).

**sexual violence**　Forced and violent assaults such as rape; usually committed by males against females.

**sexual harassment**　Offensive and unwanted behavior directed toward a person including words and actions that induce shame and fear. Most commonly used to designate actions by a higher-ranking male toward a female employee.

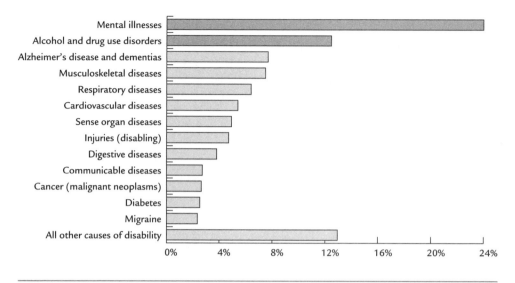

**Figure 14.2** Causes of disability in the United States, Canada, and Western Europe, 2000.

*Sources:* President's New Freedom Commission on Mental Health (2003). Achieving the Promise: Transforming Mental Health Care in America. Rockville, MD: Author, 20; and McKenzie, J., Pinger, R., & Kotecki, J. (2008). *An introduction to community health* (6th ed.). Sudbury, MA: Jones and Bartlett Publishers.

Now a disability and health team exists to support the development of guidelines for making emergency preparation, fitness and recreation sites, primary care, communication, and conferences more accessible to people with disabilities (CDC, 2008a). The team's web site is not controlled by the Centers for Disease Control, Department of Health and Human Services, or the Public Health Service. Some states have centers for universal design and the San Antonio Planning Department has a disability etiquette handbook. State and local governments provide disaster resources and emergency evacuation for people with physical disabilities. Disabilities may be physical, intellectual, emotional, or a combination of these difficulties.

**Accessible** is a term describing the suitability of a product or service for people with disabilities. **Universal design** describes products and environments that can be used re-

**accessible**  A term describing buildings and other facilities that may be easily used by people with disabilities such as those confined to a wheelchair.

**universal design**  Design of products and environments to make them useable regardless of body dimension, age, or disability status.

gardless of body dimension, age, or disability status. Using universal design prior to construction is usually superior to retrofitting environments. Accessibility is a very important biopsychosocial issue.

Biological Aspects of Disabilities

Problems with fatigue, balance, heat tolerance, sensory loss, muscle and skeletal weakness, tremors, and difficulty with vision, hearing, swallowing, and breathing may undermine overall health and prevent regular exercise among those with disabilities. For all people with disabilities, exercise should be modified or adapted to enhance health and prevent injury. Lower-limb amputations are usually due to diabetes, trauma such as war injury or automobile accidents, and congenital malformations. Exercise can be managed differently depending on the cause of the amputation (Pitetti & Pedrotty, 2003). For example, persons with diabetes should focus on cardiovascular exercise to prevent further deterioration in their health. Too-vigorous exercise may result in overuse injuries, joint pain, and falls that cause skin damage that may be slow to heal. Exercise is important for those with disabilities due to causes of amputations other than diabetes. For persons who have experienced trauma or congenital disability, exercise management may include aerobic, strength, flexibility, and functional exercises. Exercise may mean vigorous arm rather than leg movement for increasing aerobic capacity. Those with balance problems can use reclining or recumbant cycles, and guard rails when walking. When seizures are controlled, people with epilepsy may enjoy competitive contact sports. Muscle memory is affected by neurological diseases such as Parkinson's.

Exercises are usually modifiable for people with intellectual and emotional limitations. Attention deficits, motivation, and understanding may vary from day to day and require greater supervision. Some types of mental retardation are accompanied by heart defects. Coordination, along with difficulties in balance, weakness, and breathing may interfere with exercise (Fernhall, 2003). Alzheimer's disease is progressive and characterized by degeneration in both mental and physical health. Agitation, memory loss, depression, and incontinence may interfere with caregivers' efforts to maintain physical fitness in patients with Alzheimer's. A supervised short daily walk may be the maximum exercise possible. Exercise may improve mood and self-concept, and decrease depression and anxiety for people diagnosed with long-term or serious and persistent mental illness or psychiatric disability (Skrinar, 2003). Exercise is therapeutic in treating depressive disorders as well as beneficial to biological health. Some medications may interfere with exercising.

Psychosocial Aspects of Disabilities

Depression and deteriorating self-concept may follow losing control over one's life due to disabilities (see **Figure 14.3**). The emotional state of those with a mental or physical disability can vary from day to day and include angry reactions. Structured supervision is usually important. When a culture idealizes physical beauty and perfection, then prejudice and discrimination are issues for many people with noticeable physical or mental disabilities. Children with disabilities are often discouraged early in life by well-meaning but overprotective

**Figure 14.3**
Physical and mental disabilities may lead to depression.

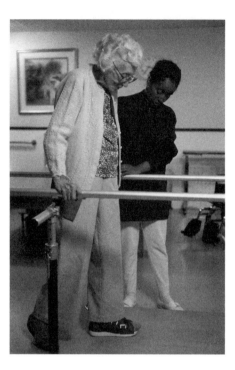

parents and caregivers. Establishing and maintaining independence rather than dependence requires major effort on the child's part and on the part of the caregivers.

## Health and Age

Illness and Injury in Children and Adolescents
The U.S. Department of Health and Human Services Healthy People 2010 includes goals specific to the health of children and adolescents (2007). Children's health issues interest health psychology researchers and developmental psychologists. Research topics include such varied areas as prenatal counseling for couples at risk of infant birth defects, childhood obesity, learning disabilities, school-based problems, and effective therapies for child abuse. **Developmental disabilities** and birth defects are a diverse group of severe and chronic conditions resulting in mental and physical impairment. These can affect learning, language

---

**developmental disabilities** A diverse group of severe and chronic conditions resulting in mental and physical impairment. These may affect learning, language development, mobility, and self-help.

development, mobility, and self-help. Developmental disabilities include cerebral palsy, autism, hearing loss, vision impairments, intellectual disabilities, and traumatic brain injury (CDC, 2008c; see **Figure 14.4**).

Childhood obesity is another important area of research interest, because obesity is a major risk factor for diabetes, cardiovascular disease, and some cancers. Overweight children and adolescents are more likely to become obese as adults (CDC, 2008c). Eighty percent of children who were overweight at ages 10 to 15 were obese at age 25 years, and 25% of obese adults were overweight as children. Data from the National Health and Nutrition Examination Survey (NHANES) surveys show that the prevalence of people who are overweight is increasing. The most recent surveys show that 14% of children aged 2–5, 19% of children ages 6–11, and 17% of those 12–19 are overweight (CDC, 2008c).

Health promotion and injury prevention are additional areas of children's health research. The leading cause of death for people from ages 1–24 is accidents. Most are motor vehicle accidents for which adults are responsible, but playground injuries, poisoning, fires, and

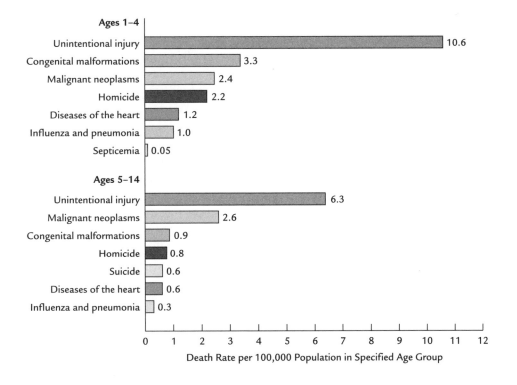

**Figure 14.4**  Leading causes of death in children aged 1–14, 2003.

*Sources:* National Center for Health Statistics; and McKenzie, J., Pinger, R., & Kotecki, J. (2008). *An introduction to community health* (6th ed.). Sudbury, MA: Jones and Bartlett Publishers.

drowning are additional causes of injury and death (DHHS, 2006). Both children and teens tend to overestimate their physical abilities, resulting in injuries (Plumert, 2004). Personality traits such as being impulsive, aggressive, daring, and careless are also linked to higher rates of injuries in children. This is especially true of children diagnosed with ADHD or **attention deficit-hyperactivity disorder** (Schwebel & Plumert, 1999; Farmer & Peterson, 1995).

Violence is a serious threat to the health and well-being of children and adolescents in the United States. Each year hundreds of thousands of children suffer abuse or neglect. For ages 5–24, the third and fourth leading causes of death are homicides and suicides (CDC, 2008d). For adolescents, risk-taking behaviors are a major health and safety problem. The teenage years are burdened with tendencies to substance abuse, motor vehicle injuries, violence, stress, depression, suicide, pregnancy, eating disorders, and sexually transmitted infections. More than 3 million young women between the ages of 14 and 19 have a sexually transmitted disease (CDC, 2008a). These include the human papillomavirus (HPV), chlamydia, herpes simplex virus, and trichomoniasis. Adolescent health is also affected by delinquency, homelessness, and academic underachievement. Youth violence includes aggressive behaviors such as verbal abuse, bullying, hitting, slapping, and fistfighting. Adolescents with chronic diseases such as diabetes are at high risk for not following medical therapies, leading to potentially life-threatening consequences. Detrimental experiences in childhood increase the probability of health problems in later life.

**The Adverse Childhood Experiences Study**  The **Adverse Childhood Experiences Study (ACE)** is an ongoing investigation of the link between childhood maltreatment and later-life health and well-being (CDC, 2008f). Over 17,000 adult members of the Kaiser Permanente Health Maintenance Organization are participating in comprehensive physical examinations and providing detailed information about their childhood experiences of abuse, neglect, and family dysfunction. To date over 30 scientific articles have been published.

The study began when researchers recognized the fact that many risk factors for chronic illness tended to cluster together. That is, people who have one risk factor such as smoking tended to have other risk factors such as alcohol abuse. The ACE Study suggests that adverse childhood experiences are a major risk factor for the leading causes of illness, death, and poor quality of life. The conceptual framework for the study takes a whole-life perspective, suggesting that adverse childhood experiences lead to social, emotional, and cognitive impairment, followed by behaviors leading to disease, disability, social problems, and early death.

**attention deficit-hyperactivity disorder (ADHD)**  A developmental disability that interferes with learning due to short attention spans and other problems.

**the Adverse Childhood Experiences Study (ACE)**  An ongoing investigation of the link between childhood maltreatment and health in later life.

**Figure 14.5**
Everyone should be aware of the effects of drugs on their bodies. Older people, who take many medications, must be especially careful.

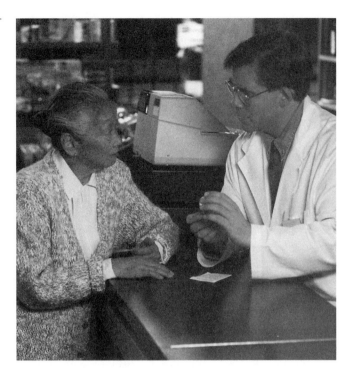

Illness and Injury in Older Adults

**Gerontology** is the science of aging and special problems of aged persons. **Geriatrics** is a medical specialty focusing on the diagnosis and treatment of diseases affecting the aged. It is sometimes difficult for medical personnel and researchers to distinguish between effects of aging and certain types of physical and persistent mental illness. By 2030 the number of Americans over 65 years of age will have more than doubled to 70 million, or 1 in every 5 persons (CDC, 2008c). This will increase demands on the public health system, including medical and social services (see **Figure 14.5**). Illness, disability, and premature death are avoidable with regular physical activity, healthy eating, avoiding tobacco use, and early detection for diseases through routine screening.

Some studies suggest that **cohort effects** may be more important than the effects of aging (Satre & Cook, 2004). Cohort effects reflect differences between generations rather

**gerontology**  The scientific study of aging or of old age.

**geriatrics**  A medical specialty dealing with health problems of the aged.

**cohort effects**  Influences on study participants reflecting generational differences. These may confound or interfere with conclusions when a study is complete.

than aging per se. For example, later generations with more education may exhibit intellectual abilities superior to earlier generations. Culture change is reflected by research attention being given to newer cohorts such as "baby boomers" and "generation X." These studies suggest that cultural changes in society are more important than age in affecting cognitive capacity.

**Ageism**, or prejudice and discrimination based on age, is common in the United States. Some sociologists suggest that being young is more valued than having the wisdom of old age. Feeling, acting, and looking young are the ideal of many. Ageism affects the health and safety of all persons regardless of gender, race, ethnicity, education, or socioeconomic status. As life expectancy increases, more research will probably focus on biological, psychological, and sociocultural factors related to aging.

**Biological Effects of Aging** Age shapes types of illness and injury. Chronic physical disorders and pain are more common in elderly populations than in younger people. Multiple medications, drug interactions, and confusion about dosage sometimes require hospitalization for the elderly. Osteoporosis, arthritis, and back pain are more common at older ages. Some ailments and accidents can be prevented by home renovations, including increased lighting, non-slippery floor coverings, convenient locations for essential items, hand rails, and lift chairs. Preventive action should include discussions of ways to avoid accidents and falls. Deafness is more characteristic of older Americans. As more and more Americans live into old age, technology for hearing aids will probably improve. Many of the elderly experience lower incomes following retirement. This interferes with healthy nutritional practices and access to medical care and medications. Economic problems add to the health problems of aging populations, especially among widowed women who are dependent on spousal Social Security or pensions. In spite of lower incomes and declining energy and strength, it is important for the elderly to be encouraged to exercise and to follow nutritious eating patterns.

**Psychosocial Aspects of Aging** The elderly are vulnerable to ageism and elder abuse. Both are harmful to biological and psychosocial health. Examples of ageism in this culture include jokes made about sexuality in old age and jokes about disabilities such as deafness and feebleness. Many elderly people are psychologically at risk due to social isolation, which causes damage to both physical and mental health. Single elders are more likely to live in age-segregated communities such as retirement centers and nursing homes. This often has demoralizing effects. Quality of life issues are especially important for elderly people who have limited ability to drive themselves to medical care and for grocery shopping. Problems with activities of daily living such as dressing, bathing, and room cleaning are more problematic for the elderly than other age groupings. Insomnia is also more characteristic of older Americans. It is not the typical problem of trying to go to sleep, but rather of staying asleep. The following day they are tired and more likely to fall or eat inadequately. Help for this type of

**ageism** Discriminatory actions, thoughts, and statements directed against people based on their age.

insomnia may be exercise by brisk walking during the day. Stress, depression, and suicide are additional hazards of aging. These often result from loss and loneliness due to deaths of spouses and longtime friends, as well as the loss of previous levels of physical activity.

## Summary

This chapter focused on disparities in health and health care related to poverty, race/ethnicity/national origin, gender, age, and disabilities. Poverty prevents easy access to health care services. Additionally, the poor are more likely to find themselves in dangerous jobs

---

### Think About It!

#### Start Now!

Taking the following actions now, while you are still young, may help you enjoy a healthier, longer life:

- Maintain a healthy weight and eat a nutritious, low-fat diet that includes plenty of whole grains, fruits, and vegetables.
- Be physically active; exercise daily.
- Do not smoke, drink too much alcohol, or abuse other drugs.
- Manage stress; take time to relax daily.
- Have regular physical examinations.
- Adopt safer sex practices.
- Do not drive while under the influence of alcohol or other drugs; always wear a seat belt in vehicles.
- Protect your skin and eyes from sunlight.
- Obtain enough sleep.
- Be concerned about your safety at home, work, or play.
- Maintain social networks with your family and friends.
- Be flexible; expect changes.
- Develop a positive attitude; have a sense of humor.
- Find opportunities to learn new skills or information.
- Get involved with living while accepting your mortality.

*Sources:* Alters, S., & Schiff, W. (2009). *Essential concepts for healthy living* (5th ed.). Sudbury, MA: Jones and Bartlett Publishers. Adapted from Kerschner, H., & Pegues, J. A. (1998). Productive aging: A quality of life agenda. *Journal of the American Dietetic Association*, 98:1445–1448; and Turner, L. W., Sizer, F. S., Whitney, E. N., & Wilks, B. B. (1992). *Life choices: Health concepts and strategies*. Minneapolis: West Publishing Co.

with little or no health care coverage. Racial and ethnic differences are frequently associated with disparities in wealth and result in inequality in health and health care. Some racial groups have specific health risks that may be genetic and/or consequences of day-to-day living conditions.

The social structure of the United States values females less than males. This results in disparities in health and health care. For centuries the main focus of medical care for women has been on reproductive health, rather than on other important causes of illness, injury, and death. People with physical, intellectual, and emotional disabilities may experience discrimination, affecting their emotional and physical health. In spite of limitations, those with a physical or psychiatric disability should be encouraged to exercise to maintain health and mobility. Age groups are also at particular risks for injury or illness. Children are at the mercy of their parents or caregivers with regard to health and health care. Adolescents are more likely than other age groups to take risks threatening to health and safety. Old age is often a time characterized by declines in income, health, energy, and even intellectual capacity. The very old are prone to falls, broken bones, heart disease, and cancers. Poverty, race/ethnicity, gender, age, and disabilities all impact biological, psychological, and social health.

## Review Questions

1. Give an overall description of special populations whose health problems are related to inequities in the U.S. culture.

2. Explain the various ways poverty affects health and health care.

3. Give examples of ways biological and psychosocial differences relate to race, ethnicity, and national origin, and affect health.

4. Enumerate ways biological, psychological, and social disparities associated with being female in the United States affect women's health.

5. Describe unique problems with health and health care for children and adolescents.

6. Discuss biological, psychological, and social variations associated with aging that affect health and health care.

7. Explain biological, psychological, and social problems in health and health care related to physical, intellectual, and emotional disabilities.

## Student Activity

Sensitivity training about special populations is usually available from student services or the counseling center. It is worthwhile to have speakers address biological and psychosocial consequences of membership in one or more marginalized groupings discussed in this chapter. In groups or as individuals, students can explore the health and health care problems of a special population. Many times students have their own personal experiences or those of some member of their families or friendship groups that relate to the information presented in this chapter. Student essays (photocopied and bound or stapled together) can be given to each class member. A general essay question on an exam might ask students to summarize what they learned from the set of student essays.

# References

Adams, P. F., Lucas, J. W., & Barnes, P. M. (2008). Summary health statistics for the U.S. population: National Health Interview Survey, 2006. National Center for Health Statistics. *Vital Health Statistics 10*(236).

Alexander, L. L., LaRosa, J. H., Bader, H., & Garfield, S. (2004). *New dimensions in women's health* (3rd ed.). Sudbury, MA: Jones and Bartlett.

Allgower, A., Wardle, J., & Steptoe, A. (2001). Depressive symptoms, social support, and personal health behaviors in young men and women. *Health Psychology, 20,* 223–227.

Boston Women's Health Collective (1973). *Our bodies, ourselves: A book for and by women.* New York: Simon and Schuster.

Brown, R. T., Mulhern, R. K., & Simonian, S. (2002). Diseases of the blood and blood-forming organs. In S. B. Johnson, N. W. Perry, Jr., & R. H. Rozensky (Eds.), *Handbook of clinical health psychology* (Vol. 1, pp. 101–141). Washington, DC: American Psychological Association.

Census Bureau, Census 2000 Brief: Overview of Race and Hispanic Origin, 2001.

Centers for Disease Control. (2005a). National diabetes fact sheet: General information and national estimates on diabetes in the United States, 2005. Atlanta, GA: U.S. Department of Health and Human Services.

Centers for Disease Control. (2005b). HIV Infection Reporting. Retrieved May 5, 2007 from http://www.cdc.gov/hiv/topics/surveillance/reporting.htm

Centers for Disease Control. (2006a). Cigarette use among adults—United States, 2005. *Mortality and Morbidity Weekly Report, 55*(42), 1145–1148.

Centers for Disease Control. (2006b). Cigarette use among high school students—United States, 1991–2005. *Mortality and Morbidity Weekly Report, 55*(26), 724–726.

Centers for Disease Control, National Center for Health Statistics. (2007). Deaths: Leading Causes for 2003. Retrieved May 5, 2007 from http://www.cdc.gov/nchs/products/pubs/pubc/hestats/leading

Centers for Disease Control. (2008a). Understanding Sexual Violence. Retrieved April 15, 2008 from http://www.cdc.gov/injury

Centers for Disease Control. (2008b). Disabilities, National Center on Birth Defects and Developmental Disabilities. Retrieved April 15, 2008 from http://www.cdc.gov/ncbddd

Centers for Disease Control. (2008c). Childhood Overweight. Retrieved April 15, 2008 from http://www.cdc.gov/nccdphp/dnpa/obesity/childhood/index.htm

Centers for Disease Control. (2008d). Healthy Youth! Health Topics: Youth. Retrieved April 15, 2008 from http://www.cdc.gov/HealthyYouth

Centers for Disease Control. (2008e). Healthy Aging for Older Adults. Retrieved August 29, 2008 from http://www.cdc.gov/aging

Centers for Disease Control. (2008f). Adverse Childhood Experiences Study. Retrieved October 26, 2008 from http://www.cdc.gov/nccdphp/ace/.

Emmons, K. M. (2000). Health behaviors in a social context. In L. F. Berkman & I. Kawachi (Eds.), *Social epidemiology* (pp. 242–266). NY: Oxford University Press.

Etaugh, C. A., & Bridges, J. S. (2004). *The psychology of women: A lifetime perspective* (2nd ed.). Boston: Pearson.

Farmer, J. E., & Peterson, L. (1995). Injury risk factors in children with attention deficit hyperactivity disorder. *Health Psychology, 14,* 325–332.

Fernhall, B. (2003). Mental retardation. In J. L. Durstine & G. E. Moore (Eds.), *ACSM exercise management for persons with chronic diseases and disabilities* (2nd ed. pp. 304–310). Champaign, IL: Human Kinetics.

Fisher, B. S., Cullen, F. T., & Turner, M. G. (2000). *The sexual victimization of college women* (Publication No.: NCH 182369). Washington,

DC: Department of Justice, National Institute of Justice.

Fisher, E. B., Brownson, R. C., Heath, A. C., Luke, D. A., & Walton, S., II. (2004). Cigarette smoking. In J. M. Raczynski & L. C. Leviton (Eds.), *Handbook of clinical health psychology: Vol. 2.* (pp. 75–120). Washington, DC: American Psychological Association.

Gallant, S. J., Keita, G. P., & Royak-Schaler, R. (Eds.). (1997). *Health care for women: Psychological, social and behavioral influences.* Washington, DC: American Psychological Association.

Healthy People 2010. Retrieved May 10, 2007 from http://www.healthypeople.gov/data/midcourse/html/introduction.htm

Ironson, G., Balbin, E., & Schneiderman, N. (2002). Health psychology and infectious diseases. In S. B. Johnson, N. W. Perry, Jr., & R. H. Rozensky (Eds.), *Handbook of clinical health psychology* (Vol. 1, pp. 5–36). Washington, DC: American Psychological Association.

Kaplan, G. A., Everson, S. A., & Lynch, J. W. (2000). The contribution of social and behavioral research to an understanding of the distribution of disease: A multilevel approach. In B. D. Smedley & S. L. Syme (Eds.), *Promoting health: Intervention strategies from social and behavioral research* (pp. 37–80). Washington, DC: National Academies Press.

Office of Minority Health and Health Disparities. (2008). Eliminating Racial and Ethnic Health Disparities. Retrieved April 15, 2008 from http://www.cdc.gov/omhd

Pitetti, K. H., & Pedrotty, M. H. (2003). Lower-limb amputation. In J. L. Durstine & G. E. Moore (Eds.), *ACSM exercise management for persons with chronic diseases and disabilities* (2nd ed., pp. 230–235). Champaign, IL: Human Kinetics.

Plumert, J. M. (2004). Accidents. In A. J. Christensen, R. Martin, & J. M. Smyth (Eds.), *Encyclopedia of health psychology* (pp. 1–3). New York: Kluwer Academic.

Ratcliff, K. S. (2002). *Women and health: Power, technology, inequality and conflict in a gendered world.* Boston: Allyn and Bacon.

Rugulie, R., Aust, B., & Syme, S. L. (2004). Epidemiology of health and illness: A socio-psycho-physiological perspective. In S. Sutton, A. Baum, & M. Johnson (Eds.), *The Sage handbook of health psychology,* (pp. 39–42). London: Sage Publications.

Satre, D. D., & Cook, B. L. (2004). Aging. In A. J. Christensen, R. Martin, & J. M. Smyth (Eds.), *Encyclopedia of health psychology* (pp. 5–8). New York: Kluwer Academic.

Skrinar, G. S. (2003). Mental illness. In J. L. Durstine & G. E. Moore (Eds.), *ACSM exercise management for persons with chronic diseases and disabilities* (2nd ed., pp. 316–319). Champaign, IL: Human Kinetics.

Schwebel, D. C., & Plumert, J. M. (1999). Longitudinal and concurrent relations between temperament, ability, estimation, and injury proneness. *Child Development, 70,* 700–712.

Snooks, M. K. (2000). Title IX of the Education Amendments of 1972. In A. M. Howard & F. M. Kavenik (Eds.), *Handbook of American women's history* (2nd ed., pp. 571–572). Thousand Oaks, CA: Sage Publications.

Stanton, A. L. & Gallant, S. J. (Eds.). (1995). *The psychology of women's health: Progress and challenges in research and application.* Washington, DC: American Psychological Association.

Thompson, R. J., Jr. & Gustafson, K. E. (1996). *Adaptation to chronic childhood illness.* Washington, DC: American Psychological Association.

Tjaden, P., & Thoennes, N. (2000). *Extent, nature, and consequence of intimate partner violence: Findings from the National Violence Against Women Survey* (Publication No.: NCJ 181867). Washington, DC: Department of Justice.

Tricard, L. M. (2008). *American women's track and field, 1981–2000.* (pp. 1–2). Jefferson, NC: McFarland.

United States Department of Health and Human Services. (2006). *National Vital Statistics Reports,* June 28, 2006, 54(19).

Williams, D. R. (1993). Race in the health of America, problems, issues and directions. *Mortality and Morbidity Weekly Report, 42* (RR-10); 9.

Wysocki, T. & Buckloh, L. M. (2002). Endocrine, metabolic, nutritional, and immune disor-ders. In S. B. Johnson, N. W. Perry, Jr., & R. H. Rozensky (Eds.), *Handbook of clinical health psychology* (Vol. 1, pp. 65–99). Washington, DC: American Psychological Association.

# Glossary

**accessible**   A term describing buildings and other facilities that may be easily used by people with disabilities such as those confined to a wheelchair.

**acute pain**   Pain that usually indicates tissue damage sending a signal of physical harm and causing enough anxiety that a person will seek medical care.

**addiction**   Physical and psychological dependence on a behavior. The term is generally applied to compulsive use of substances harmful to health, such as alcohol.

**adequacy**   Eating sufficient amounts and types of foods to consume the correct number of calories and all necessary nutrients.

**adherence**   The degree to which a person follows a medical directive or continues with a behavior change.

**Adverse Childhood Experiences Study (ACE)**   An ongoing investigation of the link between childhood maltreatment and health in later life.

**aerobic exercise**   Any form of movement that elevates the rate of heartbeats and breathing.

**affirmations**   Statements about one's ability to overcome adversity and go through life free of stress or pain.

**ageism**   Discriminatory actions, thoughts, and statements directed against people based on their age.

**alcohol abuse**   Excessive and habitual consumption of alcohol.

**alcohol dehydrogenase enzyme (ADE)**   An enzyme found in the stomach that assists in metabolizing alcohol molecules. In general, women appear to have less of the enzyme than men.

**Alcoholics Anonymous (AA)**   A worldwide self-help group providing social support for avoiding alcohol and staying sober.

**Alzheimer's disease**   A loss of cognitive ability especially memory. It usually occurs in old age and results in personality changes and confusion.

**American Stop Smoking Intervention Study (ASSIST)**   A U.S. government–funded demonstration project to help states develop strategies to reduce smoking. One goal was to change social, cultural, economic, and environmental factors that promote smoking.

**anaphylactic shock**   A serious allergic response to insect stings, foods such as peanuts and seafood, or to medicines such as penicillin; being exposed to very small amounts of these substances causes allergic persons to experience this sudden life-threatening illness.

**angina pectoris**   Recurrent chest pain caused by disease of the cardiovascular system.

**angiocardiogram**   A series of x-rays of the heart while a contrasting medium is being passed through it; used to diagnose disorders of the heart.

**angioplasty**   A medical procedure that improves blood flow to the heart by pressing accumulated plaque against the walls of the coronary arteries with a small balloon. The procedure increases the space through which blood can flow to heart muscle cells and may relieve angina.

**anonymous**   An assurance given to research participants that any data collected will not be attributed to them. Participants filling out a survey form are assured they are anonymous and no one will ever know who filled out the form.

**anorexia nervosa**   A disordered eating pattern consisting of repeated dieting and/or overexercising, with the result that body weight falls below healthy levels.

**appetite**   The desire to eat or drink.

**appraisal**   The first stage of the coping process in which persons think about a stressor or demand made upon them. People evaluate threatening situations and think about possible responses.

**arteriosclerosis**   Disorder of the arteries including the hardening of the artery walls and loss of elasticity, resulting in decreased blood flow to the heart and brain.

**arthritis**   A disorder that inflames joints resulting in swelling and pain.

**asthma**   A disorder that interferes with breathing and is characterized by wheezing. Mucus in the respiratory system results in inflammation of the bronchi.

**atherosclerosis**   Disorder of the arteries in which plaque consisting of cholesterol and other fats lines the inner arterial wall and narrows the space through which blood can flow to the heart and brain.

**atopic dermatitis (AD)**   A neurodermatitis characterized by itching, redness, oozing, crusting, scratching, and thickening of the skin, also called eczema.

**atrophy**   Wasting away and weakening of the musculoskeletal system due to lack of movement or exercise. This most noticeably occurs in muscles as people age if they do not make it a point to exercise.

**attention deficit-hyperactivity disorder (ADHD)**   A developmental disability that interferes with learning due to short attention spans and other problems.

**automated external defibrillator (AED)**   A device that analyzes heart rhythms and can tell when to administer a shock to a victim of cardiac arrest. The shock, defibrillation, may re-establish an effective heart rhythm.

**autonomic nervous system**    Part of the nervous system that affects involuntary functions of the body such as blood vessels, the heart, smooth muscles, and glands. It includes the sympathetic and parasympathetic divisions.

**avoidant coping**    Reacting to a stressor by denial or minimizing a threat rather than taking some kind of action to resolve the issue.

**behavior modification**    Interventions to encourage behaviors such as exercise or extinguish behaviors such as smoking; for example, efforts to change or shape a behavior by reinforcing that behavior with rewards.

**behavioral health**    A subfield of behavioral medicine emphasizing the maintenance of health including prevention of both physical and emotional illnesses. Behavioral medicine combines work in the biomedical and behavioral sciences.

**benign tumor**    A growth of tissue that is noncancerous or nonspreading.

**binge drinking**    Consuming more than four drinks on one occasion for men and more than three drinks on one occasion for women.

**biofeedback**    A cognitive-behavioral instructional process combining talk therapy with technology to teach individuals to gain control over anxiety, tension, or pain. Sensors placed on the body feed back information to a receiver that emits sound or light depending on muscle tension. Individuals learn to control and relax tense areas of the body to such an extent that the sound or light fades and disappears. The success of biofeedback-facilitated relaxation training (BFRT) depends on the individual following up on training sessions by frequently practicing going into relaxed states of mind and body.

**biomedical model of health**    A narrow perspective that includes the idea that illness and injury are biological problems with biomedical solutions. People who hold this view assume that when someone is ill or injured only the physical self is affected and must be treated.

**biopsychosocial model of health**    The perspective that illness and injury have biological, psychological, and sociocultural components. From this perspective diagnosis and treatment decisions should take into account all three aspects.

**blood alcohol concentration (BAC)**    The concentration of alcohol in the bloodstream.

**body composition**    Ratio of fat to muscle, bone, and water in the body. Regular exercise improves body composition by reducing fat weight.

**brachytherapy**    Medical approach to cancer using tiny radioactive seeds placed inside or near tumors to destroy them.

**bulimia nervosa**    A disordered or unhealthy pattern consisting of eating followed by vomiting or purging with laxatives.

**burnout**    A negative outcome of over-exercising or over-participation in sports. It may be related to feeling constantly pressured by oneself or others to improve physical performance. Participants may lose all sense of the purpose or fun of an exercise or sport.

**calisthenics**   A simple form of exercise using the strength and weight of one's own body to increase fitness levels. One example is the pushup, an exercise in which people lie on the ground and use their arms to push their upper body off the ground.

**cancer**   An abnormal malignant growth of cells that can invade nearby tissue and may spread throughout the body.

**carcinogens**   Substances capable of making body cells malignant or cancerous; a cancer-forming agent or a risk factor for cancer.

**cardiac arrest**   A stoppage of the heart leading to oxygen deprivation in important organs such as the lungs, brain, and kidneys.

**cardiopulmonary resuscitation (CPR)**   The provision of external massage of the heart and oxygen by another person on someone who is experiencing cardiac arrest.

**cardiovascular disease (CVD)**   Diseases of the cardiovascular system, which includes the heart and blood vessels. The system pushes blood, nutrients, oxygen, and waste products throughout the body.

**cardiovascular reactivity**   A tendency of one's heart to act in response to some factors such as fright or some other stressor.

**chemotherapy**   Disease treatment using chemicals, including drugs such as antibiotics. The most common usage refers to drugs used to treat cancer.

**cholesterol**   A waxy fat or sterol existing in animal fats and the human body that forms deposits in blood vessels, clogging arteries and contributing to heart attacks and strokes.

**chronic intractable pain**   Persistent pain that is not relieved by medications or medical procedures.

**chronic obstructive pulmonary disease (COPD)**   Nonreversible lung disease, including emphysema and bronchitis; often caused by smoking.

**chronic pain**   Pain lasting 6 months or longer; normal healing should have occurred and there should be no residual pain. One example of chronic pain is the pain of arthritis.

**clinical psychologist**   A mental health professional with a background in counseling and health psychology.

**cognition**   The act or process of knowing, and products of the process such as problem solving. In health psychology, cognitions affect perception of stressors. Cognitive restructuring refers to methods of changing ones thinking about a stressor.

**cohort effects**   Influences on study participants reflecting generational differences. These may confound or interfere with conclusions when a study is complete.

**colonoscopy**   A medical procedure to examine the interior of the colon.

**combat stress reaction (CSR)**  Name given to the reaction of some American soldiers to the stress of combat in World War II. It was viewed as a temporary or transient reaction to traumatic experiences in otherwise-normal individuals.

**community-based intervention**  A health-behavior-change program that focuses on an entire community of people rather than on one person or a small group. One example is townspeople deciding to develop and implement a campaign to prevent smoking by their young people.

**complementary health care or alternative medicine**  Therapeutic pain treatment interventions developed outside of traditional Western medical practice. Examples are acupuncture, massage, relaxation therapy, self-help groups, herbal medicine, megavitamins, chiropractics, and self-hypnosis.

**complex carbohydrate**  A food containing carbohydrates for energy along with other important nutrients and fiber. Dietary guidelines for Americans encourage intake of complex carbohydrates by increasing consumption of fruit, vegetables, whole grains, and low-fat milk. Chemically, the term refers to chains of two or more monosaccharides to differentiate them from simple carbohydrates or sugar molecules.

**confidentiality**  A promise made to participants in research that their names and answers or information will be protected from people outside of the research staff.

**continuum**  Illustrative figure such as a line with two extreme conditions of some phenomenon located at either end of the line.

**coping**  People's efforts or behaviors to meet the challenges of stressors in their lives and to alleviate distress.

**correlation**  The degree of relationship between variables. Correlations can be positive or negative. For example, the more cigarettes people smoke the more likely they are to develop lung cancer. There is a positive correlation between smoking and lung cancer.

**correlational study**  A research effort to discover relationships between variables.

**cross-sectional study**  A research design that studies participants representing all age sets and occurs over a short period of time.

**cue**  Something that motivates or incites to action, a stimulus; billboard advertising, or a delicious odor may be a cue to eat or drink something.

**culture shock**  Emotional upheaval and even illness due to significant changes in living conditions. It particularly occurs when people experience a drastic change in their surroundings due to immigration or forced migration to new geographical areas. Another example is moving from a rural area to an urban area.

**cynicism**  Belief, attitude, or viewpoint that other people cannot be trusted. It is believed to be a risk factor for cardiovascular disease. Part of the Type A personality.

**data**    Information assembled about variables. The word data is plural, and the word datum is singular. For example, the student assembled or amassed data about the variables relating to her class research project.

**deep breathing**    A stress management/relaxation technique that encourages one to give attention only to one's breathing rather than thinking about anything else.

**delirium tremens (DTs)**    Severe physical and mental disorders occurring when alcohol is withdrawn from heavy users.

**deoxyribonucleic acid (DNA)**    A large molecule found in the chromosomes of the cell nucleus that contains genetic information.

**dependent variable**    The variable that is viewed as the probable result of the independent variable. For example, in the hypothesis that auto wrecks often occur because the person driving the car has been drinking alcohol, the dependent variable is automobile wrecks.

**depressant**    A psychoactive substance that slows down the central nervous system, decreasing physical and mental activity. Depressants may relieve anxiety and promote sleep, but also impair coordination, judgment, and respiration.

**designer drugs**    Combinations of psychoactive substances that may result in unpredictable and dangerous effects such as euphoria, paranoia, and mood swings.

**developmental disabilities**    A diverse group of severe and chronic conditions resulting in mental and physical impairment. These may affect learning, language development, mobility, and self-help.

**diabetes mellitus**    A complex chronic disorder of metabolism due to lack of insulin or having insulin that the body cannot use.

**diagnosis**    Identification of a disease or injury following an evaluation of symptoms and health history.

**diastolic**    The diastole is the period between two contractions of the heart; it is the second or lower number given in blood pressure readings.

**diet**    A person's usual eating practice or pattern.

**dietary reference intakes (DRIs)**    Suggested by the Food and Nutrition Board of the National Academy of Sciences. There are targets for intake by healthy individuals and include vitamins, minerals, water, carbohydrates, fiber, fat, linoleic acid, and alpha-linolenic acid protein. The DRIs include the RDAs.

**distorted ambulation**    An abnormal walking behavior indicating pain in some area of the body.

**distraction**    Avoidance thinking or diversion that may be useful for short-term pain relief.

**domestic violence**    Coercion of a family member or partner by physical, social, or psychological action. It includes child abuse and spousal abuse.

**dose-response relationship**   Refers to the body's reaction to the dosage or amount of substances put into it. For example, the greater the number of cigarettes smoked, the greater the damage to the body.

**double-blind study**   A study designed to eliminate the expectations of participants in a study and the biases of those conducting the study. In single-blind research designs, the participants do not know if they are receiving the treatment or a placebo but the providers of the treatment do know. In a double-blind study, neither participants nor scientists know who is in the experimental group and who is in the control group.

**duration**   The length of time one exercises; gradual increases in duration are recommended to safely increase fitness levels.

**dyspnea**   Difficult or labored breathing upon movement; shortness of breath associated with lung disorders such as COPD.

**ECGs or EKGs**   Electrocardiogram; a diagnostic procedure that graphically records the electrical activity of the heart.

**emotion**   Affective consciousness including feelings such as joy, sadness, fear, and hate. In health psychology, emotional support from others is helpful in recovery from illness and injury, and emotion-focused coping is a way to manage stress.

**emotional disclosure**   Relieving stress from a traumatic event by talking with someone or writing or journaling it.

**emotion-focused coping**   Coping directed toward managing the emotions or feelings aroused by a stressor.

**endocrine system**   A network of glands that produce and secrete hormones into the bloodstream, thereby regulating activities, including growth, digestion, metabolism, and reproduction.

**epidemic**   An outbreak of a specific health problem affecting a large number of people within a geographic area.

**epidemiology**   A branch of medicine that studies the occurrence, cause, and control of diseases.

**essential hypertension (EH)**   Blood pressure considered too high for good health but with no known cause.

**exercise**   Physical activity done purposely to maintain or improve physical fitness and health.

**experiential learning**   Learning through personal experience or activity rather than through reading or being formally taught by an instructor.

**fetal alcohol spectrum disorders (FASDs)**   The leading preventable cause of mental retardation and birth defects in children whose mothers drank alcohol during their pregnancy.

**fibrosis**   The early stage of liver damage due to alcohol; cirrhosis, the later stage, makes the regeneration of liver cells impossible.

**fight-or-flight response**   The response of animals, including humans, when threatened with harm. It includes arousal by the sympathetic nervous and endocrine systems to attack or flee.

**flexibility**   The freedom to move joints through their full range of motion.

**free weight**   A quantity or mass, usually made of metal and not attached to a strength-training machine. A free weight is used to improve muscle strength by lifting or moving the weight through space for a certain number of times. One example of a free weight is the barbell.

**frequency**   The regularity or incidence of exercise, usually measured in terms of the number of days each week one exercises.

**functional support**   That part of social support that provides resources such as financial help or other aids to help us to cope with stressors.

**gate control theory of pain**   A theory of pain perception that explains pain as a sensation that can be blocked by a neural gate in the spinal cord that modifies pain signals.

**general adaptation syndrome (GAS)**   Selye's conceptualization of three stages of stress, including the alarm stage (when an animal perceives a threat and prepares to fight or flee), the resistance stage (when the animal copes with stressful situations), and the exhaustion stage (when the body begins to deteriorate under stress).

**geriatrics**   A medical specialty dealing with health problems of the aged.

**gerontology**   The scientific study of aging or of old age.

**gestational diabetes**   A form of diabetes appearing during pregnancy; it usually disappears after delivery but is a risk factor for Type II diabetes.

**guarding**   A protective behavior that may indicate a painful injury. For example, when someone breaks a bone in his arm he may hold that arm against his body with the undamaged hand to diminish movement and pain.

**guided imagery**   A therapist guides patients' thinking so they visualize or imagine a pleasant relaxing situation. Individuals learn to use their own imaginations whenever they feel stressed.

**Hans Selye**   Physiologist who injected noxious agents into rats' bodies and put them under threatening conditions. Experimental animals developed hyperactivity, atrophy of lymph glands, and peptic ulcers. He believed that the response to stress was general and included three phases.

**hardiness**   Ability to withstand stressful events and take appropriate and decisive action.

**health**   Soundness of body and mind: a state of physical, emotional, and social well-being.

**health belief model (HBM)**   One of the earliest explanations or theories of health-related behaviors; the model proposes that people will take action to protect their health if they believe they are susceptible to a serious threat, that taking action will be an effective deterrent to illness or injury, and that the barriers to taking action are worth being overcome.

**health psychology**   A specialty applying psychological principles to the scientific study of health, illness, and health-related behaviors. It is specifically aimed toward a broader understanding of health, illness, injury, recovery, and the impact of each on human life. Knowledge developed in this field includes psychological, social, and cultural influences on the development, diagnosis, treatment, and rehabilitation of ill and injured people. Health psychologists are also interested in the prevention of illness and injury and in health policy formation. It is a field of study within the general discipline of psychology.

**health risk analysis (HRA)**   A series of questions on topics that may indicate a high risk of some diseases, such as heart disease.

**heavy drinking**   Consuming more than two drinks per day for men and more than one drink per day for women.

**honorarium**   A reward in recognition of participation in a study; For example, participants in the Women's Health Study were given pencils and emery boards after filling out forms.

**hostility**   An attitude of antagonism toward others. It is believed to be a risk factor for CVD. Part of the Type A personality.

**human immunodeficiency virus/acquired immune deficiency syndrome (HIV/AIDS)**   HIV is a contagious virus that causes a life-threatening deficiency of the immune system (AIDS), leading to vulnerability to opportunistic infection and disease.

**human papillomavirus (HPV)**   A virus that may cause genital warts and/or the development of abnormal cells in the anus, cervix, penis, and vaginal tissue.

**hunger**   Hunger refers to a biological or physiological state. It is often described as an unpleasant, even painful, sense of the need to eat.

**hypertension**   A disorder of the cardiovascular system in which the blood pressure is persistently above 140/90 mg HG.

**hypothesis**   A prediction about a relationship between variables. If the hypothesis is that when people believe they have a serious disease, they will usually seek medical treatment for the disease, the independent variable is the belief, the dependent variable is the behavior, and the hypothesis is the prediction about the effect of the independent variable on the dependent variable.

**iatrogenic illness**   A condition occurring as a result of medical diagnostic procedures, medical treatments, or exposure while in a medical facility.

**illness behavior**   Actions taken by people who believe they are ill to discover causes and solutions to their situation.

**immunology**    The study of the body's response to foreign invasion.

**incidence**    A measure of frequency, or the number of times a new event occurs within a given period of time, usually a year. For example, a study might find that the incidence of new cases of the sexually transmitted disease of genital warts or HPV is over 5 million each year.

**independent variable (IV)**    The variable that is viewed as a cause affecting another variable within a hypothesis. For example, in the hypothesis that alcohol use by drivers increases the likelihood of automobile wrecks, the independent variable is alcohol use.

**injury**    Damage to some component of the body.

**intensity**    The extent to which the heart and breathing rates are elevated during exercise. Intensity can be measured by counting the number of heartbeats per minute after about 15 minutes of exercise. Mathematical formulas exist to measure intensity and to set goals for intensity according to age and desired levels of fitness.

**intervention**    An organized program designed to help people change or modify their behavior.

**ischemia**    Decreased blood supply to a body part; myocardial ischemia refers to insufficient blood flow to meet the heart's metabolic demands.

**learned resourcefulness**    Skills and intellectual qualities of persons who learn to anticipate, plan, self-regulate, cope with failure, and change coping strategies.

**leukemia**    Cancer of the blood; a malignant neoplasm of blood-forming tissue

**life expectancy**    Actuarial tables provide estimated length of life based on gender, age, and other factors. It is a calculation commonly used to assess health differences by race, ethnicity, and national origin by the U.S. Department of Health and Human Services.

**loaded question**    A question in an interview or survey that is phrased in such a way as to make a certain answer more likely. For example, asking "How often do you eat at fast food restaurants?" rather than asking, "Please give the names of the last three restaurants from which you bought a meal."

**longitudinal study**    A research design that studies the same respondents over a long period of time.

**lymphoma**    Cancer in lymph tissues.

**malignant tumor**    A growth of tissue that is damaging to the body, such as a cancer that is invasive and spreads throughout the body.

**malingering**    A deliberate feigning of symptoms such as pain or illness to try to gain some end such as attention, sympathy, or release from obligations.

**malnutrition**    Inadequate nutrient intake or taking in too few nutrients from food or by intravenous feeding. Malnutrition may lead to sickness and death. Socioeconomic levels and geographic location often result in malnutrition due to famine, war, or natural disasters resulting in the widespread lack of food products for a population. People diagnosed with anorexia nervosa often suffer from malnutrition.

**McGill-Melzack pain questionnaire (MMPQ)**   A complex and detailed set of questions used to assess people's pain.

**meditation**   A process of using the mind-body connections to improve health, including contemplation, thinking, and concentration of thoughts that may produce positive outcomes including relaxation.

**metastasis**   The spread of cancerous tissue from its original site through the lymphatic system, bloodstream, or across a body cavity.

**mind–body connection**   The idea that emotions, personality, and culture affect physical health, and that the reverse is also true. One example is a belief in the power of positive attitudes on health outcomes, such as the effectiveness of cancer treatments. The idea is that mind–body illnesses and mind–body healing are possible.

**mindfulness meditation**   An effort to relieve people from physical suffering by teaching them to focus on the present moment and on nothing else, including the past or future.

**model**   In health psychology, a model is a set of statements explaining the relationship between factors or variables contributing to some phenomenon. For example, a model may include principles constructed to explain the human behavior of regular aerobic exercise or the behavior of choosing to be vaccinated against a disease. An example is the health belief model. A model is less formal than a theory.

**moderate drinking**   Men drinking two or fewer drinks each day, and women having one drink or less each day.

**morbidity**   A proportion of illness or the ratio of persons who are ill compared to others within a geographic area. For example, a study may find that at any given time about 33% of the population is ill.

**mortality rate**   Frequency of death or the death rate associated with a health problem or geographic area; for example, a study might find that 10 out of every 1,000 people die of heart disease.

**motivator**   A factor that encourages an idea or a behavior; for example, the likelihood of improvement in their personal appearance and health may motivate people to exercise or stop smoking.

**myocardial infarction**   A heart attack that destroys that part of the heart muscle that has lost its blood supply.

**naturalistic stress**   A stressor faced outside of laboratory testing situations. One example is college students taking exams. When students take examinations their immune system may be weakened, resulting in illness.

**neoplasm**   Any abnormal development of a cell; it may be benign or malignant.

**neuromatrix model of pain**   An extension of the gate control theory that integrates the concept of stress. This explanation of pain emphasizes the biopsychosocial model of pain that is more helpful in understanding and treating pain disorders.

**neuromuscular disorder**   Illness or injury relating to nerves and muscles.

**nicotine**   A chemical stimulant found in tobacco products.

**nociception**   The perception of pain produced when body tissue is damaged; nociceptors are nerve endings that respond to painful stimuli causing the sensation of pain.

**non-random sample**   The process of taking a sample in such a way that certain members or parts are more likely to be chosen thus biasing the conclusions of a study.

**norepinephrine**   A hormone secreted by the adrenal medulla, and a neurotransmitter released at nerve endings that constricts small blood vessels, raises blood pressure, slows heart rate, increases breathing, and relaxes the smooth muscles of the intestinal tract.

**nosocomial infection**   Infection acquired during a hospital stay.

**obesity**   A body composition that includes fat at too high a percentage for good health. Obesity is usually determined by comparing one's height and weight to body mass index tables designed for this purpose. Obesity is a risk factor for many serious diseases, including heart disease and diabetes.

**objectivity**   A goal of scientists to avoid prejudice or their own biases in research.

**observational study**   A study in which no variables are manipulated as they are in experiments; the researcher is simply observing what occurs, such as watching a group of children to see how they share toys. When people know they are being observed, they may change their behavior.

**operationalization**   The process of defining a variable by stating precisely how it will be measured in a study.

**optimal**   An ideal diet.

**optimistic bias**   Part of the precaution adoption process model referring to a tendency on the part of people to be aware of a risk but not believe it applies to them.

**orthopedic disabilities**   Physical limitations due to damage to the bones, joints, muscles, ligaments, and tendons.

**osteoarthritis**   The most common form of arthritis; it occurs mainly in old age.

**osteopathic medicine**   A form of medical therapy that emphasizes the relationship of organs to the musculoskeletal system and restores body health by manipulating bones and muscles.

**osteoporosis**   A disease resulting in fragile bones due to bone loss; outcomes include fractures, back pain, and loss of height.

**pain**   A sense of discomfort and distress due to a sensation in the body.

**pain syndrome**   A combination of signs and symptoms. More than 14 pain syndromes have been identified including whiplash injuries, back pain, headaches, cancer pain, and pain from muscular dystrophy, multiple sclerosis, herpes zoster, rheumatic disease, and sickle-cell disease.

**pain threshold**   The point of perception of a pain that results in people describing a sensation as painful. Thresholds vary from person to person.

**panic disorder (PD)**   A tendency of humans to experience fear and anxiety in many situations where dangers are either imagined or real.

**parasympathetic system**   The part of the nervous system that slows the heart rate, dilates blood vessels, and relaxes sphincter muscles stimulating peristalsis and digestion.

**pathogen**   Microorganism capable of producing illness or disease.

**perceived behavioral control**   The idea that humans are more likely to intend to change their behavior if they believe they have the will and strength to do so.

**perceived exertion rate**   A simple way to assess intensity; if people can talk, they are moving at the correct rate; if people can sing, then the intensity is too low to improve fitness.

**personality**   Attributes or aspects of an individual that may be revealed through conversation and other activities. Personality is indicated by perceptions or cognitions, through emotional responses or affect, and through behaviors or actions.

**phantom limb pain**   Persistent pain perceived to be located in a part of the body that was removed or amputated. Some people experience tingling, discomfort, itching, or other sensations.

**physical activity**   Any movement or use of the musculoskeletal system.

**physical dependence**   When a decline in the usual level of a substance in the bloodstream results in unpleasant psychological and physical symptoms.

**physical health**   Positive physical functioning.

**pica**   A condition of craving and eating non-food items such as clay, chalk, and laundry starch.

**placebo**   A treatment or substance believed to be ineffective by researchers that may contribute to positive changes in research participants due to their beliefs about its effectiveness. The placebo effect must be taken into account when designing experimental research.

**placebo effect**   An outcome or result attributed to a person's belief. For example, physicians gave patients sugar pills to encourage their recovery from an illness. If the patient believed the placebo would help them, it usually did. The placebo effect is a difficulty in experimental research.

**post-traumatic stress disorder (PTSD)**   An anxiety disorder that occurs after having experienced a serious threat of death or injury to oneself or others as from an assault or from living in a war zone. It involves intense emotional reactions such as fear, helplessness, horror, and/or flashbacks of the trauma(s) and it may interfere with sleep and memory.

**precaution adoption process model (PAPM)**   Theory that emphasizes that people move backwards and forwards through stages of belief about their susceptibility to a health risk. In stage 1 people are unaware of their risk, and in stage 2 they are aware of a risk but, due to their optimistic outlook, they do not believe they are at risk. In stage 3 they accept their susceptibility and become more cautious. In stages 4 and 5 they either decide to act or decide not to do anything about the perceived risk. In stage 6 they have taken precautions about avoiding the risk. Stage 7 is maintenance of the precautionary steps.

**prevalence**   Disease rate, or the number of occurrences of a disease within a designated time period within a population. Prevalence is often expressed as a percentage. For example, a study may find that 10% of people who use tanning beds develop skin cancer.

**primary appraisal**   In their first exposure to a potential stressor, people may decide there is a threat or that the stressor is harmless, neutral, or even a positive event in their life.

**primary pain management**   Pain management for short-lived and less severe acute pain. It includes information and encouragement so patients can return to the same activity level that existed prior to the injury or disease. Pain is relieved with analgesics and this treatment allows healing.

**primary prevention**   Any effort to completely avoid a health or safety problem.

**proactive coping**   Taking actions to prevent exposure to known stressors.

**problem-focused coping**   Coping aimed toward managing a stressor.

**prognosis**   Prediction of a probable outcome of a disease or injury.

**progressive muscle relaxation (PMR)**   A stress management/relaxation technique based on first tensing and then relaxing muscle groups to gain an understanding about the way a muscle or limb feels when relaxed.

**prospective records**   Records of eating, exercise, smoking, or other behaviors written at the time the behavior occurs. Analysis makes it possible to set up a plan for changes in eating, exercise, or smoking behavior.

**prospective study**   A longitudinal research design that looks to the future by following subjects forward from a starting point, for example, a study of the children of women who drank alcohol during pregnancy.

**protein**   A large complex compound consisting of amino acids that provide nutrients to the body for growth and repair of body tissue. Examples of foods containing sizeable amounts of protein are meat, poultry, milk, eggs, fish, and some vegetables and grains. Burns, surgery, fevers, and infections require greater amounts of protein than normal to maintain health.

**psychoactive substances**   Chemical compounds affecting the nervous system, especially the brain. Such substances affect mood and perception. Examples are alcohol and nicotine.

**psychogenic pain**   A chronic pain with no currently identifiable physical basis.

**psychological health**   Positive emotional functioning.

**psychoneuroimmunology (PNI)**   A science studying the bidirectional connections between behavior and the nervous, endocrine, and immune system. Research shows the brain influences immune reactivity. For example, depression may lower immune system resistance.

**qualitative research methods**   Types of research used to assemble data on measures that are not numerical such as people's gender, their perception about their health risks, or factors affecting that perception.

**quantitative research methods**   Types of research used to assemble numerical data about a variable; one example of a quantitative variable is age.

**radiation**   Electromagnetic energy emitted as rays used for both diagnostic work and in the treatment of some cancers. Radiation may cause severe burns and even trigger cancer development.

**random sample**   The process of taking a sample in such a way that each member or part has an equal chance of being selected. For example, scientists might use a table of random numbers to select 1,000 students from among the 10,000 students in the sophomore class to be included in their study.

**reappraisal**   The third state of transactional analysis, when new information changes the original appraisal. People gain new perspectives and discover new resources.

**reciprocal determinism**   A concept that human action is influenced by people's environments and also by personal beliefs such as self-efficacy, expectations, standards, and by other cognitions or perceptions, knowledge, and thinking.

**recommended dietary allowances (RDAs)**   These specify recommendations about calories, protein, fats, fiber, and some vitamins and minerals that meet the needs of most healthy individuals by life-stage and gender. RDAs and DRIs can usually be found on the inside cover or in the appendices of most nutrition textbooks.

**recurrent pain and chronic intermittent pain**   Brief but acute pain episodes repeated over and over and distressing to patients.

**redefinition**   A stress management technique that substitutes positive constructive thoughts for frightening ones or devises positive statements about the likelihood of tolerating a stressor.

**referred pain**   Pain due to confusion of sensations within the nervous system. Referred pain is felt in one part of the body, but the injury or disease is actually in another part. Referred pain is difficult to diagnose, but experienced physicians who specialize in pain control are aware of connections among various parts of the body.

**rehabilitation psychology**    A specialty centering on helping people recover from injuries and disease. Treatment focuses on cognitive, emotional, behavioral, and social difficulties following disability.

**Reiki**    An alternative or complementary medicine that uses universal life energy to relax, and reduce stress and pain by reconnecting the mind with the body.

**relapse prevention**    Efforts to avoid a lapse or reversion to previous unhealthy behavior.

**reliability**    The quality of getting consistent results from a set of questions or observations. For example, a stress scale is reliable if it consistently identifies or separates highly stressed people from less-stressed people and predicts who will get sick and who will not.

**René Descartes**    A French philosopher and mathematician generally considered one of the first to write in terms of the body being apart from or separated from the influence of the mind (1596–1650).

**replication**    The practice of repeating scientific studies to affirm accuracy of study results.

**reps**    The number of repetitions or times a weight is moved through space.

**resilience**    Refers to an ability to maintain balance in the face of trauma and loss.

**retrospective records**    Records of past eating, exercise, or other behaviors relying on the memory of intervention participants. For example, retrospective food records usually focus on the last 3 days or the last 24 hours of eating. This provides a quick assessment of eating patterns.

**retrospective study**    A longitudinal research design that asks participants or subjects to tell about what happened in their past or looking backward.

**risk factors**    Behaviors and conditions that put people at risk of certain illnesses such as heart disease.

**sample**    A small quantity of some phenomenon taken to understand the nature of the total phenomenon. For example, a scientist may interview a sample of a hundred cancer patients about the level of their optimism to survive the disease and draw conclusions about all cancer patients.

**satiety**    A biologically based feeling that the stomach is full.

**scale**    A measurement device. In psychology it often is a series of questions by which the combined answers represent a complex concept. For example, a life-events survey may measure major stressors. A stress inventory may assess sources and the impact of stressful events in people's lives. Mood, fatigue, self-efficacy, helplessness, and other social science factors may be measured by validated sets of questions or scales.

**secondary appraisal**    The second stage of transactional analysis comes when a stressor is believed to be a threat. People think about their options and devise strategies to meet any demands being made upon them.

**secondary gain of pain**   Any benefit of pain used by persons to avoid some task or to draw attention to themselves.

**secondary pain management**   Psychosocial interventions used to promote a return to pre-pain productivity levels and to prevent further deterioration in a patient's biological and psychosocial well-being. It is used if primary pain management does not succeed.

**secondary prevention**   Screening so disease and injury are discovered at an early stage, when chances are better for healing.

**self-efficacy**   A theory of human behavior that people are more likely to change if they believe they have control over their lives and can change. People act or change behavior if their thinking or cognitions include the idea that they are capable of overcoming the barriers that are currently preventing change.

**self-selection bias**   When participants decide to opt into a social science study as a respondent or are allowed to choose between being in the experimental group or the control group, this may affect the accuracy of research results. Making the choice risks the inclusion of an important bias or prejudice that might invalidate study results. Random selection of participants makes study results more likely to be accurate.

**set**   A group of repetitions used in strength-training programs to improve fitness levels.

**sexism**   Discriminatory actions, thoughts, and statements directed against people based on their biological status as a female or male.

**sexual harassment**   Offensive and unwanted behavior directed toward a person including words and actions that induce shame and fear. Most commonly used to designate actions by a higher-ranking male toward a female employee.

**sexual violence**   Forced and violent assaults such as rape; usually committed by males against females.

**sickle-cell disease (SCD)**   A hereditary blood disease in which blood cells are abnormally shaped. It occurs mainly in people of African descent and causes a form of anemia.

**signs**   Objective indicators of an injury or illness that can be observed by medical personnel. Examples are shortness of breath, vomiting, bleeding, and bones protruding from patients' arms.

**snowball sample**   A non-random sampling process that relies on participants to recommend others they know to be included in a study, for example, interviewing people with HIV/AIDS and then asking for names of other patients to be included in the study. This study may be biased because each participant knows the other.

**social and cultural health**   Normal functioning within a culture including having friends and family members for interaction and social support.

**socialization**   The process of teaching young persons what is acceptable behavior within a society.

**social readjustment rating scale (SRRS)**   An effort to assess the effect of stressors on health.

**social structure**   The organizational components within which people live. The term includes the political, economic, family/kinship, religious, and educational systems of a nation or country.

**social support**   Efforts by others to make us feel loved and valuable, including providing tangible help and encouragement during sad times.

**somatic pain**   Pain sensations originating in the skin, ligaments, muscles, bones, or joints.

**stages of change model**   Model that suggests that people go through a series of stages or phases when altering their behavior.

**starvation**   The process of suffering from lack of food or nourishment.

**stimulant**   A psychoactive substance that speeds up or quickens central nervous system processing, increasing physical and mental activity. Stimulants may provide temporary feelings of alertness and suppress appetite. Caffeine and amphetamines are examples.

**stoic**   A person who is patient and who endures adversity including pain.

**strength training**   Exercise to increase the strength of various muscles.

**stress**   A physical and psychological reaction to a threat to physical, psychological, or social health.

**stress fractures**   Physical injuries usually resulting from repetitive impact on limbs.

**stress inoculation training (SIT)**   A form of cognitive-behavioral therapy designed to immunize people against stress. SIT consists of three stages: conceptualization, skills development and application, and coping skills, including relaxation, distraction, and redefinition.

**stress management**   Interventions or programs designed to improve people's ability to cope by increasing their knowledge and skills.

**stressor**   An event or situation perceived by persons to be a danger to their physical, psychological, or social health.

**stretching**   Gentle movements to extend and relax muscles and joints; more safely accomplished when muscles are warmed by non-vigorous exercise, but may also follow a vigorous exercise session.

**stroke**   A cerebrovascular event in which oxygen is blocked in the blood vessels of the brain. The person may experience paralysis, weakness, an inability to speak, or death.

**structural support**   That part of social support that includes networks of close social ties and connections such as marital status.

**sympathetic nervous system**   The part of the nervous system that mobilizes the body for action in response to stress by constricting blood vessels, raising blood pressure, and increasing the heart rate.

**symptoms**   Subjective indicators of pain that must be reported by patients. Pain is a symptom.

**synergistic effects**   Chemicals in tobacco interacting with other substances, increasing damage to the health of users.

**systems theory**   An approach to human events, such as injury and illness, including the idea that events occur and exist within several interconnected systems. Each system influences the others. Systems theory in health psychology includes the idea that medical providers, patients, family members, and friends need to consider the total situation and think about many different factors when dealing with an illness or injury.

**systolic**   The systole is the contraction of the heart that drives blood into the aorta and pulmonary artery; it is the top number reported in blood pressure readings.

**tenderness**   Pain perceived when the affected area is touched or pressed.

**termination**   The act of ending a behavior.

**tertiary pain management**   Intense interdisciplinary treatments to offset physical deterioration and prevent permanent disability due to pain. Psychosocial and disability management team efforts are combined.

**tertiary prevention**   Controlling complications of illness, improving patients' quality of life, and preventing death.

**theory**   In health psychology, a theory is a set of related statements or propositions from which hypotheses can be developed for research purposes; theories organize and explain observations.

**theory of planned behavior (TpB)**   According to this theory, human behavior is influenced by three kinds of beliefs. In addition to their attitude toward a behavior and the attitudes of others, people are also influenced by their perceived behavioral control. When people have resources and opportunities, they are more likely to believe they can successfully change their behavior and intend to do so.

**theory of reasoned action (TRA)**   The theory that people take action if they believe a behavior change will achieve a desirable outcome and that other people whose opinion is important to them also believe the change is desirable (the subjective norm). Humans weigh their own negative attitudes about a change against the importance of the change to others and may develop the intention to act that is followed by the actual behavior.

**tolerance**   A biologically based response to a substance. Consistent use of many substances requires larger amounts to attain the same psychogenic effects. Tolerance for pain refers to the amount of pain individuals will put up with before they ask for something to stop the sensation.

**training effect**   Aerobic exercise done on a regular basis gradually becomes easier, because the body adjusts to the rigor of the activity and is no longer stimulated at that level. One can gradually increase the vigor of exercise by moving faster or exercising for longer periods of time, resulting in a higher level of fitness.

**transactional analysis**   Lazarus and Folkman described stress as a continuing exchange between people and their environment. Reactions to stressors are based on an individual's cognitive processes or interpretations of the meaning of events and on their typical methods of coping or responding to stressors. Facing stressful situations involves a series of adjustments as people decide how to react. Lazarus and Folkman proposed that there are three steps in the transaction between an individual and a stressor.

**transcendental meditation (TM)**   A form of reflection that instructs people to choose a mantra or secret word to be repeated over and over in order to focus thoughts away from distressful ideas or pain.

**transcutaneous electrical nerve stimulation (TENS)**   A process by which electrodes are placed on the skin near the site of pain and the area is given a mild electrical shock. The theory is that the electrical shock will interfere with the transmission of the pain signal from the injury site to the brain.

**transient ischemic attacks (TIAs)**   A brief episode of insufficient blood supply to the brain.

**transtheoretical model of change**   A stage-of-change model of health-related behavior that applies several components of other theories describing the behavior change process. The stages include 1) pre-contemplation, which exists when a person is not even thinking about changing a behavior, 2) contemplation, which exists when a person thinks about making a change and weighs the pros and cons of the change, including their own attitudes and the attitudes of others, 3) the preparation stage, in which a person gets ready to implement the change he or she has been considering, 5) the action stage, in which people actually change their behavior, and 6) the maintenance stage, in which a person has successfully implemented the behavior change.

**tumor**   A growth of tissue characterized by cell increases; it may be benign or malignant.

**Type A personality**   A behavioral and emotional pattern of responding to experiences in life with a chronic sense of time urgency and free-floating hostility. It may include a competitive attitude and anger; this type of personality may be a response to insufficient self-esteem or self-confidence.

**Type I diabetes**   A complex and chronic disorder; a form of diabetes mellitus that tends to appear early in life.

**Type II diabetes**   A form of diabetes usually appearing in adulthood but now appearing in obese young people.

**universal design**   Design of products and environments to make them useable regardless of body dimension, age, or disability status.

**validity** The accuracy of a test or measurement. For example, does the question or measurement accurately assess obesity or stress or anger?

**variable** Any factor used in research that can diverge or take on more than one form, such as age or gender.

**visceral pain** Pain sensations resulting from injury or disease to an organ in the thoracic or abdominal cavities.

**visual analogue scale** A series of pictures of faces from happy to grimacing. The scale is used to determine the amount of pain in patients with limited verbal ability such as children.

**Walter Cannon** Physiologist credited with naming the fight-or-flight response as a response to stressors. During the 1930s, Cannon experimented with cats and found that the adrenal glands secreted the hormone adrenaline or epinephrine when the animals were threatened, causing physiological changes.

**weight-bearing exercises** Exercise that puts weight or stress on the muscles and bones of the feet, ankles, legs, and spine, helping to prevent osteoporosis. One weight-bearing exercise is walking. Swimming is not a weight-bearing exercise because the water supports most of the body's weight.

**withdrawal effects** Unpleasant physical and psychological symptoms due to decreases in the usual level of substances in the body of addicted persons.

**yo-yo dieting** An eating pattern of alternating limiting food intake (dieting), followed by regaining weight, followed by a repetition of dieting and weight loss. This pattern is believed to be detrimental to health because one's total percentage of body fat tends to increase each time because muscle and bone are lost due to dieting.

# INDEX

# Photo Credits

**Chapter 1**
Opener © Muriel Lasure/ShutterStock, Inc.

**Chapter 2**
Opener © Laurence Gough/ShutterStock, Inc.; 2-2 © PhotoCreate/ShutterStock, Inc.

**Chapter 3**
Opener © Photodisc

**Chapter 4**
Opener © Redbaron/Dreamstime.com; 4-1A © Photodisc; 4-1B © Photodisc; 4-2 © Kris Butler/ShutterStock, Inc.; 4-3 © Monkey Business Images/ShutterStock, Inc.

**Chapter 5**
Opener Hannamariah/ShutterStock, Inc.; 5-1 © Photodisc

**Chapter 6**
Opener © Steve Skjold/Alamy Images; 6-2 © Pixtal/SuperStock, Inc.; 6-3 © Photodisc; 6-5 © Joe Skipper/Reuters/Landov

**Chapter 7**
Opener © PhotoCreate/ShutterStock, Inc.; 7-1 © AbleStock; 7-4 © Don Hammond/ Design Pics, Inc./age fotostock

**Chapter 8**
Opener © Paul Cowan/ShutterStock, Inc.; 8-4 © Jerry Zitterman/ShutterStock, Inc.

**Chapter 9**
Opener © Don Hammond/age fotostock; 9-2 © Blend Images/Alamy Images; 9-3 © LiquidLibrary

**Chapter 10**
Opener © AbleStock; 10-1 © Ron Chapple/ Thinkstock/Creatas; 10-2 © Cora Reed/ ShutterStock, Inc.

**Chapter 11**
Opener © Simone van den Berg/ ShutterStock, Inc.

**Chapter 12**
Opener © Jupiterimages/BrandX/Alamy Images; 12-2 Courtesy of National Cancer Institute; 12-3 © Marc Pagani Photography/ShutterStock, Inc.

**Chapter 13**
Opener © Gertjan Hooijer/ShutterStock, Inc.; 13-2 © iofoto/ShutterStock, Inc., 13-3 © Bill Aron/PhotoEdit, Inc.

**Chapter 14**
Opener © Shariff Che' Lah/Dreamstime.com; 14-3 © Photodisc; 14-5 © Photodisc/Creatas